Territory, territory, territory

If there is anything truly unique and special about traditional Chinese medicine, it is the understanding and exquisitely detailed mapping of the territories of the channels, their functions and pathologies. Other dimensions such as taste and temperature are shared by nearly all indigenous medicine systems, but this gorgeous entanglement of energies, functions, tissues and physiological systems is what makes our system shine.

How did our ancient medical predecessors arrive at this intimate view of the human body and its activities, non-activities and capacities? It happened through a process of observation, contemplation, speculation, experimentation, more observation and dialogue over a very long period of time.

An environment of continuous, if not stable, language and culture allowed this observational work to flourish over the centuries that were required to bring this process into our current state of knowledge and practice. It would be a shame to exclude ourselves from this progression of development and understanding by imagining that it only happened in some glorious past. We are the ones who are carrying on this tradition, and if it is going to stay alive, we need to commit ourselves to its continued growth and maturation.

The demands of furthering this venture require us to enhance and refine ourselves, our awareness, our caring, our observational and communication skills and our basic desire to share and preserve this information so that we all can benefit. If we are able to leverage our current and future communication technologies to open up a space for an ongoing congress of observation and testing, the possibilities of where we can take this exploration are endless.

It is surprising to me that even though our professional knowledge of the channels is so highly developed in the realm of acupuncture, the clinical application of this incredible understanding of the human body seems to fall apart completely, or nearly so, when we enter the realm of traditional Chinese herbology. Somehow, we have abandoned what we know in favor of looking outward to authorities and third-hand information sources, including modern science, rather than simply applying the system that we have gone through such agonizing extensions to learn.

Yet if we choose to investigate the sources of commentary on our pharmacopoeia a little deeper, and if we have the good fortune to develop authentic and long-term relationships with truly outstanding practitioners of traditional Chinese herbology, we discover one thing again and again: these practitioners never deviate from the basics that we learn from the beginning of our studies. They master these basics and learn how to apply them in masterful ways. Every miracle cure from a magic formula that I have seen has boiled down to a single methodology, which is a very precise application of the qualities of the herbs to an incredibly detailed utilization of the channel territories.

The contrasts between channel territories and categories give us the down-and-dirty basics of where an herb is going in the body and what it's going to do once it gets there. Beyond that, the other qualities of the herbs granulate into metrics of nuance and detail that can take a formula from serviceable to awe-inspiring.

The broad strokes are here. Learn to use them well.

John Mini MSCM, LAc, Dipl Ac
Belvedere-Tiburon, California July 2021

FORWARD

Method

Although I used many resources to compile the information in this book and the other works in the Min Jie Pharmacopoeia series, of the written material, I focused on four works in English to provide non-Chinese speaking/reading practitioners the ability to investigate these sources in a deeper way. They are: Chen and Chen's *Chinese Medical Herbology and Pharmacology*, Bensky, Clavey, Stöger & Gamble's *Chinese Herbal Medicine Materia Medica*, Brand & Wiseman's *Concise Chinese Materia Medica*, and Maciocia's *The Channels of Acupuncture*. I highly recommend purchasing and studying each of these works to deepen your understanding and appreciation of Chinese herbs and energetic physiology as well as the pioneering authors of these books.

A fifth written source in Chinese was the exception, which is my own 2015 translation of the *Ben Cao Wen Da*, by Tang Rong Chuan (Tang Zong Hai). I have included material from it because this text has proven to be a fascinating and invaluable wealth of clinical insights and doorways into the processes of Taoist natural science and our understanding and utilization of Chinese herbs.

My emphasis in collecting, comparing and compressing this information was to find and include both points of agreement and points of disagreement between authors and traditions. In the footnoting if two or more sources agree, there is usually no footnote. Wherever there is a unique viewpoint, a footnote will lead you back to its origin. Anything that is not footnoted is either completely commonplace or is being written down for the first time on these pages.

What You Are Looking At

The process that I used in creating the structure of the *Formulary Companion* has no written precedent that I know of. It is an extension and expression of my own clinical methodology, which are derived from the convergence and distillation of oral teachings from several lineages that have been passed on to me in my study, work and travels as a physician of Chinese medicine.

Each entry in the *Formulary Companion* comes in the following format:

Name
Traditional Category
Taste(s)
Temperature
Channels Entered
Internal Relationships

Beyond this simple structure, you will discover that I have arranged the entries themselves in a non-traditional, but classically oriented, sequence that traverses the following pattern:

Lu
Lu/LI
Lu/LI/St
Lu/LI/St/Sp
Lu/LI/St/Sp/H
Lu/LI/St/Sp/H/SI
Lu/LI/St/Sp/H/SI/UB
Lu/LI/St/Sp/H/SI/UB/Kid
Lu/LI/St/Sp/H/SI/UB/Kid/P
Lu/LI/St/Sp/H/SI/UB/Kid/P/SJ
Lu/LI/St/Sp/H/SI/UB/Kid/P/SJ/GB
Lu/LI/St/Sp/H/SI/UB/Kid/P/SJ/GB/Liv
LI/St/Sp/H/SI/UB/Kid/P/SJ/GB/Liv
St/Sp/H/SI/UB/Kid/P/SJ/GB/Liv
Sp/H/SI/UB/Kid/P/SJ/GB/Liv
H/SI/UB/Kid/P/SJ/GB/Liv
SI/UB/Kid/P/SJ/GB/Liv
Kid/P/SJ/GB/Liv
P/SJ/GB/Liv
SJ/GB/Liv
GB/Liv
Liv

This is the familiar progression of qi flow from Jing-channel to Jing-channel set in a hierarchical order, where anything that is higher on the diamond takes priority over what is lower.

In addition to this framework, the herbs are also arranged in the following hierarchy in the occasional event of a repeated internal channel structure:

Taste-Sour, Bitter, Sweet, Bland, Acrid, Astringent, Salty
Temperature-very Cold to very Hot

And where there are any repeats beyond these criteria, I have further organized the herbs according to their structure, kingdom and power.

The remaining composition of this volume of *The Formulary Companion* organizes our pharmacopoeia into a set of flows that contrasts the herbs by name, category, tastes, temperature, channels, and internal relationships. The overall structure of this work is therefore an expanded fractal enunciation of each of its parts and vice versa.

This is the best way that I've found to reveal the innate structure in the order of the arrangement of the herbs within the categories. It allows for easy comparisons of similarity, internal organization and complexity while focusing on ease of access in the clinic. It also reinforces our understanding and depth of appreciation for the natural flow of qi each time we refer to it.

Information in this format gives you the vast majority of what you need to know about an herb, once you know how to interpret it, and forms the basis of virtually all pre-modern commentary on the herbs themselves. If you can become familiar with and master these basics, other subsequent information usually won't come as a surprise, and when it does, that surprise becomes much more valuable and memorable because of its uniqueness.

How To Use This Book

I honestly don't know what the best way for you to use this book might be. Only you can discover that on your own by using it. I can and will tell you how I use it, and how others use it, but those may or may not be the best ways for you.

I'm also not going to *explain* everything to you, because the exploration is where and how you'll learn the most from this material.

You can learn some things from written sources. Other things you work out for yourself. Still other things we can only learn together through dialogue, discussion, application, feedback and review. I look forward to the day when you can tell me how you use *The Formulary Companion*.

How I Use The Formulary Companion

I examine and diagnose the patient to determine what qualities, channels, patterns and/or combinations of patterns are at play.

My diagnosis determines an essential treatment principle.

I discern what qualities, channels, patterns and/or combinations of patterns will optimize the essential treatment principle to create the most balanced picture of health.

Keeping in mind all those who have come before us, I select an herb that most perfectly matches this optimized treatment principle.

I then select the herbs that will most elegantly complement the main herb to complete the most balanced picture.

I double-check for contraindications and toxicity, and add a little Gan Cao.

That's it.

CHANNELS BY CATEGORY

Hand Tai Yin Lung Herbs

Acrid Warm Exterior Releasing

Bai Zhi (Radix Angelicae Dahuricae, Angelica Root)
Acrid Warm Exterior Releasing
Acrid, Aromatic
Warm
Lung, Stomach, Spleen,[2] Large Intestine[3]
Name (Tai Yin, Lung/Spleen, Yang Ming, Large Intestine/Stomach), Biao/Li (Stomach/Spleen, Large Intestine/Lung), Clock Neighbor (Large Intestine/Stomach)

Xin Yi Hua, Xin Yi, Wang Chun Hua (Flos Magnoliae, Magnolia Flower)
Acrid Warm Exterior Releasing
Acrid, Aromatic
Warm
Lung, Stomach

Cong Bai, Xiang Cong (Bulbus Allii Fistulosi, Scallion, Spring Onion, Green Onion)
Acrid Warm Exterior Releasing
Acrid
Warm
Lung, Stomach

Hu Sui (Coriandri Herba cum Radice, Coriander, Cilantro)
Acrid Warm Exterior Releasing
Acrid
Warm
Lung, Stomach

Zi Su Geng (Caulis Perillae, Perilla Stem)
Acrid Warm Exterior Releasing/Regulate and Rectify Qi
Acrid, Sweet, Aromatic
Slightly Warm
Lung, Spleen, Stomach
Name (Tai Yin, Lung/Spleen), Biao/Li (Stomach/Spleen)

Sheng Jiang (Rhizoma Zingiberis Recens, Fresh Ginger Rhizome)
Acrid Warm Exterior Releasing
Acrid
Slightly Warm
Lung, Spleen, Stomach
Name (Tai Yin, Lung/Spleen), Biao/Li (Stomach/Spleen)

Xiang Ru, Hua Qi Ning, Shi Xiang Rou (Herba Elsholtziae seu Moslae, Aromatic Madder)
Acrid Warm Exterior Releasing
Acrid, Aromatic
Slightly Warm
Lung, Spleen,[4] Heart,[5] Stomach
Name (Tai Yin, Lung/Spleen), Biao/Li (Stomach/Spleen), Clock Neighbor (Spleen/Heart)

Xi He Liu, Guan Yin Liu (Cacumen Tamaricis, Tamarisk stems and leaves)
Acrid Warm Exterior Releasing
Acrid, Sweet
Warm
Lung, Stomach, Heart

Zi Su Ye (Folium Perillae, Perilla Leaf)
Acrid Warm Exterior Releasing
Acrid, Aromatic
Warm
Lung, Spleen
Name (Tai Yin, Lung/Spleen)

Gui Zhi, Liu Gui (Ramulus Cinnamomi, Cassia Twig)
Acrid Warm Exterior Releasing
Acrid, Sweet
Warm
Heart, **Lung**, Urinary Bladder
Bie Jing (Tai Yin/Tai Yang, Lung/Urinary Bladder), Clock Opposite (Lung/Urinary Bladder) + Heart

Xi Xin (Radix et Rhizoma Asari, Asarum, Chinese Wild Ginger)
Acrid Warm Exterior Releasing/Warm Interior
Acrid to extremely Acrid,[6] Aromatic
Warm, slightly Toxic*
Lung, Heart, Kidney, Du,[7] all channels[8]
Name (Shao Yin, Heart/Kidney), Branch (You/Chicken, Lung/Kidney, 5PM-6:59PM) + Du

Ma Huang, Ma Huang Cao (Herba Ephedrae, Ephedra Stem, Mormon Tea)
Acrid Warm Exterior Releasing
Acrid, slightly Bitter[9] to Bitter, no big taste[10]
Warm
Lung, Urinary Bladder, Yang Qiao[11]
Bie Jing (Tai Yin/Tai Yang, Lung/Urinary Bladder), Clock Opposite (Lung/Urinary Bladder) + Yang Qiao

Jing Jie (Herba Schizonepitae, Schizonepeta)
Acrid Warm Exterior Releasing
Acrid, Aromatic
Slightly Warm
Lung, Liver, Gall Bladder,[12] San Jiao,[13] Du[14]
Name (Shao Yang, Gall Bladder/San Jiao), Biao/Li (Gall Bladder/Liver), Clock Neighbor (San Jiao/Gall Bladder, Liver/Lung), Branch (Yin/Tiger, Gall Bladder/Lung, 3AM-4:59AM) + Du

Ji Xiang Teng (Caulis Paederiae, Paederia)
Acrid Warm Exterior Releasing
Sweet
Neutral to slightly Warm[15] to Warm
Lung, Liver
Clock Neighbor (Liver/Lung)

E Bu Shi Cao, Nue Ji Cao, Di Hu Jiao (Herba Centipedae)
Acrid Warm Exterior Releasing
Acrid
Slightly Warm[16] to Warm
Lung, Liver
Clock Neighbor (Liver/Lung)

Cang Er Zi (Fructus Xanthii, Cocklebur Fruit, Xanthium Fruit)
Acrid Warm Exterior Releasing
Sweet,[17] Bitter, Acrid
Warm, slightly Toxic*
Lung, Liver,[18] Du[19]
Clock Neighbor (Liver/Lung) + Du

Acrid Cool Exterior Releasing

Wu Tian (Radix et Folium Viticis Quinatae)
Acrid Cool Exterior Releasing
Sweet, Acrid, Bland
Cold
Lung

Shuang Liu Huang (Herba Vernoniae Patulae, Half-Spreading Ironweed)
Acrid Cool Exterior Releasing
Bitter
Neutral
Lung, Large Intestine
Biao/Li (Large Intestine/Lung)

Sheng Ma (Radix Cimicifugae, Black Cohosh Rhizome, Bugbane Rhizome)
Acrid Cool Exterior Releasing
Acrid, Sweet
Cool to slightly Cold[20]
Lung, Spleen, Stomach, Large Intestine
Name (Tai Yin, Lung/Spleen, Yang Ming, Large Intestine/Stomach), Biao/Li (Large Intestine/Lung, Stomach/Spleen), Clock Neighbor (Large Intestine/Stomach)

Sang Ye (Folium Mori, White Mulberry Leaf)
Acrid Cool Exterior Releasing
Bitter, Sweet, Acrid,[21] Aromatic
Cold
Lung, Liver, Large Intestine,[22] Stomach[23]
Name (Yang Ming, Large Intestine/Stomach), Biao/Li (Large Intestine/Lung), Bie Jing (Jue Yin/Yang Ming, Liver/Large Intestine), Clock Neighbor (Liver/Lung, Large Intestine/Stomach), Branch (Mao/Rabbit, Liver/Large Intestine, 5AM-6:59AM)

Dan Dou Chi (Semen Sojae Praeparatum, Prepared Soybean, Fermented Soybean)
Acrid Cool Exterior Releasing
Acrid, Sweet, slightly Bitter, Aromatic
Cold or Warm, depending on the type of preparation.
Lung, Stomach

Niu Bang Zi, Da Li Zi, Shu Nian Zi (Fructus Arctii, Great Burdock Seed, Arctium)
Acrid Cool Exterior Releasing
Acrid, Bitter, Aromatic
Cold
Lung, Stomach

Man Jing Zi, Jing Tiao Zi, Bai Bu Jing (Fructus Viticis, Vitex Fruit)
Acrid Cool Exterior Releasing
Acrid, Bitter
Both Cool and Warm[24]
Lung,[25] Liver, Stomach, Urinary Bladder,[26] Gall Bladder,[27] San Jiao[28]
Name (Shao Yang, Gall Bladder/San Jiao), Bie Jing (Tai Yin/Tai Yang, Lung/Urinary Bladder), Biao/Li (Gall Bladder/Liver), Clock Opposite (Lung, Urinary Bladder), Clock Neighbor (San Jiao/Gall Bladder, Liver/Lung), Qian/Hou (Front/Back, Stomach/Urinary Bladder), Branch (Yin/Tiger, Gall Bladder/Lung, 3AM-4:59AM, Hai/Pig, Urinary Bladder/San Jiao, 9PM-10:59PM)

Mao Zi Dun Tou (Herba Abutilon Indicum, Indian Abutilon)
Acrid Cool Exterior Releasing
Sweet
Neutral, slightly Toxic*
Lung, Liver, Gall Bladder, Spleen
Name (Tai Yin, Lung/Spleen), Biao/Li (Gall Bladder, Liver), Clock Neighbor (Liver/Lung), Branch (Yin/Tiger, Gall Bladder/Lung, 3AM-4:59AM, and Chou/Ox, Spleen/Liver, 1AM-2:59AM)

Fu Ping, Fu Piao, Qing Ping (Herba Spirodelae, Duckweed, Spirodela)
Acrid Cool Exterior Releasing
Acrid
Cold
Lung, Urinary Bladder
Bie Jing (Tai Yin/Tai Yang, Lung/Urinary Bladder), Clock Opposite (Lung/Urinary Bladder)

Mu Zei, Jie Gu Cao, Jie Jie Cao (Herba Equesti Hiemalis, Scouring Rush, Shave Grass, Horsetail)
Acrid Cool Exterior Releasing
Sweet
Neutral to slightly Cold
Lung, Liver, Gall Bladder[29]
Biao/Li (Gall Bladder/Liver), Clock Neighbor (Liver/Lung), Branch (Yin/Tiger, Gall Bladder/Lung, 3AM-4:59AM)

Ju Hua (Flos Chrysanthemi, Chrysanthemum Flower)
Acrid Cool Exterior Releasing
Acrid,[30] Sweet, Bitter, Aromatic[31]
Cool to slightly Cold[32]
Lung, Liver
Clock Neighbor (Liver/Lung)

Ye Ju Hua, Ku Yi (Flos Chrysanthemi Indici, Wild Chrysanthemum Flower)
Acrid Cool Exterior Releasing/Clear Heat Clean Toxin
Bitter, Acrid
Cool to slightly Cold[33]
Lung, Liver
Clock Neighbor (Liver/Lung)

Yi Zhi Xiang (Herba Vernoniae Cinereae, Vernonia)
Acrid Cool Exterior Releasing
Acrid, Bitter
Cool
Lung, Liver
Clock Neighbor (Liver/Lung)

Chan Tui, Chan Yi (Periostracum Cicadae, Cicada Moulting)
Acrid Cool Exterior Releasing
Sweet, Salty, Bland[34]
Slightly Cold[35] to Cold
Liver, **Lung**
Clock Neighbor (Liver/Lung)

Bo He (Herba Menthae, Field Mint)
Acrid Cool Exterior Releasing
Acrid, Aromatic
Cool
Lung, Liver
Clock Neighbor (Liver/Lung)

Clear Heat Purge Fire

Xia Ku Hua (Flos Prunellae)
Clear Heat Purge Fire
Acrid
Cold
Lung

Qing Guo Gen (Radix Canarium Album, White Olive Root)
Clear Heat Purge Fire
Sweet, Sour, Astringent
Cool
Lung, Stomach

Tian Hua Fen, Gua Lou Gen (Radix Trichosanthis, Trichosanthis Root, Snake Gourd Root)
Clear Heat Purge Fire
Bitter, slightly Sweet
Cold
Lung, Stomach

Shi Gao, Bai Hu, Li Shi (Gypsum Fibrosum, Gypsum)
Clear Heat Purge Fire
Acrid, Sweet
Very Cold
Lung, Stomach

Qing Guo (Fructus Canarii, Chinese White Olive)
Clear Heat Purge Fire
Sweet, Sour, Astringent[36]
Neutral
Lung, Stomach, Spleen
Name (Tai Yin, Lung/Spleen), Biao/Li (Stomach, Spleen)

Zhu Ye (Herba Phyllostachys, Bamboo Leaves)
Clear Heat Purge Fire
Sweet, Bland
Cold
Heart, Stomach, **Lung**

Lu Gen (Rhizoma Phragmitis, Reed Rhizome)
Clear Heat Purge Fire
Sweet, Bland[37]
Cold
Lung, Stomach, Heart[38]

Wu Long Cha (Folium Camellia Sinensis Fermentata, 'Oolong' Tea)
Clear Heat Purge Fire
Bitter, Sweet
Cool
Heart, **Lung**, Stomach, Small Intestine
Biao/Li (Small Intestine/Heart) + Lung, Stomach

Xi Gua (Fructus Citrulli, Watermelon Fruit)
Clear Heat Purge Fire
Sweet
Cold
Heart, Stomach, Urinary Bladder, **Lung**[39]
Bie Jing (Tai Yin/Tai Yang, Lung/Urinary Bladder), Clock Opposite (Lung/Urinary Bladder), Qian/Hou (Front/Back, Stomach/Urinary Bladder) + Heart

Shan Zhi Zi, Zhi Zi (Fructus Gardeniae, Cape Jasmine Fruit, Gardenia Fruit)
Clear Heat Purge Fire
Bitter
Cold
Heart, **Lung**, Stomach, San Jiao, Liver[40]
Clock Neighbor (Liver/Lung) + Heart, Stomach, San Jiao

Ya Zhi Cao, Zhu Ye Shui Cao, Zhu Jie Cai (Herba Commelinae, Common Dayflower)
Clear Heat Purge Fire
Sweet, Bland
Cold
Lung, Stomach, Small Intestine

Zhi Mu (Radix Anemarrhenae, Anemarrhena)
Clear Heat Purge Fire
Bitter, Sweet
Cold
Lung, Stomach, Kidney
Branch (You/Chicken, Lung/Kidney, 5PM-6:59PM) + Stomach

Da Ding Huang (Caulis Euonymi, Euonymus)
Clear Heat Purge Fire
Bitter
Cold
Liver, **Lung**
Clock Neighbor (Liver/Lung)

Clear Heat Dry Dampness

Huang Qin (Radix Scutellariae, Baical Skullcap Root, Scutellaria, Scute)
Clear Heat Dry Dampness
Bitter
Cold
Lung, Gall Bladder, Stomach, Large Intestine and possibly San Jiao[41]
Name (Yang Ming, Large Intestine/Stomach), Biao/Li (Large Intestine/Lung), Clock Neighbor (Large Intestine/Stomach), Branch (Yin/Tiger, Gall Bladder/Lung, 3AM-4:59AM), and possibly Name (Shao Yang, San Jiao/Gall Bladder), Clock Neighbor (San Jiao/Gall Bladder)

Clear Heat Cool Blood

Fu Rong (Radix Hibisci, Hibiscus Root)
Clear Heat Cool Blood
Acrid
Cool
Lung

Xuan Shen, Yuan Shen, Hei Shen (Radix Scrophulariae, Ningpo Figwort Root)
Clear Heat Cool Blood
Bitter, Sweet, Salty
Cold
Lung, Stomach, Kidney
Branch (You/Chicken, Lung/Kidney, 5PM-6:59PM) + Stomach

Dong Qing Ye (Folium Ilexis, Ilex)
Clear Heat Cool Blood
Bitter, Astringent
Cold
Lung, Heart

Clear Heat Clean Toxin

Dao Di Wu Gong (Rhizoma Helminthostachytis)
Clear Heat Clean Toxin
Bitter
Cold
Lung

Wan Nian Qing (Radix et Rhizoma Rohdeae Japonica, Rohdea Root)
Clear Heat Clean Toxin
Bitter, slightly Sweet
Cold, slightly Toxic*
Lung

She Gan, Bian Zhu, Gui San (Rhizoma Belamcandae, Belamcanda, Blackberry Lilly Rhizome)
Clear Heat Clean Toxin
Bitter, Acrid[42]
Cold
Lung

Ma Bo (Lasiosphaera seu Calvatia, Fruiting Body of the Puffball, Lasiosphaera)
Clear Heat Clean Toxin
Acrid
Neutral to Cool
Lung

Jin Guo Lan (Radix Tinosporae)
Clear Heat Clean Toxin
Bitter
Cold
Lung, Large Intestine
Biao/Li (Large Intestine/Lung)

Yu Xing Cao (Herba Houttuyniae)
Clear Heat Clean Toxin
Acrid
Cool to slightly Cold
Lung, Large Intestine[43]
Biao/Li (Large Intestine/Lung)

Bei Dou Gen (Rhizoma Menispermi, Asiatic Moonseed Rhizome)
Clear Heat Clean Toxin
Bitter
Cold
Lung, Stomach, Large Intestine
Name (Yang Ming, Large Intestine/Stomach), Biao/Li (Large Intestine/Lung), Clock Neighbor (Large Intestine/Stomach)

Ren Dong Teng (Caulis Lonicerae, Honeysuckle Vine)
Clear Heat Clean Toxin
Sweet
Neutral to slightly Cold[44] to Cold
Lung, Stomach, Large Intestine,[45] Spleen[46]
Name (Yang Ming, Large Intestine/Stomach, Tai Yin, Lung/Spleen), Biao/Li (Large Intestine/Lung, Stomach/Spleen) Clock Neighbor (Large Intestine/Stomach)

Shan Dou Gen, Dou Gen, Nan Dou Gen (Radix Sophorae Tonkinensis, Subprostrate, Sophora Root)
Clear Heat Clean Toxin
Bitter to very Bitter[47]
Cold, slightly Toxic*
Lung, Stomach,[48] Large Intestine,[49] Heart[50]
Name (Yang Ming, Large Intestine/Stomach), Biao/Li (Large Intestine/Lung), Clock Neighbor (Large Intestine/Stomach) + Heart

Jin Yin Hua (Flos Lonicerae, Honeysuckle Flower, Lonicera Flower)
Clear Heat Clean Toxin
Sweet
Cold
Lung, Stomach, Large Intestine, Heart[51]
Name (Yang Ming, Large Intestine/Stomach), Biao/Li (Large Intestine/Lung), Clock Neighbor (Large Intestine/Stomach) + Heart

Chuan Xin Lian, Lan He Lian (Herba Andrographis, Green Chiretta, Kariyat)
Clear Heat Clean Toxin
Bitter
Cold
Lung, Stomach, Large Intestine, Small Intestine
Name (Yang Ming, Large Intestine/Stomach), Biao/Li (Large Intestine/Lung), Clock Neighbor (Large Intestine/Stomach) + Small Intestine

Ban Zhi Lian (Herba Scutellariae Barbatae, Barbat Skullcap, Barbed Skullcap)
Clear Heat Clean Toxin
Acrid, slightly Bitter
Cool
Liver, **Lung**, Stomach, Kidney,[52] Large Intestine[53]
Name (Yang Ming, Large Intestine/Stomach), Bie Jing (Jue Yin/Yang Ming, Liver/Large Intestine), Biao/Li (Large Intestine/Lung), Clock Opposite (Kidney/Large Intestine), Clock Neighbor (Large Intestine/Stomach, Liver/Lung), Branch (You/Chicken, Lung/Kidney, 5PM-6:59PM, Mao/Rabbit, Liver/Large Intestine, 5AM-6:59AM)

Hu Yao Huang (Herba Leucas Mollissimae, Leucas)
Clear Heat Clean Toxin
Bitter
Cool
Large Intestine, Small Intestine, **Lung**
Biao/Li (Large Intestine/Lung) + Small Intestine

Qian Li Guang (Herba Senecionis Scandens, Climbing Groundsel, Ragwort)
Clear Heat Clean Toxin
Bitter
Cold
Lung, Liver, Large Intestine
Biao/Li (Large Intestine/Lung), Bie Jing (Jue Yin/Yang Ming, Liver/Large Intestine), Clock Neighbor (Liver/Lung), Branch (Mao/Rabbit, Liver/Large Intestine, 5AM-6:59AM)

Ban Lan Gen, Bei Ban Lan Gen (Radix Isatidis, Isatis Root)
Clear Heat Clean Toxin
Bitter
Cold
Heart, Stomach, **Lung**[54]

Da Qing Ye (Folium Isatidis, Woad Leaf, Indigo Leaf)
Clear Heat Clean Toxin
Bitter, Salty[55]
Very Cold
Heart, **Lung**, Stomach, Liver[56]
Clock Neighbor (Liver/Lung) + Heart, Stomach

Nan Ban Lan Ye, Ma Lian Ye (Folium Baphicacanthis)
Clear Heat Clean Toxin
Bitter, Salty
Cold
Lung, Stomach, Heart, Liver
Clock Neighbor (Liver/Lung) + Stomach, Heart

Long Kui, Ku Kui (Herba Solanum Nigrum, Black Nightshade)
Clear Heat Clean Toxin
Slightly Bitter, slightly Sweet[57]
Cold, non-Toxic[58] to slightly Toxic*
Lung, Urinary Bladder, Stomach[59]
Bie Jing (Tai Yin/Tai Yang, Lung/Urinary Bladder), Clock Opposite (Lung/Urinary Bladder), Qian/Hou (Front/Back, Stomach/Urinary Bladder)

Qing Dai (Indigo Naturalis)
Clear Heat Clean Toxin
Salty
Cold to very Cold[60]
Liver, **Lung**, Stomach
Clock Neighbor (Liver/Lung) + Stomach

Ban Bian Lian (Herba Lobeliae Chinensis)
Clear Heat Clean Toxin/Regulate Water Resolve Dampness
Acrid, Sweet,[61] Bland[62]
Slightly Cold[63] to Cold, Toxic*[64]
Heart, **Lung**, Small Intestine
Biao/Li (Small Intestine/Heart) + Lung

Lian Qiao (Fructus Forsythiae, Forsythia Fruit)
Clear Heat Clean Toxin
Bitter, slightly Acrid[65]
Cool to slightly Cold[66]
Lung, Heart, Gall Bladder
Bie Jing (Shao Yin/Shao Yang, Heart/Gall Bladder), Clock Opposite (Heart/Gall Bladder), Branch (Yin/Tiger, Gall Bladder/Lung, 3AM-4:59AM)

Shan Ma Ti (Radix Rauvolfiae, Devil Pepper Root)
Clear Heat Clean Toxin
Bitter
Cold, slightly Toxic*
Lung, Liver, Heart
Clock Neighbor (Liver/Lung) + Heart

Pao Zai Cao, Deng Long Cao (Herba Physalis Angulatae)
Clear Heat Clean Toxin
Bitter
Cool
Lung, Urinary Bladder, Liver, Kidney
Bie Jing (Tai Yin/Tai Yang, Lung/Urinary Bladder), Biao/Li (Urinary Bladder/Kidney), Clock Neighbor (Liver/Lung), Clock Opposite (Lung/Urinary Bladder), Branch (You/Chicken, Lung/Kidney, 5PM-6:59PM)

Dao Diao Jin Zhong, Feng Fang Ran (Melothria Maderospatana, Melothria)
Clear Heat Clean Toxin
Sweet, Bitter
Cool
Lung, Liver, Urinary Bladder
Bie Jing (Tai Yin/Tai Yang, Lung/Urinary Bladder), Clock Opposite (Lung/Urinary Bladder), Clock Neighbor (Liver/Lung)

Tu Niu Xi (Radix Achyranthes Longiflora, Native Achyranthis Root)
Clear Heat Clean Toxin/Vitalize Blood Transform Stasis
Bitter, Sour, Acrid[67]
Neutral to Cold,[68] slightly Toxic[69]
Lung, Liver, Kidney
Clock Neighbor (Liver/Lung), Branch (You/Chicken, Lung/Kidney, 5PM-6:59PM)

Ye Ju Hua, Ku Yi (Flos Chrysanthemi Indici, Wild Chrysanthemum Flower)
Acrid Cool Exterior Releasing/Clear Heat Clean Toxin
Bitter, Acrid
Cool to slightly Cold[70]
Lung, Liver
Clock Neighbor (Liver/Lung)

Zhu Zi Cao (Herba Euphorbiae Thymifoliae)
Clear Heat Clean Toxin
Sweet
Cool
Liver, **Lung**
Clock Neighbor (Liver/Lung)

Clear Deficient Heat

Bai Wei (Radix Cynanchi Atrati, Black Swallow-Wort Root)
Clear Deficient Heat
Bitter, Salty
Cold
Stomach, Liver, Kidney,[71] **Lung**,[72] Ren and Chong[73]
Clock Neighbor (Liver/Lung), Branch (You/Chicken, Lung/Kidney, 5PM-6:59PM) + Stomach, Ren, Chong

Di Gu Pi (Cortex Lycii, Wolfberry Root Cortex)
Clear Deficient Heat
Sweet, Bland, Bitter[74]
Cold
Lung, Kidney, Liver[75]
Clock Neighbor (Liver/Lung), Branch (You/Chicken, Lung/Kidney, 5PM-6:59PM)

Purgative

Mang Xiao (Natri Sulfas, Mirabilite, Glauber's Salt, Epsom Salts)
Purgative
Salty, Bitter, Acrid[76]
Cold
Lung,[77] Stomach, Large Intestine
Name (Yang Ming, Large Intestine/Stomach), Biao/Li (Large Intestine/Lung), Clock Neighbor (Large Intestine/Stomach)

Ba Dou (Fructus Crotonis, Croton)
Purgative/Cathartic
Acrid
Hot, extremely Toxic*
Stomach, Large Intestine, **Lung**[78]
Name (Yang Ming, Large Intestine/Stomach), Biao/Li (Large Intestine/Lung), Clock Neighbor (Large Intestine/Stomach)

Moist Laxative

Song Zi Ren (Semen Pini, Pine Nut)
Moist Laxative
Sweet
Warm
Lung, Liver, Large Intestine
Bie Jing (Jue Yin/Yang Ming, Liver/Large Intestine), Biao/Li (Large Intestine, Lung), Clock Neighbor (Liver/Lung), Branch (Mao/Rabbit, Liver/Large Intestine, 5AM-6:59AM)

Cathartic

Ba Dou (Fructus Crotonis, Croton)
Purgative/Cathartic
Acrid
Hot, extremely Toxic*
Stomach, Large Intestine, **Lung**[79]
Name (Yang Ming, Large Intestine/Stomach), Biao/Li (Large Intestine/Lung), Clock Neighbor (Large Intestine/Stomach)

Shang Lu (Radix Phytolaccae, Poke Root)
Cathartic
Bitter
Cold, highly Toxic*
Lung, Spleen,[80] Kidney, Large Intestine, Urinary Bladder[81]
Name (Tai Yin, Lung/Spleen), Bie Jing (Tai Yin/Tai Yang, Lung/Urinary Bladder), Biao/Li (Large Intestine/Lung, Urinary Bladder/Kidney), Clock Opposite (Kidney/Large Intestine, Lung/Urinary Bladder), Branch (You/Chicken, Lung/Kidney, 5PM-6:59PM, Shen/Monkey, Large Intestine/Urinary Bladder, 3PM-4:59PM)

Da Ji (Radix Euphorbiae seu Knoxiae)
Cathartic
Bitter, Acrid
Cold, extremely Toxic*
Spleen,[82] **Lung**,[83] Kidney, Large Intestine, Liver,[84] Gall Bladder[85]
Name (Tai Yin, Lung/Spleen), Bie Jing (Jue Yin/Yang Ming, Liver/Large Intestine), Biao/Li (Large Intestine/Lung, Gall Bladder/Liver), Clock Opposite (Kidney/Large Intestine), Clock Neighbor (Liver/Lung), Branch (Zi/Rat, Kidney/Gall Bladder, 11PM-12:59AM, Chou/Ox, Spleen/Liver, 1AM-2:59AM, Mao/Rabbit, Liver/Large Intestine, 5AM-6:59AM, and You/Chicken, Lung/Kidney, 5PM-6:59PM)

Qian Niu Zi (Semen Pharbitidis, Pharbitis, Morning Glory Seed)
Cathartic
Bitter, Acrid[86]
Cold, Toxic*
Lung, Kidney, Large Intestine, Small Intestine[87]
Biao/Li (Large Intestine/Lung), Clock Opposite (Kidney/Large Intestine), Branch (You/Chicken, Lung/Kidney, 5PM-6:59PM) + Small Intestine

Gan Sui (Radix Euphorbiae Kansui, Kan Sui Root)
Cathartic
Bitter, Sweet
Cold, Toxic*
Lung, Kidney, Large Intestine
Biao/Li (Large Intestine/Lung), Clock Opposite (Kidney/Large Intestine), Branch (You/Chicken, Lung/Kidney, 5PM-6:59PM)

Yuan Hua, Lao Shu Hua (Flos Genkwa, Genkwa Flower, Lilac Daphne Flower Bud)
Cathartic
Acrid, Bitter
Warm, Toxic*
Lung, Kidney, Large Intestine
Biao/Li (Large Intestine/Lung), Clock Opposite (Kidney/Large Intestine), Branch (You/Chicken, Lung/Kidney, 5PM-6:59PM)

Dispel Wind Dampness, Open Channels and Luo-Network Vessels and Relieve Pain

Hong Gu She (Radix Kadsura Japonicae, Kadsura)
Dispel Wind Dampness, Open Channels and Luo-Network Vessels and Relieve Pain
Acrid, Bitter
Cool
Lung, Liver, Stomach
Clock Neighbor (Liver/Lung) + Stomach

Han Fang Ji/Fen Fang Ji (Radix Stephaniae Tetandrae, Stephania Root)
Dispel Wind Dampness, Open Channels and Luo-Network Vessels and Relieve Pain
Acrid, Bitter to very Bitter[88]
Cold to very Cold[89]
Urinary Bladder, **Lung**,[90] Spleen,[91] Kidney, Yang Qiao,[92] and possibly San Jiao[93]
Name (Tai Yin, Spleen/Lung), Bie Jing (Tai Yin/Tai Yang, Lung/Urinary Bladder), Biao/Li (Urinary Bladder/Kidney), Clock Opposite (Lung/Urinary Bladder), Branch (You/Chicken, Lung/Kidney, 5PM-6:59PM), and possibly Bie Jing (Shao Yin/Shao Yang, Kidney/San Jiao), Clock Opposite (San Jiao/Spleen), Branch (Hai/Pig, Urinary Bladder/San Jiao, 9PM-10:59PM) + Yang Qiao

Mu Gua (Fructus Chaenomelis, Japanese Quince)
Dispel Wind Dampness, Open Channels and Luo-Network Vessels and Relieve Pain
Sour, not Astringent,[94] Aromatic[95]
Warm
Liver, Spleen, **Lung**[96]
Name (Tai Yin, Spleen/Lung), Clock Neighbor (Liver/Lung), Branch (Chou/Ox, Spleen/Liver, 1AM-2:59AM)

Guang Fang Ji (Radix Aristolochiae Fangchi)
Dispel Wind Dampness, Open Channels and Luo-Network Vessels and Relieve Pain
Acrid, Bitter
Cold, Toxic*
Urinary Bladder, **Lung**, Yang Qiao[97]
Bie Jing (Tai Yin/Tai Yang, Lung/Urinary Bladder), Clock Opposite (Lung/Urinary Bladder) + Yang Qiao

Chuan Shan Long, Huang Jiang, Chuan Di Long (Rhizoma Dioscoriae Nipponicae, Japanese Dioscoriae Rhizome)
Dispel Wind Dampness, Open Channels and Luo-Network Vessels and Relieve Pain
Bitter
Neutral[98] to Cool, slightly Toxic*[99]
Liver, **Lung**
Clock Neighbor (Liver/Lung)

Dispel Wind-Dampness Strengthen Sinew/Tendon and Bone

Zou Ma Tai (Rhizoma Ardisiae, Ardisia Root, Giant Leaf Ardisia Rhizome)
Dispel Wind-Dampness Strengthen Sinew/Tendon and Bone
Acrid
Neutral
Lung, Stomach, Spleen, Large Intestine
Name (Tai Yin, Lung/Spleen, Yang Ming, Large Intestine/Stomach), Biao/Li (Large Intestine/Lung, Stomach/Spleen), Clock Neighbor (Large Intestine/Stomach)

Shi Nan Teng (Ramulus Piper, Piper Vine)
Dispel Wind-Dampness Strengthen Sinew/Tendon and Bone
Acrid
Warm
Liver, **Lung**, Kidney
Clock Neighbor (Liver/Lung), Branch (You/Chicken, Lung/Kidney, 5PM-6:59PM)

Aromatic Dissolve Dampness

Hou Po, Chuan Po, Lie Po (Cortex Magnoliae Officinalis, Officinal Magnolia Bark)
Aromatic Dissolve Dampness
Bitter, Acrid, Aromatic
Warm
Large Intestine, **Lung**, Spleen, Stomach
Name (Tai Yin, Lung/Spleen and Yang Ming, Large Intestine/Stomach), Biao/Li (Large Intestine/Lung, Stomach/Spleen), Clock Neighbor (Large Intestine/Stomach)

Huo Xiang (Herba Agastache *or* Herba Pogostemonis, Patchouli)
Aromatic Dissolve Dampness
Acrid, Sweet,[100] Aromatic
Slightly Warm
Spleen, Stomach, **Lung**
Name (Tai Yin, Spleen/Lung), Biao/Li (Stomach/Spleen)

Pei Lan (Herba Eupatorii, Fortune Eupatorium)
Aromatic Dissolve Dampness
Acrid, Aromatic
Neutral
Spleen, Stomach, **Lung**
Name (Tai Yin, Spleen/Lung), Biao/Li (Stomach/Spleen)

Hong Dou Kou (Fructus Galangae, Galanga Seed)
Aromatic Dissolve Dampness/Warm Interior
Acrid, Aromatic
Warm
Spleen, Stomach,[101] **Lung**
Name (Tai Yin, Spleen/Lung), Biao/Li (Stomach/Spleen)

Bai Dou Kou (Fructus Amomi Rotundus, Round Cardamom Fruit)
Aromatic Dissolve Dampness
Intensely[102] Acrid, not Astringent,[103] Aromatic
Warm
Lung, Spleen, Stomach and possibly San Jiao[104]
Name (Tai Yin, Lung/Spleen), Biao/Li (Stomach/Spleen) and possibly Clock Opposite (Spleen/San Jiao)

Regulate Water Resolve Dampness

Dong Gua Zi (Semen Benincasae, White Gourd Seed, Winter Melon Seed)
Regulate Water Resolve Dampness
Sweet
Cool to Cold[105]
Lung, Stomach, Small Intestine, Large Intestine
Name (Yang Ming, Large Intestine/Stomach), Biao/Li (Large Intestine/Lung), Clock Neighbor (Large Intestine/Stomach) + Small Intestine

Ze Qi (Herba Euphorbiae Helioscopiae, Euphorbia, Sun Spurge)
Regulate Water Resolve Dampness/Transform Phlegm
Sweet, Bitter, Acrid
Cool to slightly Cold,[106] slightly Toxic[107] to Toxic*
Large Intestine, Small Intestine, **Lung**
Biao/Li (Large Intestine/Lung) + Small Intestine

Tong Cao (Medulla Tetrapanacis, Rice Paper Pith)
Regulate Water Resolve Dampness
Sweet, Bland
Cool to slightly Cold[108]
Lung, Stomach

Yi Yi Ren (Semen Coicis, Job's Tears)
Regulate Water Resolve Dampness
Sweet, Bland
Cool to slightly Cold
Spleen, Stomach, **Lung**, Kidney[109]
Name (Tai Yin, Spleen/Lung), Biao/Li (Stomach/Spleen), Branch (You/Chicken, Lung/Kidney, 5PM-6:59PM)

Cha Ye (Folium Theae, Tea Leaves)
Regulate Water Resolve Dampness
Bitter, Sweet
Cool
Heart, **Lung**, Stomach

Fu Ling, Yun Ling (Poria, Hoelen, China Root)
Regulate Water Resolve Dampness
Sweet, Bland
Neutral
Heart, Spleen, Kidney, **Lung**[110]
Name (Shao Yin, Heart/Kidney, Tai Yin, Spleen/Lung), Clock Neighbor (Spleen/Heart)

Deng Xin Cao (Medulla Junci, Juncus, Rush Pith)
Regulate Water Resolve Dampness
Sweet, Bland
Cool to slightly Cold[111]
Heart, **Lung**, Small Intestine
Biao/Li (Small Intestine/Heart) + Lung

Ban Bian Lian (Herba Lobeliae Chinensis)
Clear Heat Clean Toxin/Regulate Water Resolve Dampness
Acrid, Sweet,[112] Bland[113]
Slightly Cold[114] to Cold, Toxic*[115]
Heart, **Lung**, Small Intestine
Biao/Li (Small Intestine/Heart) + Lung

Chuan Mu Tong (Caulis Clematidis Armandii, Armand's Clematis)
Regulate Water Resolve Dampness
Bitter, Bland[116]
Cold
Urinary Bladder, Heart, **Lung**,[117] Small Intestine
Name (Tai Yang, Small Intestine/Urinary Bladder), Bie Jing (Tai Yin/Tai Yang, Lung/Urinary Bladder), Biao/Li (Small Intestine/Heart), Clock Opposite (Lung/Urinary Bladder), Clock Neighbor (Small Intestine/Urinary Bladder)

Dong Gua Pi (Exocarpium Benincasae, White Gourd Rind, Winter Melon Rind)
Regulate Water Resolve Dampness
Sweet, Bland[118]
Slightly Cold
Lung, Small Intestine

Che Qian Zi (Semen Plantaginis, Plantago Seed, Plantain Seed)
Regulate Water Resolve Dampness
Sweet, Bland[119]
Cold
Kidney, Urinary Bladder, Liver, **Lung**, Small Intestine[120]
Name (Tai Yang, Small Intestine/Urinary Bladder), Bie Jing (Tai Yin/Tai Yang, Lung/Urinary Bladder), Biao/Li (Urinary Bladder/Kidney), Clock Opposite (Lung/Urinary Bladder, Liver/Small Intestine), Clock Neighbor (Small Intestine/Urinary Bladder, Liver/Lung), Branch (You/Chicken, Lung/Kidney, 5PM-6:59PM)

Che Qian Cao (Herba Plantaginis)
Regulate Water Resolve Dampness
Sweet
Cold
Liver, Kidney, **Lung**, Small Intestine
Clock Opposite (Liver/Small Intestine), Clock Neighbor (Liver/Lung), Branch (You/Chicken, Lung/Kidney, 5PM-6:59PM)

Shi Wei, Shi Lan, Fei Xin Cao (Folium Pyrrosiae, Pyrrosia, Japanese Felt Fern)
Regulate Water Resolve Dampness
Bitter, Sweet
Cool to slightly Cold[121]
Urinary Bladder, **Lung**
Bie Jing (Tai Yin/Tai Yang, Lung/Urinary Bladder), Clock Opposite (Urinary Bladder/Lung)

Bai Long Chuan Hua Tou (Radix Clerodendron Paniculatum, Clerodendron, Scarlet Glory Bower)
Regulate Water Resolve Dampness
Slightly Bitter
Warm
Lung, Liver, Kidney
Clock Neighbor (Liver/Lung), Branch (You/Chicken, Lung/Kidney, 5PM-6:59PM)

Liu Zhi Huang (Herba Solidaginis, Solidago)
Regulate Water Resolve Dampness
Bitter, Sweet
Cold
Lung, Liver, Kidney
Clock Neighbor (Liver/Lung), Branch (You/Chicken, Lung/Kidney, 5PM-6:59PM)

Shan Pu Tao (Radix Vitis Amurensis, Viticis)
Regulate Water Resolve Dampness
Sweet
Cold
Lung, Liver, Kidney
Clock Neighbor (Liver/Lung), Branch (You/Chicken, Lung/Kidney, 5PM-6:59PM)

Ma Ti Jin (Herba Dichondrae Repentis, Dichondra)
Regulate Water Resolve Dampness
Bitter, Acrid
Cool
Liver, **Lung**
Clock Neighbor (Liver/Lung)

Aromatic Dissolve Dampness

Hong Dou Kou (Fructus Galangae, Galanga Seed)
Aromatic Dissolve Dampness/Warm Interior
Acrid, Aromatic
Warm
Spleen, Stomach,[122] **Lung**
Name (Tai Yin, Spleen/Lung), Biao/Li (Stomach/Spleen)

Warm Interior

Hong Dou Kou (Fructus Galangae, Galanga Seed)
Aromatic Dissolve Dampness/Warm Interior
Acrid, Aromatic
Warm
Spleen, Stomach,[123] **Lung**
Name (Tai Yin, Spleen/Lung), Biao/Li (Stomach/Spleen)

Gan Jiang (Rhizoma Zingiberis, Dried Ginger Root)
Warm Interior
Acrid, Aromatic
Hot
Heart, **Lung**, Spleen, Stomach
Name (Tai Yin, Lung/Spleen), Biao/Li (Stomach/Spleen), Clock Neighbor (Spleen/Heart)

Jiao Mu (Semen Zanthoxyli, Zanthoxylum Seed, Sichuan Peppercorn Seed)
Warm Interior
Bitter
Cold, Toxic*
Spleen, Urinary Bladder, **Lung**, Kidney
Name (Tai Yin, Spleen/Lung), Bie Jing (Tai Yin/Tai Yang, Lung/Urinary Bladder), Biao/Li (Urinary Bladder/Kidney), Clock Opposite (Lung/Urinary Bladder), Branch (You/Chicken, Lung/Kidney, 5PM-6:59PM)

Xi Xin (Radix et Rhizoma Asari, Asarum, Chinese Wild Ginger)
Acrid Warm Exterior Releasing/Warm Interior
Acrid to extremely Acrid,[124] Aromatic
Warm, slightly Toxic*
Lung, Heart, Kidney, Du,[125] all channels[126]
Name (Shao Yin, Heart/Kidney), Branch (You/Chicken, Lung/Kidney, 5PM-6:59PM) + Du

Dou Chi Jiang (Rhizoma et Radix Litsae, Cubeb Rhizome and Root)
Warm Interior
Acrid, Aromatic
Warm
Liver, **Lung**
Clock Neighbor (Liver/Lung)

Regulate and Rectify Qi

Wan Dian Jin (Radix Ilicis Asprellae, Ilex)
Regulate and Rectify Qi
Bland
Cool
Lung

Xie Bai, Xiao Suan, Ye Suan (Bulbus Alli Macrostemonis, Chive Bulb)
Regulate and Rectify Qi
Acrid, Bitter, Aromatic
Warm
Large Intestine, Stomach, **Lung**
Name (Yang Ming, Large Intestine/Stomach), Biao/Li (Large Intestine/Lung), Clock Neighbor (Large Intestine/Stomach)

Ju Hong, Yun Pi, Yun Hong (Exocarpium Citri Rubrum, Tangerine Flavedo)
Regulate and Rectify Qi
Bitter, Acrid, Aromatic
Warm
Lung, Stomach

Shi Di, Shi Ding, Shi Zi Ba (Calyx Kaki, Persimmon Calyx)
Regulate and Rectify Qi
Bitter, Astringent[127]
Neutral
Lung,[128] Stomach

Hua Ju Hong, Hua Pi, You Pi Ju Hong (Exocarpium Citri Grandis, Pumelo Peel)
Regulate and Rectify Qi
Bitter, Acrid, Aromatic
Warm
Lung, Spleen, Stomach
Name (Tai Yin, Lung/Spleen), Biao/Li (Stomach/Spleen)

Chen Pi, Ju Pi, Hong Pi (Pericarpium Citri Reticulatae, Aged Tangerine Peel)
Regulate and Rectify Qi
Acrid, Bitter, Aromatic
Warm
Lung, Spleen, Stomach[129]
Name (Tai Yin, Lung/Spleen), Biao/Li (Stomach/Spleen)

Zi Su Geng (Caulis Perillae, Perilla Stem)
Acrid Warm Exterior Releasing/Regulate and Rectify Qi
Acrid, Sweet, Aromatic
Slightly Warm
Lung, Spleen, Stomach
Name (Tai Yin, Lung/Spleen), Biao/Li (Stomach/Spleen)

Tan Xiang (Lignum Santali Albi, Sandalwood)
Regulate and Rectify Qi
Acrid, Aromatic
Warm
Spleen, Stomach, **Lung**
Name (Tai Yin, Spleen/Lung), Biao/Li (Stomach/Spleen)

Fo Shou (Fructus Citri Sarcodactylis, Finger Citron Fruit, Buddha's Hand Citron)
Regulate and Rectify Qi
Acrid, Bitter, Aromatic
Warm
Liver, **Lung**, Stomach, Spleen
Name (Tai Yin, Lung/Spleen), Biao/Li (Stomach/Spleen), Clock Neighbor (Liver/Lung), Branch (Chou/Ox, Spleen/Liver, 1AM-2:59AM)

Tian Xian Teng, Ma Dou Ling Teng (Herba Aristolochiae, Aristolochia, Dutchman's Pipe)
Regulate and Rectify Qi
Bitter
Warm, Toxic*
Heart, **Lung**, Spleen, Kidney
Name (Shao Yin, Heart/Kidney, Tai Yin, Spleen/Lung)
Clock Neighbor (Spleen/Heart), Branch (You/Chicken, Lung/Kidney, 5PM-6:59PM)

Wu Yao, Tai Wu Yao, Tai Wu (Radix Linderae, Lindera Root)
Regulate and Rectify Qi
Acrid, Aromatic[130]
Warm
Urinary Bladder, Kidney, **Lung**, Spleen
Name (Tai Yin, Lung/Spleen), Bie Jing (Tai Yin/Tai Yang, Lung/Urinary Bladder), Biao/Li (Urinary Bladder/Kidney), Clock Opposite (Lung/Urinary Bladder), Branch (You/Chicken, Lung/Kidney, 5PM-6:59PM)

Xiang Yuan (Fructus Citri, Citron)
Regulate and Rectify Qi
Acrid, slightly Bitter, Sour, Aromatic
Warm
Liver, Spleen, **Lung**
Name (Tai Yin, Spleen/Lung), Clock Neighbor (Liver/Lung), Branch (Chou/Ox, Spleen/Liver, 1AM-2:59AM)

Tu Mu Xiang, Qi Mu Xiang (Radix Inulae)
Regulate and Rectify Qi
Acrid, Bitter
Warm
Lung, Liver, Spleen
Name (Tai Yin, Lung/Spleen), Clock Neighbor (Liver/Lung) Branch (Chou/Ox, Spleen/Liver, 1AM-2:59AM)

Ju Luo, Ju Si, Ju Jin (Citri Reticulatae Fructus Fasciculus Vascularis, Tangerine Pith, White Vein Network of Orange Peel)
Regulate and Rectify Qi
Sweet, Bitter
Neutral
Liver, **Lung**
Clock Neighbor (Liver/Lung)

Digestive

Lai Fu Zi (Semen Raphani, Radish/Daikon/Turnip Seeds)
Digestive
Acrid, Sweet
Neutral
Spleen, Stomach, **Lung**
Name (Tai Yin, Spleen/Lung), Biao/Li (Stomach/Spleen)

Expel Parasites

Fei Zi (Semen Torreyae, Torreya Seeds)
Expel Parasites
Sweet, Astringent[131]
Neutral, relatively Non-Toxic[132]
Lung, Large Intestine, Stomach[133]
Name (Yang Ming, Large Intestine/Stomach), Biao/Li (Large Intestine/Lung), Clock Neighbor (Large Intestine/Stomach)

Da Suan (Bulbus Alli Sativi, Garlic)
Expel Parasites/External Application
Acrid, Sweet[134]
Neutral to Warm
Spleen, Stomach, **Lung**, Large Intestine[135]
Name (Tai Yin, Spleen/Lung, Yang Ming, Large Intestine/Stomach), Biao/Li (Stomach/Spleen, Large Intestine/Lung), Clock Neighbor (Large Intestine/Stomach)

Chang Shan (Radix Dichroae, Dichroa Root)
Expel Parasites/Emetic
Acrid, Bitter
Cold, Toxic*
Lung, Heart, Liver
Clock Neighbor (Liver/Lung) + Heart

Stop Bleeding

Wan Nian Song (Herba Selaginellae, Selaginella)
Stop Bleeding
Acrid
Neutral
Lung, Large Intestine
Biao/Li (Large Intestine/Lung)

Zong Lu Tan (Trachycarpi Petiolus Carbonisatus, Charred Trachycarpus Petiole)
Stop Bleeding
Bitter, Astringent
Neutral
Lung, Liver, Large Intestine, Spleen[136]
Name (Tai Yin, Lung/Spleen), Bie Jing (Jue Yin/Yang Ming, Liver/Large Intestine), Biao/Li (Large Intestine/Lung), Clock Neighbor (Liver/Lung), Branch (Mao/Rabbit, Liver/Large Intestine, 5AM-6:59AM)

Zong Lu Pi (Fibra Stipulae Trachicarpi, Trachycarpus Stipule Fiber)
Stop Bleeding
Bitter, Sour, Astringent[137]
Neutral
Liver, **Lung**, Large Intestine
Bie Jing (Jue Yin/Yang Ming, Liver/Large Intestine), Biao/Li (Large Intestine/Lung), Clock Neighbor (Liver/Lung), Branch (Mao/Rabbit, Liver/Large Intestine, 5AM-6:59AM)

Ce Bai Ye (Cacumen Platycadi, Biota Leaves, Arborvitae Leaf)
Stop Bleeding
Bitter, Astringent
Cool[138] to slightly Cold
Lung, Liver, Large Intestine
Bie Jing (Jue Yin/Yang Ming, Liver/Large Intestine), Biao/Li (Large Intestine/Lung), Branch (Mao/Rabbit, Liver/Large Intestine, 5AM-6:59AM)

Bai Mao Gen (Rhizoma Imperatae, Wolly Grass Rhizome, Cogon Rhizome)
Stop Bleeding
Sweet
Cold
Lung, Stomach, Urinary Bladder, Small Intestine[139]
Name (Tai Yang, Small Intestine/Urinary Bladder), Bie Jing (Tai Yin/Tai Yang, Lung/Urinary Bladder), Clock Opposite (Lung/Urinary Bladder), Clock Neighbor (Small Intestine/Urinary Bladder), Qian/Hou (Front/Back, Stomach/Urinary Bladder)

Zhu Fan Hua Tou, Su Xiang (Rhizoma Mirabilidis, Mirabilis)
Stop Bleeding
Sweet, Bitter, Astringent
Neutral
Lung, Stomach, Urinary Bladder
Bie Jing (Tai Yin/Tai Yang, Lung/Urinary Bladder), Clock Opposite (Lung/Urinary Bladder), Qian/Hou (Front/Back, Stomach/Urinary Bladder)

Bai Ji, Bai Gen, Gan Gen (Rhizoma Bletillae, Bletilla Rhizome)
Stop Bleeding
Bitter, Sweet, Astringent
Cool to slightly Cold[140]
Lung, Stomach, Liver
Clock Neighbor (Liver/Lung) + Stomach

Zi Zhu, Zi Zhu Cao (Folium Callicarpae, Callicarpa Leaf, Beauty-Berry Leaf)
Stop Bleeding
Bitter, Astringent
Cool
Liver, **Lung**, Stomach
Clock Neighbor (Liver/Lung) + Stomach

Ou Jie (Nodus Nelumbinis Rhizomatis, Lotus Rhizome Nodes)
Stop Bleeding/Astringe, Stabilize and Bind
Sweet, Astringent
Neutral
Lung, Stomach, Liver
Clock Neighbor (Liver/Lung) + Stomach

Xian He Cao, Tuo Li Cao, Lang Ya Cao (Herba Agrimoniae, Agrimony Grass)
Stop Bleeding
Bitter, Astringent
Neutral
Lung, Liver, Spleen
Name (Tai Yin, Lung/Spleen), Clock Neighbor (Liver/Lung), Branch (Chou/Ox, Spleen/Liver, 1AM-2:59AM)

Vitalize Blood Transform Stasis

Tao Ren (Semen Persicae, Peach Kernel)
Vitalize Blood Transform Stasis
Bitter, Sweet[141]
Neutral, slightly Toxic*
Heart, Large Intestine, Liver, **Lung**
Bie Jing (Jue Yin/Yang Ming, Liver/Large Intestine), Biao/Li (Large Intestine/Lung), Clock Neighbor (Liver/Lung), Branch (Mao/Rabbit, Liver/Large Intestine, 5AM-6:59AM) + Heart

Jin Bu Huan, Qian Ceng Ta (Herba Lycopodii Serrati, Lycopodium)
Vitalize Blood Transform Stasis
Acrid, Sweet
Neutral
Lung, Liver, Large Intestine
Bie Jing (Jue Yin/Yang Ming, Liver/Large Intestine), Biao/Li (Large Intestine/Lung), Clock Neighbor (Liver/Lung), Branch (Mao/Rabbit, Liver/Large Intestine, 5AM-6:59AM)

Wa Leng Zi (Concha Arcae, Cockle Shell, Ark Shell)
Vitalize Blood Transform Stasis/Transform Phlegm/External Application
Salty
Neutral
Liver, Stomach, **Lung**, Spleen[142]
Name (Tai Yin, Lung/Spleen), Biao/Li (Stomach/Spleen), Clock Neighbor (Liver/Lung), Branch (Chou/Ox, Spleen/Liver, 1AM-2:59AM)

Yu Jin (Radix Curcumae, Aromatic Tumeric Tuber)
Vitalize Blood Transform Stasis
Acrid, Bitter, Aromatic
Cold
Heart, Liver, Gall Bladder, **Lung**[143]
Bie Jing (Shao Yin/Shao Yang, Heart/Gall Bladder), Biao/Li (Gall Bladder/Liver), Clock Opposite (Heart/Gall Bladder), Clock Neighbor (Liver/Lung), Branch (Yin/Tiger, Gall Bladder/Lung, 3AM-4:59AM)

Tu Niu Xi (Radix Achyranthes Longiflora, Native Achyranthis Root)
Clear Heat Clean Toxin/Vitalize Blood Transform Stasis
Bitter, Sour, Acrid[144]
Neutral to Cold,[145] slightly Toxic[146]
Lung, Liver, Kidney
Clock Neighbor (Liver/Lung), Branch (You/Chicken, Lung/Kidney, 5PM-6:59PM)

Hu Zhang (Rhizoma Polygoni Cuspidati, Bushy Knotweed Rhizome, Japanese Knotweed Rhizome, Giant Knotweed Rhizome)
Vitalize Blood Transform Stasis
Bitter
Cold
Liver, Gall Bladder, **Lung**
Biao/Li (Gall Bladder/Liver), Clock Neighbor (Liver/Lung), Branch (Yin/Tiger, Gall Bladder/Lung, 3AM-4:59AM)

Transform Phlegm

Bai Qian, Cao Bai Qian, E Bai Qian (Rhizoma Cynanchi Stauntonii, Willow Leaf Swallow-Wort)
Transform Phlegm
Acrid, Sweet, Bitter[147]
Slightly Cold to Neutral to slightly Warm[148]
Lung

Jie Geng, Bai Yao (Radix Platycodonis, Balloon Flower Root, Chinese Bell Flower Root)
Transform Phlegm
Bitter, Acrid
Neutral
Lung

Pang Da Hai, Da Hai Zi (Semen Sterculiae Lychnophorae, Boat Sterculia Seed)
Transform Phlegm
Sweet
Cold
Lung, Large Intestine
Biao/Li (Large Intestine/Lung)

Zao Jiao, Zao Jia, Xuan Dao (Fructus Gleditsiae, Chinese Honeylocust Fruit, Gleditsia)
Transform Phlegm
Acrid, Salty[149]
Warm, slightly Toxic*
Large Intestine, **Lung**
Biao/Li (Large Intestine/Lung)

Gua Lou Shi, Quan Gua Lou, Gua Lou (Fructus Trichosanthis, Snake Gourd Fruit)
Transform Phlegm
Sweet, slightly Bitter[150]
Cold
Large Intestine, **Lung**, Stomach
Name (Yang Ming, Large Intestine/Stomach), Biao/Li (Large Intestine/Lung), Clock Neighbor (Large Intestine/Stomach)

Gua Lou Pi (Pericarpium Trichosanthis, Trichosanthis Peel, Snake Gourd Peel)
Transform Phlegm
Sweet
Cold
Large Intestine, **Lung**, Stomach
Name (Yang Ming, Large Intestine/Stomach), Biao/Li (Large Intestine/Lung), Clock Neighbor (Large Intestine/Stomach)

Gua Lou Ren (Semen Trichosanthis, Trichosanthes Seed, Snake Gourd Seed)
Transform Phlegm
Sweet
Cold
Large Intestine, **Lung**, Stomach
Name (Yang Ming, Large Intestine/Stomach), Biao/Li (Large Intestine/Lung), Clock Neighbor (Large Intestine/Stomach)

Xuan Fu Hua, Jin Fei Hua, Jin Fu Hua (Flos Inulae, Inula Flower)
Transform Phlegm
Bitter, Acrid, Salty
Slightly Warm
Large Intestine, **Lung**, Stomach, Spleen, Liver[151]
Name (Yang Ming, Large Intestine/Stomach, Tai Yin, Lung/Spleen), Bie Jing (Jue Yin/Yang Ming, Liver/Large Intestine), Biao/Li (Large Intestine/Lung, Stomach/Spleen), Clock Neighbor (Large Intestine/Stomach, Liver/Lung), Branch (Chou/Ox, Spleen/Liver, 1AM-2:59AM and Mao/Rabbit, Liver/Large Intestine, 5AM-6:59AM)

Bi Qi, Di Li, Wu Yu, Ma Ti (Rhizoma Eleocharitis, Water Chestnut)
Transform Phlegm
Sweet
Slightly Cold
Lung, Liver,[152] Stomach, Large Intestine
Name (Yang Ming, Large Intestine/Stomach), Bie Jing (Jue Yin/Yang Ming, Liver/Large Intestine), Biao/Li (Large Intestine/Lung), Clock Neighbor (Large Intestine/Stomach, Liver/Lung), Branch (Mao/Rabbit, Liver/Large Intestine, 5AM-6:59AM)

Luo Han Guo (Fructus Momordicae, Momordica Fruit)
Transform Phlegm/Relieve Cough and Wheezing/Panting
Sweet
Cool
Lung, Large Intestine, Spleen[153]
Name (Tai Yin, Lung/Spleen), Biao/Li (Large Intestine, Lung)

Ze Qi (Herba Euphorbiae Helioscopiae, Euphorbia, Sun Spurge)
Regulate Water Resolve Dampness/Transform Phlegm
Sweet, Bitter, Acrid
Cool to slightly Cold,[154] slightly Toxic[155] to Toxic*
Large Intestine, Small Intestine, **Lung**
Biao/Li (Large Intestine/Lung) + Small Intestine

Ge Qiao, Ge Ke, Hai Ge Ke Fen (Concha Meretricis seu Cyclinae, Clam Shell)
Transform Phlegm
Bitter,[156] Salty
Neutral[157] to Cold
Lung, Stomach

Zhi Ban Xia, Ban Xia (Rhizoma Pinelliae preparatum)
Transform Phlegm
Acrid
Warm, Toxic* if unprocessed
Spleen, Stomach, **Lung**
Name (Tai Yin, Spleen/Lung), Biao/Li (Stomach/Spleen)

Bai Jie Zi, Huang Jie Zi, Jie Cai Zi (Semen Sinapis, White Mustard Seed)
Transform Phlegm
Acrid
Warm
Lung, Stomach,[158] Spleen[159]
Name (Tai Yin, Lung/Spleen), Biao/Li (Stomach/Spleen)

Zhi Bai Fu Zi, Bai Fu Zi (Rhizoma Typhonii preparatum, Typhonium)
Transform Phlegm
Acrid, Sweet
Warm, Toxic*
Spleen, Stomach, **Lung**,[160] Liver[161]
Name (Tai Yin, Spleen/Lung), Biao/Li (Stomach/Spleen), Clock Neighbor (Liver/Lung), Branch (Chou/Ox, Spleen/Liver, 1AM-2:59AM)

Wa Leng Zi (Concha Arcae, Cockle Shell, Ark Shell)
Vitalize Blood Transform Stasis/Transform Phlegm/External Application
Salty
Neutral
Liver, Stomach, **Lung**, Spleen[162]
Name (Tai Yin, Lung/Spleen), Biao/Li (Stomach/Spleen), Clock Neighbor (Liver/Lung), Branch (Chou/Ox, Spleen/Liver, 1AM-2:59AM)

Zhu Li (Succus Bambusae, Dried Bamboo Sap)
Transform Phlegm
Sweet, Bitter[163]
Cold
Heart, **Lung**, Stomach, Liver[164]
Clock Neighbor (Liver/Lung) + Heart, Stomach

Hai Zao (Sargassum, Seaweed, Gulfweed)
Transform Phlegm
Bitter,[165] Salty
Cold
Liver, Kidney, Stomach,[166] **Lung**[167]
Clock Neighbor (Liver/Lung), Branch (You/Chicken, Lung/Kidney, 5PM-6:59PM) + Stomach

Zhu Ru (Caulis Bambusae in Taenia, Bamboo Shavings)
Transform Phlegm
Sweet, Bitter[168]
Cool to slightly Cold[169]
Lung, Stomach, Gall Bladder
Branch (Yin/Tiger, Gall Bladder/Lung, 3AM-4:59AM) + Stomach

Si Gua Luo (Retinervus Luffae Fructus, Dried Vegetable Sponge)
Transform Phlegm/External Application
Sweet
Neutral to Cold[170]
Lung, Stomach, Liver
Clock Neighbor (Liver/Lung) + Stomach

Jin Meng Shi (Micae Lapis Aureus, Vermiculite Schist)
Transform Phlegm
Sweet, Salty
Neutral
Liver, **Lung**, Stomach
Clock Neighbor (Liver/Lung) + Stomach

Zao Jiao Ci, Tian Ding, Zao Ci, Zao Ding (Spina Gleditsiae, Spine of Honeylocust Plant)
Transform Phlegm
Acrid
Warm
Liver, Stomach, **Lung**[171]
Clock Neighbor (Liver/Lung) + Stomach

Dan Nan Xing, Dan Xing (Arisaema cum Bile)
Transform Phlegm
Cool, slightly Toxic*
Liver, **Lung**,[172] Spleen,[173] Gall Bladder[174]
Name (Tai Yin, Spleen/Lung), Biao/Li (Gall Bladder/Liver), Clock Neighbor (Liver/Lung), Branch (Chou/Ox, Spleen/Liver, 1AM-2:59AM and Yin/Tiger, Gall Bladder/Lung, 3AM-4:59AM)

Zhi Tian Nan Xing, Tian Nan Xing (Rhizoma Arisaematis preparatum, prepared Arisaema, Jack in the Pulpit)
Transform Phlegm
Bitter, very Acrid
Warm, Toxic*
Liver, **Lung**, Spleen
Name (Tai Yin, Spleen/Lung), Clock Neighbor (Liver/Lung), Branch (Chou/Ox, Spleen/Liver, 1AM-2:59AM)

Zhe Bei Mu, Da Bei Mu (Bulbus Fritillariae Thunbergii, Thunbergy Fritillary Bulb)
Transform Phlegm
Bitter
Cold
Heart, **Lung**

Chuan Bei Mu (Bulbus Fritillarie Cirrhosae, Sichuan Fritillaria Bulb, Tendrilled Fritillaria Bulb)
Transform Phlegm
Bitter, Sweet
Cool to slightly Cold[175]
Heart, **Lung**

Fu Shi, Shi Hua (Pumex, Pumice) and Fu Hai Shi, Hai Fu Shi, Fu Shui Shi (Os Costaziae, Costaziae Skeletons)
Transform Phlegm
Salty
Cold
Lung, Kidney[176]
Branch (You/Chicken, Lung/Kidney, 5PM-6:59PM)

Qian Hu (Radix Peucedani, Hogfennel Root)
Transform Phlegm
Bitter, Acrid
Cool to slightly Cold[177]
Lung, Liver,[178] Gall Bladder[179]
Biao/Li (Gall Bladder/Liver), Clock Neighbor (Liver/Lung), Branch (Yin/Tiger, Gall Bladder/Lung, 3AM-4:59AM)

Huang Yao Zi (Herba Dioscoriae Bulbiferae)
Transform Phlegm
Bitter, Sweet[180]
Neutral[181] to Cold, Toxic*
Lung, Liver
Clock Neighbor (Liver/Lung)

Ming Dang Shen, Ming Shen (Radix Changii, Changium root)
Transform Phlegm
Sweet, slightly Bitter
Cool
Lung, Liver
Clock Neighbor (Liver/Lung)

Qing Meng Shi, Meng Shi (Lapis Micae seu Chloriti, Chlorite Schist, Mica Schist)
Transform Phlegm
Salty, Sweet
Neutral
Lung, Liver
Clock Neighbor (Liver/Lung)

Relieve Cough and Wheezing/Panting

Bai Bu (Radix Stemonae, Stemona Root)
Relieve Cough and Wheezing/Panting
Sweet, Bitter
Slightly Cold[182] to Neutral to slightly Warm[183]
Lung

Zi Wan (Radix Asteris, Purple Aster Root)
Relieve Cough and Wheezing/Panting
Bitter, Sweet, Acrid[184]
Slightly Warm
Lung

Yin Guo Ye, Yin Xing Ye (Folium Ginkgo, Gingko Leaf)
Relieve Cough and Wheezing/Panting
Sweet,[185] Bitter, Astringent
Neutral
Lung

Xing Ren, Bei Xing, Ku Xing Ren (Semen Armeniacae Amarum, Apricot Seed)
Relieve Cough and Wheezing/Panting
Bitter
Slightly Warm, slightly Toxic*
Lung, Large Intestine
Biao/Li (Large Intestine, Lung)

Ma Dou Ling (Fructus Aristolochiae, Birthwort Fruit)
Relieve Cough and Wheezing/Panting
Bitter, slightly Acrid
Cold, slightly Toxic*
Lung, Large Intestine
Biao/Li (Large Intestine, Lung)

Zi Su Zi, Su Zi (Fructus Perillae, Purple Perilla Fruit)
Relieve Cough and Wheezing/Panting
Acrid, Aromatic
Warm
Lung, Large Intestine
Biao/Li (Large Intestine, Lung)

Luo Han Guo (Fructus Momordicae, Momordica Fruit)
Transform Phlegm/Relieve Cough and Wheezing/Panting
Sweet
Cool
Lung, Large Intestine, Spleen[186]
Name (Tai Yin, Lung/Spleen), Biao/Li (Large Intestine, Lung)

Pi Pa Ye, Liu Jie Ye (Folium Eriobotryae, Eriobotrya Leaf, Loquat Leaf)
Relieve Cough and Wheezing/Panting
Bitter
Neutral[187] to Cool to slightly Cold[188]
Lung, Stomach

Zhong Ru Shi (Stalactitum, Stalactite Tip)
Relieve Cough and Wheezing/Panting/Tonify Yang
Sweet, Acrid[189]
Warm
Lung, Kidney, Stomach
Branch (You/Chicken, Lung/Kidney, 5PM-6:59PM) + Stomach

Li Lu (Radix et Rhizoma Veratri, Lack False Hellebore, Vanity Grass)
Relieve Cough and Wheezing/Panting/Emetic
Acrid, Bitter
Cold, extremely Toxic*
Lung, Liver, Stomach
Clock Neighbor (Liver/Lung) + Stomach

Yang Jin Hua (Flos Daturae, Datura Flower)
Relieve Cough and Wheezing
Acrid
Warm, Toxic*
Lung, Liver, Heart, Spleen
Name (Tai Yin, Lung/Spleen), Clock Neighbor (Liver/Lung, Spleen/Heart), Branch (Chou/Ox, Spleen/Liver, 1AM-2:59AM)

Kuan Dong Hua, Dong Hua, Jiu Jiu Hua (Flos Farfarae, Coltsfoot Flower)
Relieve Cough and Wheezing/Panting
Acrid, slightly Bitter,[190] Sweet[191]
Warm
Lung, Heart,[192] Liver[193]
Clock Neighbor (Liver/Lung) + Heart

Ting Li Zi (Semen Descurainiae seu Lepidii, Descurainia seed, Lepidium Seed)
Relieve Cough and Wheezing/Panting
Acrid, Bitter
Very Cold
Lung, Urinary Bladder
Bie Jing (Tai Yin/Tai Yang, Lung/Urinary Bladder), Clock Opposite (Lung/Urinary Bladder)

Sang Bai Pi, Sang Pi (Cortex Mori, Mulberry Bark)
Relieve Cough and Wheezing/Panting
Sweet
Cold
Lung, Urinary Bladder[194]
Bie Jing (Tai Yin/Tai Yang, Lung/Urinary Bladder), Clock Opposite (Lung/Urinary Bladder)

Bai Guo, Yin Xing (Semen Ginkgo, Ginkgo Nut)
Relieve Cough and Wheezing/Panting/Astringe, Stabilize and Bind
Sweet, Bitter, Astringent
Neutral, slightly Toxic*
Lung, Kidney[195]
Branch (You/Chicken, Lung/Kidney, 5PM-6:59PM)

Zi Jin Niu, Ai Di Cha, Ping Di Mu (Herba Ardisiae Japonicae, Japanese Ardisia)
Relieve Cough and Wheezing/Panting
Bitter, Acrid
Neutral
Lung, Liver
Clock Neighbor (Liver/Lung)

Mu Hu Die, Yu Hu Die, Gu Zhi Hua (Semen Oroxyli, Oroxylum Seeds)
Relieve Cough and Wheezing/Panting
Sweet, Bland
Cool
Liver, **Lung**
Clock Neighbor (Liver/Lung)

Nourish and Calm Shen

He Huan Hua, Ye He Hua, Ye He Mi (Flos Albiziae, Mimosa Flower)
Nourish and Calm Shen
Sweet
Neutral
Liver, Stomach, Spleen,[196] Heart,[197] **Lung**[198]
Name (Tai Yin, Lung/Spleen), Biao/Li (Stomach/Spleen), Clock Neighbor (Spleen/Heart, Liver/Lung), Branch (Chou/Ox, Spleen/Liver, 1AM-2:59AM)

Yuan Zhi (Radix Polygalae, Senega Root)
Nourish and Calm Shen
Acrid, Bitter
Slightly Warm
Lung, Heart, Kidney[199]
Name (Shao Yin, Heart/Kidney), Branch (You/Chicken, Lung/Kidney, 5PM-6:59PM)

Ling Zhi, Zhi, Ling Zhi Cao (Ganoderma, Reishi Mushroom)
Nourish and Calm Shen
Sweet
Neutral
Heart, Liver, **Lung**
Clock Neighbor (Liver/Lung) + Heart

Long Chi (Fossilia Mastodi Dentis, fossilized teeth)
Calm Shen Sedative
Sweet, Astringent
Cool
Heart, Liver, **Lung**[200]
Clock Neighbor (Liver/Lung) + Heart

Calm Liver Extinguish Wind

Di Long, Qiu Yin (Pheretima, Earthworm)
Calm Liver Extinguish Wind
Salty
Cold
Liver, Spleen, Kidney,[201] Urinary Bladder, **Lung**[202]
Name (Tai Yin, Spleen/Lung), Bie Jing (Tai Yin/Tai Yang, Lung/Urinary Bladder), Biao/Li (Urinary Bladder/Kidney), Clock Opposite (Lung/Urinary Bladder), Clock Neighbor (Liver/Lung), Branch (Chou/Ox, Spleen/Liver, 1AM-2:59AM)

Jiang Can, Bai Jiang Can, Tian Cong (Bombyx Batryticatus, Mummified Silkworm)
Calm Liver Extinguish Wind
Salty, Acrid
Neutral to slightly Warm[203]
Liver, **Lung**
Clock Neighbor (Liver/Lung)

Open Orifices

Bing Pian, Long Nao Bing Pian (Borneolum, Borneolum Syntheticum, Borneol)
Open Orifices
Acrid, Bitter, Aromatic
Slightly Cold[204] to Hot[205]
Heart, Spleen, **Lung**
Name (Tai Yin, Spleen/Lung), Clock Neighbor (Spleen/Heart)

Tonify Qi

Sha Ji, Cu Liu Guo (Fructus Hippophae, Sea Buckthorn Fruit, Swallow Thorn Fruit)
Tonify Qi
Sour, slightly Sweet, Astringent
Warm
Lung, Spleen, Stomach, Large Intestine, Liver, Small Intestine[206]
Name (Tai Yin, Lung/Spleen, Yang Ming, Large Intestine/Stomach), Bie Jing (Jue Yin/Yang Ming, Liver/Large Intestine, Tai Yin/Tai Yang, Spleen/Small Intestine), Biao/Li (Large Intestine/Lung, Stomach/Spleen), Clock Opposite (Liver/Small Intestine), Clock Neighbor (Liver/Lung, Large Intestine/Stomach), Branch (Chou/Ox, Spleen/Liver, 1AM-2:59AM, Mao/Rabbit, Liver/Large Intestine, 5AM-6:59AM, Si/Snake, Small Intestine/Spleen, 9AM-10:59AM, Wei/Sheep, Spleen/Small Intestine, 1PM-2:59PM)

Feng Mi (Mel, Honey)
Tonify Qi
Sweet
Neutral
Spleen, **Lung**, Large Intestine
Name (Tai Yin, Spleen/Lung), Biao/Li (Large Intestine/Lung)

Yi Tang (Saccharum Granorum, Maltosum, Malt Sugar, Maltose)
Tonify Qi
Sweet
Slightly Warm[207] to Warm
Spleen, Stomach, **Lung**
Name (Tai Yin, Spleen/Lung), Biao/Li (Stomach/Spleen)

Gan Cao (Radix Glycyrrhizae, Licorice Root)
Tonify Qi
Sweet
Neutral
Spleen, Stomach, **Lung**, Heart, Dai,[208] some sources indicate that it enters all channels.
Name (Tai Yin, Spleen/Lung), Biao/Li (Stomach/Spleen), Clock Neighbor (Spleen/Heart) + Dai, some sources indicate that Gan Cao enters all channels and therefore creates every relationship.

Tai Zi Shen (Radix Psuedostellariae, Pseudostellaria)
Tonify Qi
Sweet, slightly Bitter
Neutral to slightly Cold[209]
Lung, Spleen
Name (Tai Yin, Spleen/Lung)

Dong Yang Shen (Radix Ginseng Japonica, Japanese Ginseng)
Tonify Qi
Sweet, slightly Bitter
Cool
Spleen, **Lung**
Name (Tai Yin, Spleen/Lung)

Dang Shen (Radix Codonopsis, Codonopsis Root)
Tonify Qi
Sweet
Neutral
Spleen, **Lung**
Name (Tai Yin, Spleen/Lung)

Hong Qi (Radix Hedysari, Many Inflorescenced Sweetvetch)
Tonify Qi
Sweet
Warm
Lung, Spleen
Name (Tai Yin, Lung/Spleen)

Hong Jing Tian, Qi Ye Dan (Herba Rhodiolae, Rhodiola)
Tonify Qi
Sweet, Astringent[210]
Cold
Spleen, **Lung**
Name (Tai Yin, Spleen/Lung)

Jiao Gu Lan, Qi Dan Ye, Long Xu Teng (Rhizoma seu Herba Gynostemmatis)
Tonify Qi
Sweet,[211] slightly Bitter
Cold
Spleen,[212] **Lung**, Heart[213]
Name (Tai Yin, Spleen/Lung), Clock Neighbor (Spleen/Heart)

Xi Yang Shen, Hua Qi Shen (Radix Panacis Quinquefoli, American Ginseng Root)
Tonify Qi/Tonify Yin
Sweet, slightly Bitter[214] to Bitter to very Bitter[215]
Cold
Kidney, Heart, **Lung**, Spleen[216]
Name (Shao Yin, Kidney/Heart, Tai Yin, Spleen/Lung), Clock Neighbor (Spleen/Heart), Branch (You/Chicken, Lung/Kidney, 5PM-6:59PM)

Ren Shen (Radix Ginseng, Ginseng Root)
Tonify Qi
Sweet, slightly Bitter
Slightly Warm
Lung, Spleen, Heart,[217] Kidney[218]
Name (Tai Yin, Lung/Spleen, Shao Yin, Kidney/Heart), Clock Neighbor (Spleen/Heart), Branch (You/Chicken, Lung/Kidney, 5PM-6:59PM)

Ci Wu Jia, Wu Jia Shen (Radix et Caulis Acanthopanacis Senticosi, Siberian Ginseng, Eleutherococcus Ginseng)
Tonify Qi
Acrid, slightly Bitter
Warm
Spleen, Kidney, Heart, **Lung**[219]
Name (Tai Yin, Spleen/Lung, Shao Yin, Kidney/Heart), Clock Neighbor (Spleen/Heart), Branch (You/Chicken, Lung/Kidney, 5PM-6:59PM)

Shan Yao, Huai Shan Yao, Huai Shan, Shan Shu (Rhizoma Dioscoriae, Chinese Yam)
Tonify Qi
Sweet, Sour,[220] slightly Astringent
Neutral
Kidney, **Lung**, Spleen, Dai[221]
Name (Tai Yin, Lung/Spleen), Branch (You/Chicken, Lung/Kidney, 5PM-6:59PM) + Dai

Huang Qi (Radix Astragali, Astragalus Root, Milk Vetch Root)
Tonify Qi
Sweet
Slightly Warm
Spleen, **Lung**, San Jiao[222]
Name (Tai Yin, Spleen/Lung), Clock Opposite (Spleen/San Jiao)

Tonify Yang

Hu Tao Ren, He Tao Ren, Hu Tao Rou (Semen Juglandis, Walnut Nut)
Tonify Yang
Sweet, Astringent[223]
Warm
Kidney, **Lung**, Large Intestine
Biao/Li (Large Intestine/Lung), Clock Opposite (Kidney/Large Intestine), Branch (You/Chicken, Lung/Kidney, 5PM-6:59PM)

Zhong Ru Shi (Stalactitum, Stalactite Tip)
Relieve Cough and Wheezing/Panting/Tonify Yang
Sweet, Acrid[224]
Warm
Lung, Kidney, Stomach
Branch (You/Chicken, Lung/Kidney, 5PM-6:59PM) + Stomach

Dong Chong Xia Cao, Dong Chong Cao (Cordyceps, Caterpillar Fungus, Aweto)
Tonify Yang
Sweet
Neutral to Warm
Lung, Kidney
Branch (You/Chicken, Lung/Kidney, 5PM-6:59PM)

Ge Jie, Xian Dan (Gecko, Tokay)
Tonify Yang
Salty
Neutral
Lung, Kidney
Branch (You/Chicken, Lung/Kidney, 5PM-6:59PM)

Zi He Che (Placenta Hominis, Human Placenta)
Tonify Yang
Sweet, Salty
Warm
Kidney, **Lung**, Liver
Clock Neighbor (Liver/Lung), Branch (You/Chicken, Lung/Kidney, 5PM-6:59PM)

Tonify Blood

Gou Qi Zi, Di Gu Zi (Fructus Lycii, Chinese Wolfberry Fruit, Matrimony Vine Fruit, Boxthorn Fruit)
Tonify Blood/Tonify Yin
Sweet
Neutral
Liver, Kidney, **Lung**
Clock Neighbor (Liver/Lung), Branch (You/Chicken, Lung/Kidney, 5PM-6:59PM)

E Jiao, Lu Pi Jiao (Colla Corii Asini, Donkey-Hide Glue, Gelatin)
Tonify Blood
Sweet
Neutral
Lung, Liver, Kidney
Clock Neighbor (Liver/Lung), Branch (You/Chicken, Lung/Kidney, 5PM-6:59PM)

Tonify Yin

Bei Sha Shen (Radix Glehniae, Glehniae)
Tonify Yin
Sweet, slightly Bitter[225]
Cool to slightly Cold[226]
Lung, Stomach

Nan Sha Shen (Radix Adenophorae, Adenophora, Four Leaf Lady Bell Root)
Tonify Yin
Sweet, slightly Bitter, Bland[227]
Cool
Lung, Stomach

Yu Zhu (Rhizoma Polygonati Odorati, Polygonatum, Solomon's Seal Rhizome)
Tonify Yin
Sweet
Neutral to slightly Cold[228]
Lung, Stomach

Bai Mu Er, Yin Er (Fructifactio Tremellae Fuciformis, Tremella, White Wood Ear)
Tonify Yin
Sweet, Bland
Neutral
Lung, Stomach

Mai Men Dong, Mai Dong (Radix Ophiopogonis, Ophiopogon Tuber)
Tonify Yin
Sweet, slightly Bitter
Cool to slightly Cold[229]
Spleen,[230] **Lung**,[231] Stomach, Heart
Name (Tai Yin, Spleen/Lung), Biao/Li (Stomach/Spleen), Clock Neighbor (Spleen/Heart)

Tian Men Dong, Tian Dong (Radix Asparagi, Asparagus Tuber)
Tonify Yin
Sweet, Bitter
Cold to very Cold
Lung, Kidney, Stomach[232]
Branch (You/Chicken, Lung/Kidney, 5PM-6:59PM) + Stomach

Xi Yang Shen, Hua Qi Shen (Radix Panacis Quinquefoli, American Ginseng Root)
Tonify Qi/Tonify Yin
Sweet, slightly Bitter[233] to Bitter to very Bitter[234]
Cold
Kidney, Heart, **Lung**, Spleen[235]
Name (Shao Yin, Kidney/Heart, Tai Yin, Spleen/Lung), Clock Neighbor (Spleen/Heart), Branch (You/Chicken, Lung/Kidney, 5PM-6:59PM)

Huang Jing, Mi Pu (Rhizoma Polygonati, Siberian Solomon Seal Rhizome)
Tonify Yin
Sweet
Neutral
Spleen, **Lung**, Kidney
Name (Tai Yin, Spleen/Lung), Branch (You/Chicken, Lung/Kidney, 5PM-6:59PM)

Bai He (Bulbus Lilii, Lilly Bulb)
Tonify Yin
Sweet, slightly Bitter,[236] Bland[237]
Neutral[238] to Cool to slightly Cold[239]
Lung, Heart

Gou Qi Zi, Di Gu Zi (Fructus Lycii, Chinese Wolfberry Fruit, Matrimony Vine Fruit, Boxthorn Fruit)
Tonify Blood/Tonify Yin
Sweet
Neutral
Liver, Kidney, **Lung**
Clock Neighbor (Liver/Lung), Branch (You/Chicken, Lung/Kidney, 5PM-6:59PM)

Astringe, Stabilize and Bind

Ye Ying Pi (Pericarpium Prunus Pseudocerasus)
Astringe, Stabilize and Bind
Sour, Bitter
Cool
Lung

Ma Huang Gen, Ku Chun Cai (Radix Ephedrae, Ephedra Root)
Astringe, Stabilize and Bind
Sweet, Astringent[240]
Neutral
Lung

He Zi, Ke Zi, He Li, He Li Le (Fructus Chebulae, Black Myrobalan Fruit, Terminalia, Chebula)
Astringe, Stabilize and Bind
Sour, Bitter, Astringent
Neutral
Lung, Stomach,[241] Large Intestine
Name (Yang Ming, Large Intestine/Stomach), Biao/Li (Large Intestine/Lung), Clock Neighbor (Large Intestine/Stomach)

Chun Gen Pi, Chun Pi (Cortex Ailanthi, Ailanthus Bark, Tree of Heaven Bark, Chinese Sumac Bark)
Astringe, Stabilize and Bind
Bitter, Astringent
Cold
Large Intestine, Stomach,[242] Liver, **Lung**[243]
Name (Yang Ming, Large Intestine/Stomach), Bie Jing (Jue Yin/Yang Ming, Liver/Large Intestine), Biao/Li (Large Intestine/Lung), Clock Neighbor (Large Intestine/Stomach, Liver/Lung), Branch (Mao/Rabbit, Liver/Large Intestine, 5AM-6:59AM)

Wu Mei (Fructus Mume, Mume Fruit, Smoked Plum)
Astringe, Stabilize and Bind
Sour, Astringent
Neutral to Warm[244]
Liver, Spleen, **Lung**, Large Intestine
Name (Tai Yin, Spleen/Lung), Bie Jing (Jue Yin/Yang Ming, Liver/Large Intestine), Biao/Li (Large Intestine/Lung), Clock Neighbor (Liver/Lung), Branch (Chou/Ox, Spleen/Liver, 1AM-2:59AM, Mao/Rabbit, Liver/Large Intestine, 5AM-6:59AM)

Ying Su Ke (Pericarpium Papaveris, Opium Poppy Husk)
Astringe, Stabilize and Bind
Sour, Astringent
Neutral, Toxic*
Kidney, Large Intestine, **Lung**
Biao/Li (Large Intestine/Lung), Clock Opposite (Kidney/Large Intestine), Branch (You/Chicken, Lung/Kidney, 5PM-6:59PM)

Wu Bei Zi, Wen Ge, Bai Chong Chong (Galla Chinensis, Gallnut of Chinese Sumac)
Astringe, Stabilize and Bind
Salty, Sour, Astringent
Cold, slightly Toxic*[245]
Lung, Large Intestine, Kidney
Biao/Li (Large Intestine/Lung), Clock Opposite (Kidney/Large Intestine), Branch (You/Chicken, Lung/Kidney, 5PM-6:59PM)

Ou Jie (Nodus Nelumbinis Rhizomatis, Lotus Rhizome Nodes)
Stop Bleeding/Astringe, Stabilize and Bind
Sweet, Astringent
Neutral
Lung, Stomach, Liver
Clock Neighbor (Liver/Lung) + Stomach

Wu Wei Zi (Fructus Schisandrae Chinensis, Schizandra Fruit)
Astringe, Stabilize and Bind
Sour, Sweet,[246] Acrid,[247] Bitter,[248] Salty,[249] Astringent
Warm
Kidney, **Lung**, Heart, Dai[250]
Name (Shao Yin, Kidney/Heart), Branch (You/Chicken, Lung/Kidney, 5PM-6:59PM) + Dai

Bai Guo, Yin Xing (Semen Ginkgo, Ginkgo Nut)
Relieve Cough and Wheezing/Panting/Astringe, Stabilize and Bind
Sweet, Bitter, Astringent
Neutral, slightly Toxic*
Lung, Kidney[251]
Branch (You/Chicken, Lung/Kidney, 5PM-6:59PM)

Nuo Dao Gen, Nuo Dao Gen Xu (Radix Oryzae Glutinosae, Glutinous Rice Root)
Astringe, Stabilize and Bind
Sweet, Acrid[252]
Neutral
Lung, Liver, Kidney[253]
Clock Neighbor (Liver/Lung), Branch (You/Chicken, Lung/Kidney, 5PM-6:59PM)

Emetic

Li Lu (Radix et Rhizoma Veratri, Lack False Hellebore, Vanity Grass)
Relieve Cough and Wheezing/Panting/Emetic
Acrid, Bitter
Cold, extremely Toxic*
Lung, Liver, Stomach
Clock Neighbor (Liver/Lung) + Stomach

Chang Shan (Radix Dichroae, Dichroa Root)
Expel Parasites/Emetic
Acrid, Bitter
Cold, Toxic*
Lung, Heart, Liver
Clock Neighbor (Liver/Lung) + Heart

Shu Qi (Folium Dichroae, Dichroa Leaves)
Emetic
Acrid, Bitter
Cold to Warm,[254] Toxic*
Lung, Heart, Liver
Clock Neighbor (Liver/Lung) + Heart

External Application

Er Cha, Hai Er Cha, Wu Die Ni (Catechu, Black Catechu, Black Cutch, Cutch)
External Application
Bitter, Astringent
Cool to slightly Cold[255]
Lung

Da Suan (Bulbus Alli Sativi, Garlic)
Expel Parasites/External Application
Acrid, Sweet[256]
Neutral to Warm
Spleen, Stomach, **Lung**, Large Intestine[257]
Name (Tai Yin, Spleen/Lung, Yang Ming, Large Intestine/Stomach), Biao/Li (Stomach/Spleen, Large Intestine/Lung), Clock Neighbor (Large Intestine/Stomach)

Ming Fan, Bai Fan, Ku Fan (Alumen, Alum)
External Application
Sour, Bitter,[258] Astringent
Cold, Toxic*
Lung, Liver, Spleen, Stomach,[259] Large Intestine[260]
Name (Tai Yin, Spleen/Lung, Yang Ming, Large Intestine/Stomach), Bie Jing (Jue Yin/Yang Ming, Liver/Large Intestine), Clock Neighbor (Liver/Lung, Large Intestine/Stomach), Biao/Li (Stomach/Spleen, Large Intestine/Lung), Branch (Chou/Ox, Spleen/Liver, 1AM-2:59AM, Mao/Rabbit, Liver/Large Intestine, 5AM-6:59AM)

Xiong Huang (Realgar)
External Application
Acrid, Bitter
Neutral to Warm, Toxic*
Heart, Liver, Kidney,[261] Stomach,[262] **Lung**,[263] Large Intestine[264]
Name (Shao Yin, Heart/Kidney, Yang Ming, Large Intestine/Stomach), Bie Jing (Jue Yin/Yang Ming, Liver/Large Intestine), Biao/Li (Large Intestine/Lung), Clock Opposite (Kidney/Large Intestine), Clock Neighbor (Large Intestine/Stomach, Liver/Lung), Branch (Mao/Rabbit, Liver/Large Intestine, 5AM-6:59AM, You/Chicken, Lung, Kidney, 5PM-6:59PM)

Peng Sha, Yue Shi (Borax)
External Application
Sweet, Salty, Bitter[265]
Cool to slightly Cold,[266] Toxic*
Lung, Stomach

Wa Leng Zi (Concha Arcae, Cockle Shell, Ark Shell)
Vitalize Blood Transform Stasis/Transform Phlegm/External Application
Salty
Neutral
Liver, Stomach, **Lung**, Spleen[267]
Name (Tai Yin, Lung/Spleen), Biao/Li (Stomach/Spleen), Clock Neighbor (Liver/Lung), Branch (Chou/Ox, Spleen/Liver, 1AM-2:59AM)

Si Gua Luo (Retinervus Luffae Fructus, Dried Vegetable Sponge)
Transform Phlegm/External Application
Sweet
Neutral to Cold[268]
Lung, Stomach, Liver
Clock Neighbor (Liver/Lung) + Stomach

Lu Feng Fang, Feng Fang (Nidus Vespae, Wasp Nest)
External Application
Sweet
Neutral, Toxic*
Stomach, **Lung**,[269] Liver[270]
Clock Neighbor (Liver/Lung) + Stomach

Tu Jing Pi, Tu Jin Pi (Cortex Psuedolaricis, Golden Larch Bark)
External Application
Acrid, Bitter[271]
Warm, Toxic
Lung, Spleen
Name (Tai Yin, Lung/Spleen)

Hand Yang Ming Large Intestine Herbs

Acrid Warm Exterior Releasing

Bai Zhi (Radix Angelicae Dahuricae, Angelica Root)
Acrid Warm Exterior Releasing
Acrid, Aromatic
Warm
Lung, Stomach, Spleen,[272] **Large Intestine**[273]
Name (Tai Yin, Lung/Spleen, Yang Ming, Large Intestine/Stomach), Biao/Li (Stomach/Spleen, Large Intestine/Lung), Clock Neighbor (Large Intestine/Stomach)

Acrid Cool Exterior Releasing

Shuang Liu Huang (Herba Vernoniae Patulae, Half-Spreading Ironweed)
Acrid Cool Exterior Releasing
Bitter
Neutral
Lung, **Large Intestine**
Biao/Li (Large Intestine/Lung)

Sheng Ma (Radix Cimicifugae, Black Cohosh Rhizome, Bugbane Rhizome)
Acrid Cool Exterior Releasing
Acrid, Sweet
Cool to slightly Cold[274]
Lung, Spleen, Stomach, **Large Intestine**
Name (Tai Yin, Lung/Spleen, Yang Ming, Large Intestine/Stomach), Biao/Li (Large Intestine/Lung, Stomach/Spleen), Clock Neighbor (Large Intestine/Stomach)

Sang Ye (Folium Mori, White Mulberry Leaf)
Acrid Cool Exterior Releasing
Bitter, Sweet, Acrid,[275] Aromatic
Cold
Lung, Liver, **Large Intestine**,[276] Stomach[277]
Name (Yang Ming, Large Intestine/Stomach), Biao/Li (Large Intestine/Lung), Bie Jing (Jue Yin/Yang Ming, Liver/Large Intestine), Clock Neighbor (Liver/Lung, Large Intestine/Stomach), Branch (Mao/Rabbit, Liver/Large Intestine, 5AM-6:59AM)

Ge Gen (Radix Puerariae, Kudzu Root, Pueraria)
Acrid Cool Exterior Releasing
Sweet, Acrid, slightly Bitter[278]
Cool
Spleen, Stomach, Tai Yang,[279] **Yang Ming**[280]
Biao/Li (Stomach/Spleen), possibly Name (Yang Ming Large Intestine/Stomach) and Clock Neighbor (Large Intestine/Stomach) if Yang Ming[281] really means the entire Yang Ming Jing-channel, and possibly Name (Tai Yang, Small Intestine/Urinary Bladder), Bie Jing (Spleen, Small Intestine), Clock Neighbor (Small Intestine/Urinary Bladder) and Qian/Hou (Front/Back, Stomach/Urinary Bladder) if Tai Yang[282] really means the entire Tai Yang Jing-channel.

Clear Heat Purge Fire

Shi Lian Zi (Herba Sinocrassulae Indicae, Indian Sinocrassula)
Clear Heat Purge Fire
Bitter
Cold
Large Intestine, Urinary Bladder, Stomach
Name (Yang Ming, Large Intestine/Stomach), Clock Neighbor (Large Intestine/Stomach), Qian/Hou (Front/Back, Stomach/Urinary Bladder), Branch (Shen/Monkey, Large Intestine/Urinary Bladder, 3PM-4:59PM)

Jue Ming Zi, Cao Jue Ming (Semen Cassiae, Cassia Seeds, Foetid Cassia Seeds)
Clear Heat Purge Fire/Calm Liver Extinguish Wind
Sweet, Bitter, Salty[283]
Cool to slightly Cold
Liver, **Large Intestine**, Kidney[284]
Bie Jing (Jue Yin/Yang Ming, Liver/Large Intestine), Clock Opposite (Kidney/Large Intestine), Branch (Mao/Rabbit, Liver/Large Intestine, 5AM-6:59AM)

Clear Heat Dry Dampness

Huang Qin (Radix Scutellariae, Baical Skullcap Root, Scutellaria, Scute)
Clear Heat Dry Dampness
Bitter
Cold
Lung, Gall Bladder, Stomach, **Large Intestine** and possibly San Jiao[285]
Name (Yang Ming, Large Intestine/Stomach) Biao/Li (Large Intestine/Lung), Clock Neighbor (Large Intestine/Stomach), Branch (Yin/Tiger, Gall Bladder/Lung, 3AM-4:59AM), and possibly Name (Shao Yang, San Jiao/Gall Bladder), Clock Neighbor (San Jiao/Gall Bladder)

Ku Shen, Ku Shen Gen, Ku Gu (Radix Sophorae Flavescentis, Flavescent Sophora Root)
Clear Heat Dry Dampness
Bitter to extremely Bitter[286]
Cold
Heart, Liver, Stomach, **Large Intestine**, Urinary Bladder, Small Intestine[287]
Name (Yang Ming, Large Intestine/Stomach, Tai Yang, Small Intestine/Urinary Bladder), Bie Jing (Jue Yin/Yang Ming, Liver/Large Intestine), Biao/Li (Small Intestine/Heart), Clock Opposite (Liver/Small Intestine), Clock Neighbor (Large Intestine/Stomach, Small Intestine/Urinary Bladder), Qian/Hou (Front/Back, Stomach/Urinary Bladder), Branch (Shen/Monkey, Large Intestine/Urinary Bladder, 3PM-4:59PM and Mao/Rabbit, Liver/Large Intestine, 5AM-6:59AM)

Huang Lian (Rhizoma Coptidis, Goldthread Rhizome, Coptis Root)
Clear Heat Dry Dampness
Very Bitter, purely Bitter[288]
Very Cold
Heart, Liver, Stomach, **Large Intestine**, Du[289]
Name (Yang Ming, Large Intestine/Stomach), Bie Jing (Jue Yin/Yang Ming, Liver/Large Intestine), Clock Neighbor (Large Intestine/Stomach), Branch (Mao/Rabbit, Liver/Large Intestine, 5AM-6:59AM) + Heart, Du

Qin Pi (Cortex Fraxini, Bark of Korean Ash Branch)
Clear Heat Dry Dampness/Clear Heat Clean Toxin
Bitter, Acrid,[290] Astringent[291]
Cold
Gall Bladder, Liver, **Large Intestine**, Stomach[292]
Name (Yang Ming, Large Intestine/Stomach), Bie Jing (Jue Yin/Yang Ming, Liver/Large Intestine), Biao/Li (Gall Bladder/Liver), Clock Neighbor (Large Intestine/Stomach), Branch (Mao/Rabbit, Liver/Large Intestine, 5AM-6:59AM)

Ji Xue Cao, Beng Da Wan (Herba Centellae, Gotu Kola, Pennywort)
Clear Heat Dry Dampness/Clear Heat Clean Toxin
Acrid, Bitter
Cold
Liver, Spleen, Kidney, Small Intestine, **Large Intestine**
Bie Jing (Jue Yin/Yang Ming, Liver/Large Intestine, Tai Yin/Tai Yang, Spleen/Small Intestine), Clock Opposite (Liver/Small Intestine, Kidney/Large Intestine), Branch (Chou/Ox, Spleen/Liver, 1AM-2:59AM, Si/Snake, Small Intestine/Spleen, 9AM-10:59AM, Wei/Sheep, Spleen/Small Intestine, 1PM-2:59PM, Mao/Rabbit, Liver/Large Intestine, 5AM-6:59AM)

Huang Bai, Huang Bo (Cortex Phellodendri, Amur Cork Tree Bark, Phellodendron Bark)
Clear Heat Dry Dampness
Bitter
Cold
Kidney, Urinary Bladder, **Large Intestine**
Biao/Li (Urinary Bladder/Kidney), Clock Opposite (Kidney/Large Intestine), Branch (Shen/Monkey, Large Intestine/Urinary Bladder, 3PM-4:59PM)

Clear Heat Cool Blood

Ji Guan Hua (Flos Celosiae Cristatae, Cock's Comb Flower)
Clear Heat Cool Blood/Astringe, Stabilize and Bind
Sweet, Astringent[293]
Cool
Large Intestine, Liver, Kidney[294]
Bie Jing (Jue Yin/Yang Ming, Liver/Large Intestine), Clock Opposite (Kidney/Large Intestine), Branch (Mao/Rabbit, Liver/Large Intestine, 5AM-6:59AM)

Clear Heat Clean Toxin

Jin Guo Lan (Radix Tinosporae)
Clear Heat Clean Toxin
Bitter
Cold
Lung, **Large Intestine**
Biao/Li (Large Intestine/Lung)

Yu Xing Cao (Herba Houttuyniae)
Clear Heat Clean Toxin
Acrid
Cool to slightly Cold
Lung, **Large Intestine**[295]
Biao/Li (Large Intestine/Lung)

Bei Dou Gen (Rhizoma Menispermi, Asiatic Moonseed Rhizome)
Clear Heat Clean Toxin
Bitter
Cold
Lung, Stomach, **Large Intestine**
Name (Yang Ming, Large Intestine/Stomach), Biao/Li (Large Intestine/Lung), Clock Neighbor (Large Intestine/Stomach)

Ren Dong Teng (Caulis Lonicerae, Honeysuckle Vine)
Clear Heat Clean Toxin
Sweet
Neutral to slightly Cold[296] to Cold
Lung, Stomach, **Large Intestine**,[297] Spleen[298]
Name (Yang Ming, Large Intestine/Stomach, Tai Yin, Lung/Spleen), Biao/Li (Large Intestine/Lung, Stomach/Spleen) Clock Neighbor (Large Intestine/Stomach)

Shan Dou Gen, Dou Gen, Nan Dou Gen (Radix Sophorae Tonkinensis, Subprostrate, Sophora Root)
Clear Heat Clean Toxin
Bitter to very Bitter[299]
Cold, slightly Toxic*
Lung, Stomach,[300] **Large Intestine**,[301] Heart[302]
Name (Yang Ming, Large Intestine/Stomach), Biao/Li (Large Intestine/Lung), Clock Neighbor (Large Intestine/Stomach) + Heart

Jin Yin Hua (Flos Lonicerae, Honeysuckle Flower, Lonicera Flower)
Clear Heat Clean Toxin
Sweet
Cold
Lung, Stomach, **Large Intestine**, Heart[303]
Name (Yang Ming, Large Intestine/Stomach), Biao/Li (Large Intestine/Lung), Clock Neighbor (Large Intestine/Stomach) + Heart

Chuan Xin Lian, Lan He Lian (Herba Andrographis, Green Chiretta, Kariyat)
Clear Heat Clean Toxin
Bitter
Cold
Lung, Stomach, **Large Intestine**, Small Intestine
Name (Yang Ming, Large Intestine/Stomach), Biao/Li (Large Intestine/Lung), Clock Neighbor (Large Intestine/Stomach) + Small Intestine

Ban Zhi Lian (Herba Scutellariae Barbatae, Barbat Skullcap, Barbed Skullcap)
Clear Heat Clean Toxin
Acrid, slightly Bitter
Cool
Liver, Lung, Stomach, Kidney,[304] **Large Intestine**[305]
Name (Yang Ming, Large Intestine/Stomach), Bie Jing (Jue Yin/Yang Ming, Liver/Large Intestine), Biao/Li (Large Intestine/Lung), Clock Opposite (Kidney/Large Intestine), Clock Neighbor (Large Intestine/Stomach, Liver/Lung), Branch (You/Chicken, Lung/Kidney, 5PM-6:59PM, Mao/Rabbit, Liver/Large Intestine, 5AM-6:59AM)

Hu Yao Huang (Herba Leucas Mollissimae, Leucas)
Clear Heat Clean Toxin
Bitter
Cool
Large Intestine, Small Intestine, Lung
Biao/Li (Large Intestine/Lung) + Small Intestine

Qian Li Guang (Herba Senecionis Scandens, Climbing Groundsel, Ragwort)
Clear Heat Clean Toxin
Bitter
Cold
Lung, Liver, **Large Intestine**
Biao/Li (Large Intestine/Lung), Bie Jing (Jue Yin/Yang Ming, Liver/Large Intestine), Clock Neighbor (Liver/Lung), Branch (Mao/Rabbit, Liver/Large Intestine, 5AM-6:59AM)

Bai Tou Weng (Radix Pulsatillae, Chinese Anemone Root, Pulsatilla)
Clear Heat Clean Toxin
Bitter
Cold
Large Intestine, Stomach[306]
Name (Yang Ming, Large Intestine/Stomach), Clock Neighbor (Large Intestine/Stomach)

Lou Lu (Radix Rhapontici, Rhaponticum Root)
Clear Heat Clean Toxin
Bitter, Salty[307]
Cold
Stomach, **Large Intestine**[308]
Name (Yang Ming, Large Intestine/Stomach), Clock Neighbor (Large Intestine/Stomach)

Bai Hua She She Cao (Herba Oldenlandia, Heydyotis)
Clear Heat Clean Toxin
Slightly Bitter, Sweet
Cold
Stomach, **Large Intestine**, Small Intestine, Liver[309]
Name (Yang Ming, Large Intestine/Stomach), Bie Jing (Jue Yin/Yang Ming, Liver/Large Intestine), Clock Opposite (Liver/Small Intestine), Clock Neighbor (Large Intestine/Stomach), Branch (Mao/Rabbit, Liver/Large Intestine, 5AM-6:59AM)

Qin Pi (Cortex Fraxini, Bark of Korean Ash Branch)
Clear Heat Dry Dampness/Clear Heat Clean Toxin
Bitter, Acrid,[310] Astringent[311]
Cold
Gall Bladder, Liver, **Large Intestine**, Stomach[312]
Name (Yang Ming, Large Intestine/Stomach), Bie Jing (Jue Yin/Yang Ming, Liver/Large Intestine), Biao/Li (Gall Bladder/Liver), Clock Neighbor (Large Intestine/Stomach), Branch (Mao/Rabbit, Liver/Large Intestine, 5AM-6:59AM)

Bai Jiang Cao (Herba cum Radice Patriniae, Patrinia, Thlaspi)
Clear Heat Clean Toxin
Acrid, Bitter, Salty[313]
Cool to slightly Cold
Stomach, **Large Intestine**, Liver
Name (Yang Ming, Large Intestine/Stomach), Bie Jing (Yang Ming/Jue Yin, Large Intestine/Liver), Clock Neighbor (Large Intestine/Stomach), Branch (Mao/Rabbit, Liver/Large Intestine, 5AM-6:59AM)

Quan Shen (Rhizoma Bistortae)
Clear Heat Clean Toxin
Bitter, Astringent
Cool, slightly Toxic*
Liver, Stomach, **Large Intestine**
Name (Yang Ming, Large Intestine/Stomach), Bie Jing (Jue Yin/Yang Ming, Liver/Large Intestine), Clock Neighbor (Large Intestine/Stomach), Branch (Mao/Rabbit, Liver/Large Intestine, 5AM-6:59AM)

Ji Xue Cao, Beng Da Wan (Herba Centellae, Gotu Kola, Pennywort)
Clear Heat Dry Dampness/Clear Heat Clean Toxin
Acrid, Bitter
Cold
Liver, Spleen, Kidney, Small Intestine, **Large Intestine**
Bie Jing (Jue Yin/Yang Ming, Liver/Large Intestine, Tai Yin/Tai Yang, Spleen/Small Intestine), Clock Opposite (Liver/Small Intestine, Kidney/Large Intestine), Branch (Chou/Ox, Spleen/Liver, 1AM-2:59AM, Si/Snake, Small Intestine/Spleen, 9AM-10:59AM, Wei/Sheep, Spleen/Small Intestine, 1PM-2:59PM, Mao/Rabbit, Liver/Large Intestine, 5AM-6:59AM)

Feng Wei Cao, Feng Huang Cao (Herba Pteris, Chinese Brake, Huguenot Fern, Spider Brake)
Clear Heat Clean Toxin
Bitter
Cold
Large Intestine, Urinary Bladder
Branch (Shen/Monkey, Large Intestine/Urinary Bladder, 3PM-4:59PM)

Ma Chi Xian, Chang Shou Cai, Wu Xing Cai (Herba Portulacae, Purslane, Portulaca)
Clear Heat Clean Toxin
Sour
Cold
Large Intestine, Liver, and possibly San Jiao[314]
Bie Jing (Jue Yin/Yang Ming, Liver/Large Intestine), Branch (Mao/Rabbit, Liver/Large Intestine, 5AM-6:59AM) + possibly San Jiao

Cha Chi Huang (Herba Stellariae Aquaticae)
Clear Heat Clean Toxin
Acrid, slightly Bitter
Neutral
Liver, **Large Intestine**, San Jiao
Bie Jing (Jue Yin/Yang Ming, Liver/Large Intestine), Branch (Mao/Rabbit, Liver/Large Intestine, 5AM-6:59AM) + San Jiao

Ya Dan Zi, Ku Dan Zi, Ku Zi, Ku Shen Zi (Fructus Bruceae, Java Brucea Fruit, Brucea)
Clear Heat Clean Toxin
Bitter
Cold, slightly to very Toxic*
Large Intestine, Liver
Bie Jing (Jue Yin/Yang Ming, Liver/Large Intestine), Branch (Mao/Rabbit, Liver/Large Intestine, 5AM-6:59AM)

Wei Ling Cai, Tian Qing Di Bai, Fan Bai Cao (Herba Potentillae Chinensis, Chinese Sliverweed, Chinese Cinquefoil)
Clear Heat Clean Toxin
Bitter
Neutral[315] to Cold
Liver, **Large Intestine**
Bie Jing (Jue Yin/Yang Ming, Liver/Large Intestine), Branch (Mao/Rabbit, Liver/Large Intestine, 5AM-6:59AM)

Hong Teng, Da Xue Teng (Caulis Sargentodoxae, Sargentodoxa Vine)
Clear Heat Clean Toxin
Bitter
Neutral
Large Intestine, Liver[316]
Bie Jing (Jue Yin/Yang Ming, Liver/Large Intestine), Branch (Mao/Rabbit, Liver/Large Intestine, 5AM-6:59AM)

Clear Deficient Heat

Hu Huang Lian, Hu Lian (Rhizoma Picrorhizae, Picrorhiza, Figwort Rhizome)
Clear Deficient Heat
Bitter, Astringing[317]
Cold
Heart, Liver, Stomach, **Large Intestine**
Name (Yang Ming, Large Intestine, Stomach), Bie Jing (Jue Yin/Yang Ming, Liver/Large Intestine), Clock Neighbor (Large Intestine, Stomach), Branch (Mao/Rabbit, Liver/Large Intestine, 5AM-6:59AM) + Heart

Purgative

Mang Xiao (Natri Sulfas, Mirabilite, Glauber's Salt, Epsom Salts)
Purgative
Salty, Bitter, Acrid[318]
Cold
Lung,[319] Stomach, **Large Intestine**
Name (Yang Ming, Large Intestine/Stomach), Biao/Li (Large Intestine/Lung), Clock Neighbor (Large Intestine/Stomach)

Ba Dou (Fructus Crotonis, Croton)
Purgative/Cathartic
Acrid
Hot, extremely Toxic*
Stomach, **Large Intestine**, Lung[320]
Name (Yang Ming, Large Intestine/Stomach), Biao/Li (Large Intestine/Lung), Clock Neighbor (Large Intestine/Stomach)

Fan Xie Ye (Folium Sennae, Senna Leaf)
Purgative
Bitter, Sweet[321]
Cold
Large Intestine

Da Huang (Radix et Rhizoma Rhei, Rhubarb Root and Rhizome)
Purgative
Bitter to very Bitter[322] to purely Bitter,[323] Aromatic[324]
Cold to very Cold[325]
Spleen, Stomach, **Large Intestine**, Liver, Heart, Du[326]
Name (Yang Ming, Large Intestine/Stomach), Bie Jing (Jue Yin/Yang Ming, Liver/Large Intestine), Biao/Li (Stomach/Spleen), Clock Neighbor (Spleen/Heart, Large Intestine/Stomach), Branch (Chou/Ox, Spleen/Liver, 1AM-2:59AM and Mao/Rabbit, Liver/Large Intestine, 5AM-6:59AM) + Du

Lu Hui, Xiang Dan (Aloe, Dried Aloe Leaf Juice)
Purgative
Very Bitter
Very Cold
Liver, **Large Intestine**, Stomach[327]
Name (Yang Ming, Large Intestine/Stomach), Bie Jing (Jue Yin/Yang Ming, Liver/Large Intestine), Clock Neighbor (Large Intestine/Stomach), Branch (Mao/Rabbit, Liver/Large Intestine, 5AM-6:59AM)

Moist Laxative

Song Zi Ren (Semen Pini, Pine Nut)
Moist Laxative
Sweet
Warm
Lung, Liver, **Large Intestine**
Bie Jing (Jue Yin/Yang Ming, Liver/Large Intestine), Biao/Li (Large Intestine, Lung), Clock Neighbor (Liver/Lung), Branch (Mao/Rabbit, Liver/Large Intestine, 5AM-6:59AM)

Huo Ma Ren (Semen Cannabis, Hemp Seeds)
Moist Laxative
Sweet
Neutral, slightly Toxic*
Spleen, Stomach, **Large Intestine**
Name (Yang Ming, Large Intestine/Stomach), Biao/Li (Stomach/Spleen), Clock Neighbor (Large Intestine/Stomach)

Cathartic

Ba Dou (Fructus Crotonis, Croton)
Purgative/Cathartic
Acrid
Hot, extremely Toxic*
Stomach, **Large Intestine**, Lung[328]
Name (Yang Ming, Large Intestine/Stomach), Biao/Li (Large Intestine/Lung), Clock Neighbor (Large Intestine/Stomach)

Shang Lu (Radix Phytolaccae, Poke Root)
Cathartic
Bitter
Cold, highly Toxic*
Lung, Spleen,[329] Kidney, **Large Intestine**, Urinary Bladder[330]
Name (Tai Yin, Lung/Spleen), Bie Jing (Tai Yin/Tai Yang, Lung/Urinary Bladder), Biao/Li (Large Intestine/Lung, Urinary Bladder/Kidney), Clock Opposite (Kidney/Large Intestine, Lung/Urinary Bladder), Branch (You/Chicken, Lung/Kidney, 5PM-6:59PM, Shen/Monkey, Large Intestine/Urinary Bladder, 3PM-4:59PM)

Da Ji (Radix Euphorbiae seu Knoxiae)
Cathartic
Bitter, Acrid
Cold, extremely Toxic*
Spleen,[331] Lung,[332] Kidney, **Large Intestine**, Liver,[333] Gall Bladder[334]
Name (Tai Yin, Lung/Spleen), Bie Jing (Jue Yin/Yang Ming, Liver/Large Intestine), Biao/Li (Large Intestine/Lung, Gall Bladder/Liver), Clock Opposite (Kidney/Large Intestine), Clock Neighbor (Liver/Lung), Branch (Zi/Rat, Kidney/Gall Bladder, 11PM-12:59AM, Chou/Ox, Spleen/Liver, 1AM-2:59AM, Mao/Rabbit, Liver/Large Intestine, 5AM-6:59AM, and You/Chicken, Lung/Kidney, 5PM-6:59PM)

Qian Niu Zi (Semen Pharbitidis, Pharbitis, Morning Glory Seed)
Cathartic
Bitter, Acrid[335]
Cold, Toxic*
Lung, Kidney, **Large Intestine**, Small Intestine[336]
Biao/Li (Large Intestine/Lung), Clock Opposite (Kidney/Large Intestine), Branch (You/Chicken, Lung/Kidney, 5PM-6:59PM) + Small Intestine

Gan Sui (Radix Euphorbiae Kansui, Kan Sui Root)
Cathartic
Bitter, Sweet
Cold, Toxic*
Lung, Kidney, **Large Intestine**
Biao/Li (Large Intestine/Lung), Clock Opposite (Kidney/Large Intestine), Branch (You/Chicken, Lung/Kidney, 5PM-6:59PM)

Yuan Hua, Lao Shu Hua (Flos Genkwa, Genkwa Flower, Lilac Daphne Flower Bud)
Cathartic
Acrid, Bitter
Warm, Toxic*
Lung, Kidney, **Large Intestine**
Biao/Li (Large Intestine/Lung), Clock Opposite (Kidney/Large Intestine), Branch (You/Chicken, Lung/Kidney, 5PM-6:59PM)

Dispel Wind Dampness, Open Channels and Luo-Network Vessels and Relieve Pain

Lao Guan Cao (Herba Erodi seu Geranii, Geranium, Common Heron's Bill Herb)
Dispel Wind Dampness, Open Channels and Luo-Network Vessels and Relieve Pain
Acrid, Bitter
Neutral
Liver, **Large Intestine**, Kidney,[337] Spleen[338]
Bie Jing (Jue Yin/Yang Ming, Liver/Large Intestine), Clock Opposite (Kidney/Large Intestine), Branch (Mao/Rabbit, Liver/Large Intestine, 5AM-6:59AM, Chou/Ox, Spleen/Liver, 1AM-2:59AM)

Ma An Teng (Herba Ipomoea Pes-caprae, Beach Morning Glory)
Dispel Wind Dampness, Open Channels and Luo-Network Vessels and Relieve Pain
Acrid, Bitter
Neutral
Liver, Kidney, **Large Intestine**
Bie Jing (Jue Yin/Yang Ming, Liver/Large Intestine), Clock Opposite (Kidney/Large Intestine), Branch (Mao/Rabbit, Liver/Large Intestine, 5AM-6:59AM)

Dispel Wind-Dampness Strengthen Sinew/Tendon and Bone

Zou Ma Tai (Rhizoma Ardisiae, Ardisia Root, Giant Leaf Ardisia Rhizome)
Dispel Wind-Dampness Strengthen Sinew/Tendon and Bone
Acrid
Neutral
Lung, Stomach, Spleen, **Large Intestine**
Name (Tai Yin, Lung/Spleen, Yang Ming, Large Intestine/Stomach), Biao/Li (Large Intestine/Lung, Stomach/Spleen), Clock Neighbor (Large Intestine/Stomach)

Aromatic Dissolve Dampness

Hou Po, Chuan Po, Lie Po (Cortex Magnoliae Officinalis, Officinal Magnolia Bark)
Aromatic Dissolve Dampness
Bitter, Acrid, Aromatic
Warm
Large Intestine, Lung, Spleen, Stomach
Name (Tai Yin, Lung/Spleen and Yang Ming, Large Intestine/Stomach), Biao/Li (Large Intestine/Lung, Stomach/Spleen), Clock Neighbor (Large Intestine/Stomach)

Regulate Water Resolve Dampness

Dong Gua Zi (Semen Benincasae, White Gourd Seed, Winter Melon Seed)
Regulate Water Resolve Dampness
Sweet
Cool to Cold[339]
Lung, Stomach, Small Intestine, **Large Intestine**
Name (Yang Ming, Large Intestine/Stomach), Biao/Li (Large Intestine/Lung), Clock Neighbor (Large Intestine/Stomach) + Small Intestine

Ze Qi (Herba Euphorbiae Helioscopiae, Euphorbia, Sun Spurge)
Regulate Water Resolve Dampness/Transform Phlegm
Sweet, Bitter, Acrid
Cool to slightly Cold,[340] slightly Toxic[341] to Toxic*
Large Intestine, Small Intestine, Lung
Biao/Li (Large Intestine/Lung) + Small Intestine

Dong Kui Guo (Fructus Malvae, Mallow Fruit, Cluster Mallow Fruit)
Regulate Water Resolve Dampness
Sweet
Cold
Urinary Bladder, Small Intestine, Stomach,[342] **Large Intestine**[343]
Name (Tai Yang, Small Intestine/Urinary Bladder, Yang Ming, Large Intestine/Stomach), Clock Neighbor (Large Intestine/Stomach, Small Intestine/Urinary Bladder), Qian/Hou (Front/Back, Stomach/Urinary Bladder), Branch (Shen/Monkey, Large Intestine/Urinary Bladder, 3PM-4:59PM)

Dong Kui Zi (Semen Malvae, Malva, Mallow Seed, Whorled Mallow Seed)
Regulate Water Resolve Dampness
Sweet
Cold
Urinary Bladder, **Large Intestine**, Small Intestine
Name (Tai Yang, Small Intestine/Urinary Bladder), Clock Neighbor (Small Intestine/Urinary Bladder), Branch (Shen/Monkey, Large Intestine/Urinary Bladder, 3PM-4:59PM)

Qing Ma Zi, Bai Ma Zi, Kui Zi (Semen Abutili, Abutilon Seed, Indian Mallow Seed)
Regulate Water Resolve Dampness
Bitter
Neutral
Urinary Bladder, **Large Intestine**, Liver
Bie Jing (Yang Ming/Jue Yin, Large Intestine/Liver), Branch (Shen/Monkey, Large Intestine/Urinary Bladder, 3PM-4:59PM and Mao/Rabbit, Liver/Large Intestine, 5AM-6:59AM)

Ding Shu Xiu (Herba Elephantopus Scaber, Elephantopi)
Regulate Water Resolve Dampness
Sweet, Bitter
Cold
Liver, Kidney, **Large Intestine**
Bie Jing (Jue Yin/Yang Ming, Liver/Large Intestine), Clock Opposite (Kidney/Large Intestine), Branch (Mao/Rabbit, Liver/Large Intestine, 5AM-6:59AM)

Warm Interior

Hu Jiao, Bai Hu Jiao, Hei Hu Jiao (Fructus Piper, Black Pepper, White Pepper)
Warm Interior
Acrid, Aromatic
Hot
Stomach, **Large Intestine**
Name (Yang Ming, Large Intestine/Stomach), Clock Neighbor (Large Intestine/Stomach)

Bi Ba, Bi Bo (Fructus Piperis Longi, Long Pepper)
Warm Interior
Acrid, Aromatic
Hot
Stomach, **Large Intestine**, Spleen[344]
Name (Yang Ming, Large Intestine/Stomach), Biao/Li (Stomach/Spleen), Clock Neighbor (Large Intestine/Stomach)

Regulate and Rectify Qi

Xie Bai, Xiao Suan, Ye Suan (Bulbus Alli Macrostemonis, Chive Bulb)
Regulate and Rectify Qi
Acrid, Bitter, Aromatic
Warm
Large Intestine, Stomach, Lung
Name (Yang Ming, Large Intestine/Stomach), Biao/Li (Large Intestine/Lung), Clock Neighbor (Large Intestine/Stomach)

Zhi Ke, Zhi Qiao (Fructus Aurantii, Ripened Bitter Orange)
Regulate and Rectify Qi
Bitter, Acrid, Aromatic
Cool to slightly Cold[345]
Large Intestine, Spleen, Stomach
Name (Yang Ming, Large Intestine/Stomach), Biao/Li (Stomach/Spleen), Clock Neighbor (Large Intestine/Stomach)

Zhi Shi (Fructus Aurantii Immaturus, Immature Bitter Orange)
Regulate and Rectify Qi
Bitter, Acrid, Aromatic
Warm[346] to Cool to slightly Cold[347]
Large Intestine, Spleen, Stomach
Name (Yang Ming, Large Intestine/Stomach), Biao/Li (Stomach/Spleen) Clock Neighbor (Large Intestine/Stomach)

Da Fu Pi (Pericarpium Arecae, Areca Peel, Betel Husk)
Regulate and Rectify Qi
Acrid
Slightly Warm
Large Intestine, Small Intestine, Spleen, Stomach
Name (Yang Ming, Large Intestine/Stomach), Bie Jing (Tai Yin/Tai Yang, Spleen/Small Intestine), Biao/Li (Stomach/Spleen), Clock Neighbor (Large Intestine/Stomach), Branch (Si/Snake, Small Intestine/Spleen, 9AM-10:59AM, Wei/Sheep, Spleen/Small Intestine, 1PM-2:59PM)

Dao Dou (Semen Canavaliae, Sword Bean)
Regulate and Rectify Qi
Sweet
Warm
Stomach, Spleen,[348] Kidney, **Large Intestine**[349]
Name (Yang Ming, Large Intestine/Stomach), Biao/Li (Stomach/Spleen), Clock Opposite (Kidney/Large Intestine), Clock Neighbor (Large Intestine/Stomach)

Mu Xiang (Radix Aucklandiae, Costus Root)
Regulate and Rectify Qi
Acrid, Bitter, slightly Astringent,[350] Aromatic
Warm
Gall Bladder, **Large Intestine**, Spleen, Stomach, San Jiao[351]
Name (Yang Ming, Large Intestine/Stomach, Shao Yang, Gall Bladder/San Jiao), Biao/Li (Stomach/Spleen), Clock Opposite (Spleen/San Jiao), Clock Neighbor (Large Intestine/Stomach, San Jiao/Gall Bladder)

Digestive

Hong Qu (Monascus, Red Yeast Rice)
Digestive
Sweet, Acrid
Warm
Spleen, Liver, **Large Intestine**
Bie Jing (Jue Yin/Yang Ming, Liver/Large Intestine), Branch (Chou/Ox, Spleen/Liver, 1AM-2:59AM and Mao/Rabbit, Liver/Large Intestine, 5AM-6:59AM)

Expel Parasites

Fei Zi (Semen Torreyae, Torreya Seeds)
Expel Parasites
Sweet, Astringent[352]
Neutral, relatively Non-Toxic[353]
Lung, **Large Intestine**, Stomach[354]
Name (Yang Ming, Large Intestine/Stomach), Biao/Li (Large Intestine/Lung), Clock Neighbor (Large Intestine/Stomach)

Da Suan (Bulbus Alli Sativi, Garlic)
Expel Parasites/External Application
Acrid, Sweet[355]
Neutral to Warm
Spleen, Stomach, Lung, **Large Intestine**[356]
Name (Tai Yin, Spleen/Lung, Yang Ming, Large Intestine/Stomach), Biao/Li (Stomach/Spleen, Large Intestine/Lung), Clock Neighbor (Large Intestine/Stomach)

Lei Wan (Omphalia, Fruiting Body of Omphalia)
Expel Parasites
Bitter
Cold, slightly Toxic*[357]
Stomach, **Large Intestine**
Name (Yang Ming, Large Intestine/Stomach), Clock Neighbor (Large Intestine/Stomach)

Bing Lang, Hai Nan Zi, Bing Men (Semen Arecae, Betel Nut, Areca Seeds)
Expel Parasites
Acrid, Bitter
Warm
Large Intestine, Stomach
Name (Yang Ming, Large Intestine/Stomach), Clock Neighbor (Large Intestine/Stomach)

Nan Gua Zi, Nan Gua Ren (Semen Cucurbitae Moschatae, Pumpkin Seed)
Expel Parasites
Sweet
Neutral
Stomach, **Large Intestine**
Name (Yang Ming, Large Intestine/Stomach), Clock Neighbor (Large Intestine/Stomach)

He Cao Ya (Gemma Agrimoniae, Agrimonia, Hairy-Vein Agrimonia Bud)
Expel Parasites
Bitter, Astringent
Cool
Liver, Small Intestine, **Large Intestine**
Bie Jing (Jue Yin/Yang Ming, Liver/Large Intestine), Clock Opposite (Liver, Small Intestine)
Branch (Mao/Rabbit, Liver/Large Intestine, 5AM-6:59AM)

Stop Bleeding

Wan Nian Song (Herba Selaginellae, Selaginella)
Stop Bleeding
Acrid
Neutral
Lung, **Large Intestine**
Biao/Li (Large Intestine/Lung)

Zong Lu Tan (Trachycarpi Petiolus Carbonisatus, Charred Trachycarpus Petiole)
Stop Bleeding
Bitter, Astringent
Neutral
Lung, Liver, **Large Intestine**, Spleen[358]
Name (Tai Yin, Lung/Spleen), Bie Jing (Jue Yin/Yang Ming, Liver/Large Intestine), Biao/Li (Large Intestine/Lung), Clock Neighbor (Liver/Lung), Branch (Mao/Rabbit, Liver/Large Intestine, 5AM-6:59AM)

Zong Lu Pi (Fibra Stipulae Trachicarpi, Trachycarpus Stipule Fiber)
Stop Bleeding
Bitter, Sour, Astringent[359]
Neutral
Liver, Lung, **Large Intestine**
Bie Jing (Jue Yin/Yang Ming, Liver/Large Intestine), Biao/Li (Large Intestine/Lung), Clock Neighbor (Liver/Lung), Branch (Mao/Rabbit, Liver/Large Intestine, 5AM-6:59AM)

Ce Bai Ye (Cacumen Platycadi, Biota Leaves, Arborvitae Leaf)
Stop Bleeding
Bitter, Astringent
Cool[360] to slightly Cold
Lung, Liver, **Large Intestine**
Biao/Li (Large Intestine/Lung), Bie Jing (Jue Yin/Yang Ming, Liver/Large Intestine), Branch (Mao/Rabbit, Liver/Large Intestine, 5AM-6:59AM)

San Qi, Tian Qi (Radix Notoginseng, Pseudoginseng Root)
Stop Bleeding
Sweet, slightly Bitter
Warm
Liver, Stomach,[361] Spleen,[362] **Large Intestine**,[363] Pericardium[364]
Name (Yang Ming, Large Intestine/Stomach and Jue Yin, Liver/Pericardium), Bie Jing (Jue Yin/Yang Ming, Pericardium/Stomach and Liver/Large Intestine), Biao/Li (Stomach/Spleen), Clock Opposite (Pericardium/Stomach), Clock Neighbor (Large Intestine/Stomach), Branch (Chou/Ox, Spleen/Liver, 1AM-2:59AM, Mao/Rabbit, Liver/Large Intestine, 5AM-6:59AM and Shu/Dog, Stomach/Pericardium, 7PM-8:59PM)

Di Yu (Radix Sanguisorbae, Bloodwort Root, Burnet Root)
Stop Bleeding
Bitter, Sour, Astringent[365]
Cool to Cold[366]
Liver, **Large Intestine**, Stomach
Name (Yang Ming, Large Intestine/Stomach), Bie Jing (Jue Yin/Yang Ming, Liver/Large Intestine), Clock Neighbor (Large Intestine/Stomach), Branch (Mao/Rabbit, Liver/Large Intestine, 5AM-6:59AM)

Huai Jiao (Fructus Sophorae, Sophora Fruit)
Stop Bleeding
Bitter, Aromatic[367]
Cold
Liver, Gall Bladder, **Large Intestine**
Bie Jing (Jue Yin/Yang Ming, Liver/Large Intestine), Biao/Li (Gall Bladder/Liver), Branch (Mao/Rabbit, Liver/Large Intestine, 5AM-6:59AM)

Huai Hua, Huai Mi, Huai Hua Mi (Flos Sophorae, Pagoda Tree Bud)
Stop Bleeding
Bitter
Cool to slightly Cold[368]
Liver, **Large Intestine**
Bie Jing (Jue Yin/Yang Ming, Liver/Large Intestine), Branch (Mao/Rabbit, Liver/Large Intestine, 5AM-6:59AM)

Vitalize Blood Transform Stasis

Tao Ren (Semen Persicae, Peach Kernel)
Vitalize Blood Transform Stasis
Bitter, Sweet[369]
Neutral, slightly Toxic*
Heart, **Large Intestine**, Liver, Lung
Bie Jing (Jue Yin/Yang Ming, Liver/Large Intestine), Biao/Li (Large Intestine/Lung), Clock Neighbor (Liver/Lung), Branch (Mao/Rabbit, Liver/Large Intestine, 5AM-6:59AM) + Heart

Jin Bu Huan, Qian Ceng Ta (Herba Lycopodii Serrati, Lycopodium)
Vitalize Blood Transform Stasis
Acrid, Sweet
Neutral
Lung, Liver, **Large Intestine**
Bie Jing (Jue Yin/Yang Ming, Liver/Large Intestine), Biao/Li (Large Intestine/Lung), Clock Neighbor (Liver/Lung), Branch (Mao/Rabbit, Liver/Large Intestine, 5AM-6:59AM)

Transform Phlegm

Pang Da Hai, Da Hai Zi (Semen Sterculiae Lychnophorae, Boat Sterculia Seed)
Transform Phlegm
Sweet
Cold
Lung, **Large Intestine**
Biao/Li (Large Intestine/Lung)

Gua Lou Shi, Quan Gua Lou, Gua Lou (Fructus Trichosanthis, Snake Gourd Fruit)
Transform Phlegm
Sweet, slightly Bitter[370]
Cold
Large Intestine, Lung, Stomach
Name (Yang Ming, Large Intestine/Stomach), Biao/Li (Large Intestine/Lung), Clock Neighbor (Large Intestine/Stomach)

Gua Lou Pi (Pericarpium Trichosanthis, Trichosanthis Peel, Snake Gourd Peel)
Transform Phlegm
Sweet
Cold
Large Intestine, Lung, Stomach
Name (Yang Ming, Large Intestine/Stomach), Biao/Li (Large Intestine/Lung), Clock Neighbor (Large Intestine/Stomach)

Gua Lou Ren (Semen Trichosanthis, Trichosanthes Seed, Snake Gourd Seed)
Transform Phlegm
Sweet
Cold
Large Intestine, Lung, Stomach
Name (Yang Ming, Large Intestine/Stomach), Biao/Li (Large Intestine/Lung), Clock Neighbor (Large Intestine/Stomach)

Xuan Fu Hua, Jin Fei Hua, Jin Fu Hua (Flos Inulae, Inula Flower)
Transform Phlegm
Bitter, Acrid, Salty
Slightly Warm
Large Intestine, Lung, Stomach, Spleen, Liver[371]
Name (Yang Ming, Large Intestine/Stomach, Tai Yin, Lung/Spleen), Bie Jing (Jue Yin/Yang Ming, Liver/Large Intestine), Biao/Li (Large Intestine/Lung, Stomach/Spleen), Clock Neighbor (Large Intestine/Stomach, Liver/Lung), Branch (Chou/Ox, Spleen/Liver, 1AM-2:59AM and Mao/Rabbit, Liver/Large Intestine, 5AM-6:59AM)

Bi Qi, Di Li, Wu Yu, Ma Ti (Rhizoma Eleocharitis, Water Chestnut)
Transform Phlegm
Sweet
Slightly Cold
Lung, Liver,[372] Stomach, **Large Intestine**
Name (Yang Ming, Large Intestine/Stomach), Bie Jing (Jue Yin/Yang Ming, Liver/Large Intestine), Biao/Li (Large Intestine/Lung), Clock Neighbor (Large Intestine/Stomach, Liver/Lung), Branch (Mao/Rabbit, Liver/Large Intestine, 5AM-6:59AM)

Luo Han Guo (Fructus Momordicae, Momordica Fruit)
Transform Phlegm/Relieve Cough and Wheezing/Panting
Sweet
Cool
Lung, **Large Intestine**, Spleen[373]
Name (Tai Yin, Lung/Spleen), Biao/Li (Large Intestine, Lung)

Ze Qi (Herba Euphorbiae Helioscopiae, Euphorbia, Sun Spurge)
Regulate Water Resolve Dampness/Transform Phlegm
Sweet, Bitter, Acrid
Cool to slightly Cold,[374] slightly Toxic[375] to Toxic*
Large Intestine, Small Intestine, Lung
Biao/Li (Large Intestine/Lung) + Small Intestine

Relieve Cough and Wheezing/Panting

Xing Ren, Bei Xing, Ku Xing Ren (Semen Armeniacae Amarum, Apricot Seed)
Relieve Cough and Wheezing/Panting
Bitter
Slightly Warm, slightly Toxic*
Lung, **Large Intestine**
Biao/Li (Large Intestine, Lung)

Ma Dou Ling (Fructus Aristolochiae, Birthwort Fruit)
Relieve Cough and Wheezing/Panting
Bitter, slightly Acrid
Cold, slightly Toxic*
Lung, **Large Intestine**
Biao/Li (Large Intestine, Lung)

Zi Su Zi, Su Zi (Fructus Perillae, Purple Perilla Fruit)
Relieve Cough and Wheezing/Panting
Acrid, Aromatic
Warm
Lung, **Large Intestine**
Biao/Li (Large Intestine, Lung)

Luo Han Guo (Fructus Momordicae, Momordica Fruit)
Transform Phlegm/Relieve Cough and Wheezing/Panting
Sweet
Cool
Lung, **Large Intestine**, Spleen[376]
Name (Tai Yin, Lung/Spleen), Biao/Li (Large Intestine, Lung)

Nourish and Calm Shen

Bai Zi Ren (Semen Platycadi, Arbor-Vitae Seed, Biota)
Nourish and Calm Shen
Sweet, Acrid,[377] Aromatic[378]
Neutral to Cool[379]
Heart, Kidney, **Large Intestine**
Name (Shao Yin, Kidney/Heart), Clock Opposite (Kidney/Large Intestine)

Calm Liver Extinguish Wind

Jue Ming Zi, Cao Jue Ming (Semen Cassiae, Cassia Seeds, Foetid Cassia Seeds)
Clear Heat Purge Fire/Calm Liver Extinguish Wind
Sweet, Bitter, Salty[380]
Cool to slightly Cold
Liver, **Large Intestine**, Kidney[381]
Bie Jing (Jue Yin/Yang Ming, Liver/Large Intestine), Clock Opposite (Kidney/Large Intestine), Branch (Mao/Rabbit, Liver/Large Intestine, 5AM-6:59AM)

Open Orifices

Shui Chang Pu, Bai Chang Pu (Rhizoma Acori Calami, Calamus, Sweetflag Rhizome)
Open Orifices
Bitter, Acrid, slightly Toxic*
Warm
Heart, Liver, Stomach, Spleen,[382] **Large Intestine**[383]
Name (Yang Ming, Large Intestine/Stomach), Bie Jing (Jue Yin/Yang Ming, Liver/Large Intestine), Biao/Li (Stomach/Spleen), Clock Neighbor (Spleen/Heart, Large Intestine/Stomach), Branch (Chou/Ox, Spleen/Liver, 1AM-2:59AM and Mao/Rabbit, Liver/Large Intestine, 5AM-6:59AM)

Tonify Qi

Sha Ji, Cu Liu Guo (Fructus Hippophae, Sea Buckthorn Fruit, Swallow Thorn Fruit)
Tonify Qi
Sour, slightly Sweet, Astringent
Warm
Lung, Spleen, Stomach, **Large Intestine**, Liver, Small Intestine[384]
Name (Tai Yin, Lung/Spleen, Yang Ming, Large Intestine/Stomach), Bie Jing (Jue Yin/Yang Ming, Liver/Large Intestine, Tai Yin/Tai Yang, Spleen/Small Intestine), Biao/Li (Large Intestine/Lung, Stomach/Spleen), Clock Opposite (Liver/Small Intestine), Clock Neighbor (Liver/Lung, Large Intestine/Stomach), Branch (Chou/Ox, Spleen/Liver, 1AM-2:59AM, Mao/Rabbit, Liver/Large Intestine, 5AM-6:59AM, Si/Snake, Small Intestine/Spleen, 9AM-10:59AM, Wei/Sheep, Spleen/Small Intestine, 1PM-2:59PM)

Feng Mi (Mel, Honey)
Tonify Qi
Sweet
Neutral
Spleen, Lung, **Large Intestine**
Name (Tai Yin, Spleen/Lung), Biao/Li (Large Intestine/Lung)

Tonify Yang

Hu Tao Ren, He Tao Ren, Hu Tao Rou (Semen Juglandis, Walnut Nut)
Tonify Yang
Sweet, Astringent[385]
Warm
Kidney, Lung, **Large Intestine**
Biao/Li (Large Intestine/Lung), Clock Opposite (Kidney/Large Intestine), Branch (You/Chicken, Lung/Kidney, 5PM-6:59PM)

Yin Yang Huo, Xian Ling Pi (Herba Epimedii, Arial Parts of Epimedium, Horny Goat Weed)
Tonify Yang
Acrid, Sweet, Aromatic[386]
Warm
Kidney, Liver, and possibly **Large Intestine**, Stomach and San Jiao[387]
Possibly Name (Yang Ming, Large Intestine/Stomach), Bie Jing (Jue Yin/Yang Ming, Liver/Large Intestine, Shao Yin/Shao Yang, Kidney/San Jiao), Clock Opposite (Kidney/Large Intestine), Clock Neighbor (Large Intestine/Stomach), Branch (Mao/Rabbit, Liver/Large Intestine, 5AM-6:59AM)

Rou Cong Rong, Cong Rong, Da Yun (Herba Cistanches, Fleshy Stem of Broomrape)
Tonify Yang
Sweet, Salty
Warm
Kidney, **Large Intestine**
Clock Opposite (Kidney/Large Intestine)

Suo Yang, Di Mao Qiu (Herba Cynomorii, Fleshy Stem of Cynomorium)
Tonify Yang
Sweet
Warm
Liver, Kidney, **Large Intestine**
Bie Jing (Jue Yin/Yang Ming, Liver/Large Intestine), Clock Opposite (Kidney/Large Intestine), Branch (Mao/Rabbit, Liver/Large Intestine, 5AM-6:59AM)

Tonify Blood

Sheng He Shou Wu (Radix Polygoni Multiflori Recens, Fresh Fleeceflower Root)
Tonify Blood
Bitter, Sweet, Astringent, not Astringent[388]
Neutral to Cold[389]
Liver, Heart, **Large Intestine**
Bie Jing (Jue Yin/Yang Ming, Liver/Large Intestine), Branch (Mao/Rabbit, Liver/Large Intestine, 5AM-6:59AM) + Heart

Tonify Yin

Hei Zhi Ma, Hu Ma Zi, Hu Ma Ren, Zhi Ma (Semen Sesame Nigrum, Black Sesame Seed)
Tonify Yin
Sweet, Aromatic[390]
Neutral
Liver, Kidney, **Large Intestine**[391]
Bie Jing (Jue Yin/Yang Ming, Liver/Large Intestine), Clock Opposite (Kidney/Large Intestine), Branch (Mao/Rabbit, Liver/Large Intestine, 5AM-6:59AM)

Astringe, Stabilize and Bind

He Zi, Ke Zi, He Li, He Li Le (Fructus Chebulae, Black Myrobalan Fruit, Terminalia, Chebula)
Astringe, Stabilize and Bind
Sour, Bitter, Astringent
Neutral
Lung, Stomach,[392] **Large Intestine**
Name (Yang Ming, Large Intestine/Stomach), Biao/Li (Large Intestine/Lung), Clock Neighbor (Large Intestine/Stomach)

Chun Gen Pi, Chun Pi (Cortex Ailanthi, Ailanthus Bark, Tree of Heaven Bark, Chinese Sumac Bark)
Astringe, Stabilize and Bind
Bitter, Astringent
Cold
Large Intestine, Stomach,[393] Liver, Lung[394]
Name (Yang Ming, Large Intestine/Stomach), Bie Jing (Jue Yin/Yang Ming, Liver/Large Intestine), Biao/Li (Large Intestine/Lung), Clock Neighbor (Large Intestine/Stomach, Liver/Lung), Branch (Mao/Rabbit, Liver/Large Intestine, 5AM-6:59AM)

Wu Mei (Fructus Mume, Mume Fruit, Smoked Plum)
Astringe, Stabilize and Bind
Sour, Astringent
Neutral to Warm[395]
Liver, Spleen, Lung, **Large Intestine**
Name (Tai Yin, Spleen/Lung), Bie Jing (Jue Yin/Yang Ming, Liver/Large Intestine), Biao/Li (Large Intestine/Lung), Clock Neighbor (Liver/Lung), Branch (Chou/Ox, Spleen/Liver, 1AM-2:59AM, Mao/Rabbit, Liver/Large Intestine, 5AM-6:59AM)

Ying Su Ke (Pericarpium Papaveris, Opium Poppy Husk)
Astringe, Stabilize and Bind
Sour, Astringent
Neutral, Toxic*
Kidney, **Large Intestine**, Lung
Biao/Li (Large Intestine/Lung), Clock Opposite (Kidney/Large Intestine), Branch (You/Chicken, Lung/Kidney, 5PM-6:59PM)

Wu Bei Zi, Wen Ge, Bai Chong Chong (Galla Chinensis, Gallnut of Chinese Sumac)
Astringe, Stabilize and Bind
Salty, Sour, Astringent
Cold, slightly Toxic*[396]
Lung, **Large Intestine**, Kidney
Biao/Li (Large Intestine/Lung), Clock Opposite (Kidney/Large Intestine), Branch (You/Chicken, Lung/Kidney, 5PM-6:59PM)

Shi Liu Pi, Shi Liu Ke, An Shi Liu (Pericarpium Granati, Pomegranate Husk)
Astringe, Stabilize and Bind
Sour, Sweet,[397] Astringent
Slightly Cooling[398] to Warm, slightly Toxic*
Stomach,[399] **Large Intestine**
Name (Yang Ming, Large Intestine/Stomach), Clock Neighbor (Large Intestine/Stomach)

Yu Yu Liang (Limonitum)
Astringe, Stabilize and Bind
Sweet, slightly Salty,[400] Bland,[401] Astringent
Neutral
Large Intestine, Stomach
Name (Yang Ming, Large Intestine/Stomach), Clock Neighbor (Large Intestine/Stomach)

Chi Shi Zhi (Halloysitum Rubrum, Red Halloysite)
Astringe, Stabilize and Bind
Sweet, Sour, Astringent[402]
Warm
Stomach, **Large Intestine**, Spleen[403]
Name (Yang Ming, Large Intestine/Stomach), Biao/Li (Stomach/Spleen), Clock Neighbor (Large Intestine/Stomach)

Rou Dou Kou (Semen Mystericae, Nutmeg Seeds)
Astringe, Stabilize and Bind
Acrid, Astringent, Aromatic
Warm
Large Intestine, Spleen, Stomach
Name (Yang Ming, Large Intestine/Stomach), Biao/Li (Stomach/Spleen), Clock Neighbor (Large Intestine/Stomach)

Jin Ying Zi (Fructus Rosae Laevigatae, Cherokee Rosehip)
Astringe, Stabilize and Bind
Sour, Astringent
Neutral to Warm[404]
Kidney, Urinary Bladder, **Large Intestine**
Biao/Li (Urinary Bladder/Kidney), Clock Opposite (Kidney/Large Intestine), Branch (Shen/Monkey, Large Intestine/Urinary Bladder, 3PM-4:59PM)

Ji Guan Hua (Flos Celosiae Cristatae, Cock's Comb Flower)
Clear Heat Cool Blood/Astringe, Stabilize and Bind
Sweet, Astringent[405]
Cool
Large Intestine, Liver, Kidney[406]
Bie Jing (Jue Yin/Yang Ming, Liver/Large Intestine), Clock Opposite (Kidney/Large Intestine), Branch (Mao/Rabbit, Liver/Large Intestine, 5AM-6:59AM)

External Application

Da Suan (Bulbus Alli Sativi, Garlic)
Expel Parasites/External Application
Acrid, Sweet[407]
Neutral to Warm
Spleen, Stomach, Lung, **Large Intestine**[408]
Name (Tai Yin, Spleen/Lung, Yang Ming, Large Intestine/Stomach), Biao/Li (Stomach/Spleen, Large Intestine/Lung), Clock Neighbor (Large Intestine/Stomach)

Ming Fan, Bai Fan, Ku Fan (Alumen, Alum)
External Application
Sour, Bitter,[409] Astringent
Cold, Toxic*
Lung, Liver, Spleen, Stomach,[410] **Large Intestine**[411]
Name (Tai Yin, Spleen/Lung, Yang Ming, Large Intestine/Stomach), Bie Jing (Jue Yin/Yang Ming, Liver/Large Intestine), Clock Neighbor (Liver/Lung, Large Intestine/Stomach), Biao/Li (Stomach/Spleen, Large Intestine/Lung), Branch (Chou/Ox, Spleen/Liver, 1AM-2:59AM, Mao/Rabbit, Liver/Large Intestine, 5AM-6:59AM)

Xiong Huang (Realgar)
External Application
Acrid, Bitter
Neutral to Warm, Toxic*
Heart, Liver, Kidney,[412] Stomach,[413] Lung,[414] **Large Intestine**[415]
Name (Shao Yin, Heart/Kidney, Yang Ming, Large Intestine/Stomach), Bie Jing (Jue Yin/Yang Ming, Liver/Large Intestine), Biao/Li (Large Intestine/Lung), Clock Opposite (Kidney/Large Intestine), Clock Neighbor (Large Intestine/Stomach, Liver/Lung), Branch (Mao/Rabbit, Liver/Large Intestine, 5AM-6:59AM, You/Chicken, Lung, Kidney, 5PM-6:59PM)

Mu Bie Zi (Semen Momordicae, Momordica Seed)
External Application
Bitter, slightly Sweet
Warm, Toxic*
Large Intestine, Liver, Stomach
Name (Yang Ming, Large Intestine/Stomach), Bie Jing (Jue Yin/Yang Ming, Liver/Large Intestine), Clock Neighbor (Large Intestine/Stomach), Branch (Mao/Rabbit, Liver/Large Intestine, 5AM-6:59AM)

Qing Fen (Calomelas, Calomel)
External Application
Acrid, Bland[416]
Cold, very Toxic*
Liver, Kidney, **Large Intestine**,[417] Small Intestine[418]
Bie Jing (Jue Yin/Yang Ming, Liver/Large Intestine), Clock Opposite (Liver/Small Intestine, Kidney/Large Intestine), Branch (Mao/Rabbit, Liver/Large Intestine, 5AM-6:59AM)

Liu Huang (Sulfur)
External Application
Sour, Sweet[419]
Warm to Hot,[420] Toxic*
Kidney, **Large Intestine**, Pericardium[421]
Clock Opposite (Kidney/Large Intestine), Clock Neighbor (Kidney, Pericardium)

Foot Yang Ming Stomach Herbs

Acrid Warm Exterior Releasing

Bai Zhi (Radix Angelicae Dahuricae, Angelica Root)
Acrid Warm Exterior Releasing
Acrid, Aromatic
Warm
Lung, **Stomach**, Spleen,[422] Large Intestine[423]
Name (Tai Yin, Lung/Spleen, Yang Ming, Large Intestine/Stomach), Biao/Li (Stomach/Spleen, Large Intestine/Lung), Clock Neighbor (Large Intestine/Stomach)

Xin Yi Hua, Xin Yi, Wang Chun Hua (Flos Magnoliae, Magnolia Flower)
Acrid Warm Exterior Releasing
Acrid, Aromatic
Warm
Lung, **Stomach**

Cong Bai, Xiang Cong (Bulbus Allii Fistulosi, Scallion, Spring Onion, Green Onion)
Acrid Warm Exterior Releasing
Acrid
Warm
Lung, **Stomach**

Hu Sui (Coriandri Herba cum Radice, Coriander, Cilantro)
Acrid Warm Exterior Releasing
Acrid
Warm
Lung, **Stomach**

Zi Su Geng (Caulis Perillae, Perilla Stem)
Acrid Warm Exterior Releasing/Regulate and Rectify Qi
Acrid, Sweet, Aromatic
Slightly Warm
Lung, Spleen, **Stomach**
Name (Tai Yin, Lung/Spleen), Biao/Li (Stomach/Spleen)

Sheng Jiang (Rhizoma Zingiberis Recens, Fresh Ginger Rhizome)
Acrid Warm Exterior Releasing
Acrid
Slightly Warm
Lung, Spleen, **Stomach**
Name (Tai Yin, Lung/Spleen), Biao/Li (Stomach/Spleen)

Xiang Ru, Hua Qi Ning, Shi Xiang Rou (Herba Elsholtziae seu Moslae, Aromatic Madder)
Acrid Warm Exterior Releasing
Acrid, Aromatic
Slightly Warm
Lung, Spleen,[424] Heart,[425] **Stomach**
Name (Tai Yin, Lung/Spleen), Biao/Li (Stomach/Spleen), Clock Neighbor (Spleen/Heart)

Xi He Liu, Guan Yin Liu (Cacumen Tamaricis, Tamarisk stems and leaves)
Acrid Warm Exterior Releasing
Acrid, Sweet, Salty[426]
Warm
Lung, **Stomach**, Heart

Acrid Cool Exterior Releasing

Sheng Ma (Radix Cimicifugae, Black Cohosh Rhizome, Bugbane Rhizome)
Acrid Cool Exterior Releasing
Acrid, Sweet
Cool to slightly Cold[427]
Lung, Spleen, **Stomach**, Large Intestine
Name (Tai Yin, Lung/Spleen, Yang Ming, Large Intestine/Stomach), Biao/Li (Large Intestine/Lung, Stomach/Spleen), Clock Neighbor (Large Intestine/Stomach)

Sang Ye (Folium Mori, White Mulberry Leaf)
Acrid Cool Exterior Releasing
Bitter, Sweet, Acrid,[428] Aromatic
Cold
Lung, Liver, Large Intestine,[429] **Stomach**[430]
Name (Yang Ming, Large Intestine/Stomach), Biao/Li (Large Intestine/Lung), Bie Jing (Jue Yin/Yang Ming, Liver/Large Intestine), Clock Neighbor (Liver/Lung, Large Intestine/Stomach), Branch (Mao/Rabbit, Liver/Large Intestine, 5AM-6:59AM)

Dan Dou Chi (Semen Sojae Praeparatum, Prepared Soybean, Fermented Soybean)
Acrid Cool Exterior Releasing
Acrid, Sweet, slightly Bitter, Aromatic
Cold or Warm depending on the type of preparation
Lung, **Stomach**

Niu Bang Zi, Da Li Zi, Shu Nian Zi (Fructus Arctii, Great Burdock Seed, Arctium)
Acrid Cool Exterior Releasing
Acrid, Bitter, Aromatic
Cold
Lung, **Stomach**

Man Jing Zi, Jing Tiao Zi, Bai Bu Jing (Fructus Viticis, Vitex Fruit)
Acrid Cool Exterior Releasing
Acrid, Bitter
Both Cool and Warm[431]
Lung,[432] Liver, **Stomach**, Urinary Bladder,[433] Gall Bladder,[434] San Jiao[435]
Name (Shao Yang, Gall Bladder/San Jiao), Bie Jing (Tai Yin/Tai Yang, Lung/Urinary Bladder), Biao/Li (Gall Bladder/Liver), Clock Opposite (Lung, Urinary Bladder), Clock Neighbor (San Jiao/Gall Bladder, Liver/Lung), Qian/Hou (Front/Back, Stomach/Urinary Bladder), Branch (Yin/Tiger, Gall Bladder/Lung, 3AM-4:59AM, Hai/Pig, Urinary Bladder/San Jiao, 9PM-10:59PM)

Ge Gen (Radix Puerariae, Kudzu Root, Pueraria)
Acrid Cool Exterior Releasing
Sweet, Acrid, slightly Bitter[436]
Cool
Spleen, **Stomach**, Tai Yang,[437] **Yang Ming**[438]
Biao/Li (Stomach/Spleen), possibly Name (Yang Ming Large Intestine/Stomach) and Clock Neighbor (Large Intestine/Stomach) if Yang Ming[439] really means the entire Yang Ming Jing-channel, and possibly Name (Tai Yang, Small Intestine/Urinary Bladder), Bie Jing (Spleen, Small Intestine), Clock Neighbor (Small Intestine/Urinary Bladder) and Qian/Hou (Front/Back, Stomach/Urinary Bladder) if Tai Yang[440] really means the entire Tai Yang Jing-channel.

Ge Hua (Flos Pueriae, Kudzu Flower)
Acrid Cool Exterior Releasing
Sweet
Neutral
Stomach
Branch (Chen/Dragon, Stomach/Stomach, 7AM-8:59AM)

Da Dou Juan, Dou Juan, Da Dou Huang Juan (Sojae Semen Germinatum, Dried Soybean Sprout)
Acrid Cool Exterior Releasing
Sweet, Bland
Neutral
Spleen, **Stomach**
Biao/Li (Stomach/Spleen)

Clear Heat Purge Fire

Qing Guo Gen (Radix Canarium Album, White Olive Root)
Clear Heat Purge Fire
Sweet, Sour, Astringent
Cool
Lung, **Stomach**

Tian Hua Fen, Gua Lou Gen (Radix Trichosanthis, Trichosanthis Root, Snake Gourd Root)
Clear Heat Purge Fire
Bitter, slightly Sweet
Cold
Lung, **Stomach**

Shi Gao, Bai Hu, Li Shi (Gypsum Fibrosum, Gypsum)
Clear Heat Purge Fire
Acrid, Sweet
Very Cold
Lung, **Stomach**

Qing Guo (Fructus Canarii, Chinese White Olive)
Clear Heat Purge Fire
Sweet, Sour, Astringent[441]
Neutral
Lung, **Stomach**, Spleen
Name (Tai Yin, Lung/Spleen), Biao/Li (Stomach, Spleen)

Zhu Ye (Herba Phyllostachys, Bamboo Leaves)
Clear Heat Purge Fire
Sweet, Bland
Cold
Heart, **Stomach**, Lung

Lu Gen (Rhizoma Phragmitis, Reed Rhizome)
Clear Heat Purge Fire
Sweet, Bland[442]
Cold
Lung, **Stomach**, Heart[443]

Wu Long Cha (Folium Camellia Sinensis Fermentata, 'Oolong' Tea)
Clear Heat Purge Fire
Bitter, Sweet
Cool
Heart, Lung, **Stomach**, Small Intestine
Biao/Li (Small Intestine/Heart) + Lung, Stomach

Xi Gua (Fructus Citrulli, Watermelon Fruit)
Clear Heat Purge Fire
Sweet
Cold
Heart, **Stomach**, Urinary Bladder, Lung[444]
Bie Jing (Tai Yin/Tai Yang, Lung/Urinary Bladder), Clock Opposite (Lung/Urinary Bladder), Qian/Hou (Front/Back, Stomach/Urinary Bladder) + Heart

Shan Zhi Zi, Zhi Zi (Fructus Gardeniae, Cape Jasmine Fruit, Gardenia Fruit)
Clear Heat Purge Fire
Bitter
Cold
Heart, Lung, **Stomach**, San Jiao, Liver[445]
Clock Neighbor (Liver/Lung) + Heart, Stomach, San Jiao

Ya Zhi Cao, Zhu Ye Shui Cao, Zhu Jie Cai (Herba Commelinae, Common Dayflower)
Clear Heat Purge Fire
Sweet, Bland
Cold
Lung, **Stomach**, Small Intestine

Zhi Mu (Radix Anemarrhenae, Anemarrhena)
Clear Heat Purge Fire
Bitter, Sweet
Cold
Lung, **Stomach**, Kidney
Branch (You/Chicken, Lung/Kidney, 5PM-6:59PM) + Stomach

Shi Lian Zi (Herba Sinocrassulae Indicae, Indian Sinocrassula)
Clear Heat Purge Fire
Bitter
Cold
Large Intestine, Urinary Bladder, **Stomach**
Name (Yang Ming, Large Intestine/Stomach), Clock Neighbor (Large Intestine/Stomach), Qian/Hou (Front/Back, Stomach/Urinary Bladder), Branch (Shen/Monkey, Large Intestine/Urinary Bladder, 3PM-4:59PM)

Lu Cha (Folium Camellia Sinensis, Green Tea)
Clear Heat Purge Fire
Bitter
Cold
Stomach
Branch (Chen/Dragon, Stomach/Stomach, 7AM-8:59AM)

Dan Zhu Ye (Herba Lophatheri, Lophatherum)
Clear Heat Purge Fire
Sweet, Bland
Cold
Heart, **Stomach**, Small Intestine
Biao/Li (Small Intestine/Heart) + Stomach

Xi Gua Pi (Exocarpium Citrulli, Watermelon Rind)
Clear Heat Purge Fire
Sweet
Cold
Heart, **Stomach**, Urinary Bladder
Qian/Hou (Front/Back, Stomach/Urinary Bladder) + Heart

Han Shui Shi, Yan Jing Shi (Glauberitum, Calcitum, Calcite)
Clear Heat Purge Fire
Acrid,[446] Salty
Very Cold
Stomach, Kidney

Gu Jing Cao (Flos Eriocauli, Pipewort Scapus and Inflorescence)
Clear Heat Purge Fire
Sweet, Acrid[447]
Cool[448] to Neutral to Warm[449]
Liver, **Stomach**

Clear Heat Dry Dampness

Huang Qin (Radix Scutellariae, Baical Skullcap Root, Scutellaria, Scute)
Clear Heat Dry Dampness
Bitter
Cold
Lung, Gall Bladder, **Stomach**, Large Intestine and possibly San Jiao[450]
Name (Yang Ming, Large Intestine/Stomach) Biao/Li (Large Intestine/Lung), Clock Neighbor (Large Intestine/Stomach), Branch (Yin/Tiger, Gall Bladder/Lung, 3AM-4:59AM), and possibly Name (Shao Yang, San Jiao/Gall Bladder), Clock Neighbor (San Jiao/Gall Bladder)

Ku Shen, Ku Shen Gen, Ku Gu (Radix Sophorae Flavescentis, Flavescent Sophora Root)
Clear Heat Dry Dampness
Bitter to extremely Bitter[451]
Cold
Heart, Liver, **Stomach**, Large Intestine, Urinary Bladder, Small Intestine[452]
Name (Yang Ming, Large Intestine/Stomach, Tai Yang, Small Intestine/Urinary Bladder), Bie Jing (Jue Yin/Yang Ming, Liver/Large Intestine), Biao/Li (Small Intestine/Heart), Clock Opposite (Liver/Small Intestine), Clock Neighbor (Large Intestine/Stomach, Small Intestine/Urinary Bladder), Qian/Hou (Front/Back, Stomach/Urinary Bladder), Branch (Shen/Monkey, Large Intestine/Urinary Bladder, 3PM-4:59PM and Mao/Rabbit, Liver/Large Intestine, 5AM-6:59AM)

Huang Lian (Rhizoma Coptidis, Goldthread Rhizome, Coptis Root)
Clear Heat Dry Dampness
Very Bitter, purely Bitter[453]
Very Cold
Heart, Liver, **Stomach**, Large Intestine, Du[454]
Name (Yang Ming, Large Intestine/Stomach), Bie Jing (Jue Yin/Yang Ming, Liver/Large Intestine), Clock Neighbor (Large Intestine/Stomach), Branch (Mao/Rabbit, Liver/Large Intestine, 5AM-6:59AM) + Heart, Du

Qin Pi (Cortex Fraxini, Bark of Korean Ash Branch)
Clear Heat Dry Dampness/Clear Heat Clean Toxin
Bitter, Acrid,[455] Astringent[456]
Cold
Gall Bladder, Liver, Large Intestine, **Stomach**[457]
Name (Yang Ming, Large Intestine/Stomach), Bie Jing (Jue Yin/Yang Ming, Liver/Large Intestine), Biao/Li (Gall Bladder/Liver), Clock Neighbor (Large Intestine/Stomach), Branch (Mao/Rabbit, Liver/Large Intestine, 5AM-6:59AM)

Long Dan Cao, Long Dan, Dan Cao (Radix Gentianae, Chinese Gentian Root, Gentiana)
Clear Heat Dry Dampness
Bitter, Astringing[458]
Cold
Liver, Gall Bladder, **Stomach**, Urinary Bladder[459]
Biao/Li (Gall Bladder/Liver), Qian/Hou (Front/Back, Stomach/Urinary Bladder)

Clear Heat Cool Blood

Xuan Shen, Yuan Shen, Hei Shen (Radix Scrophulariae, Ningpo Figwort Root)
Clear Heat Cool Blood
Bitter, Sweet, Salty
Cold
Lung, **Stomach**, Kidney
Branch (You/Chicken, Lung/Kidney, 5PM-6:59PM) + Stomach

Shui Niu Jiao (Bubali Cornu, Water Buffalo Horn)
Clear Heat Cool Blood
Salty, Bitter[460]
Cold
Heart, Liver, **Stomach**

Clear Heat Clean Toxin

Bei Dou Gen (Rhizoma Menispermi, Asiatic Moonseed Rhizome)
Clear Heat Clean Toxin
Bitter
Cold
Lung, **Stomach**, Large Intestine
Name (Yang Ming, Large Intestine/Stomach), Biao/Li (Large Intestine/Lung), Clock Neighbor (Large Intestine/Stomach)

Ren Dong Teng (Caulis Lonicerae, Honeysuckle Vine)
Clear Heat Clean Toxin
Sweet
Neutral to slightly Cold[461] to Cold
Lung, **Stomach**, Large Intestine,[462] Spleen[463]
Name (Yang Ming, Large Intestine/Stomach, Tai Yin, Lung/Spleen), Biao/Li (Large Intestine/Lung, Stomach/Spleen) Clock Neighbor (Large Intestine/Stomach)

Shan Dou Gen, Dou Gen, Nan Dou Gen (Radix Sophorae Tonkinensis, Subprostrate, Sophora Root)
Clear Heat Clean Toxin
Bitter to very Bitter[464]
Cold, slightly Toxic*
Lung, **Stomach**,[465] Large Intestine,[466] Heart[467]
Name (Yang Ming, Large Intestine/Stomach), Biao/Li (Large Intestine/Lung), Clock Neighbor (Large Intestine/Stomach) + Heart

Jin Yin Hua (Flos Lonicerae, Honeysuckle Flower, Lonicera Flower)
Clear Heat Clean Toxin
Sweet
Cold
Lung, **Stomach**, Large Intestine, Heart[468]
Name (Yang Ming, Large Intestine/Stomach), Biao/Li (Large Intestine/Lung), Clock Neighbor (Large Intestine/Stomach) + Heart

Chuan Xin Lian, Lan He Lian (Herba Andrographis, Green Chiretta, Kariyat)
Clear Heat Clean Toxin
Bitter
Cold
Lung, **Stomach**, Large Intestine, Small Intestine
Name (Yang Ming, Large Intestine/Stomach), Biao/Li (Large Intestine/Lung), Clock Neighbor (Large Intestine/Stomach) + Small Intestine

Ban Zhi Lian (Herba Scutellariae Barbatae, Barbat Skullcap, Barbed Skullcap)
Clear Heat Clean Toxin
Acrid, slightly Bitter
Cool
Liver, Lung, **Stomach**, Kidney,[469] Large Intestine[470]
Name (Yang Ming, Large Intestine/Stomach), Bie Jing (Jue Yin/Yang Ming, Liver/Large Intestine), Biao/Li (Large Intestine/Lung), Clock Opposite (Kidney/Large Intestine), Clock Neighbor (Large Intestine/Stomach, Liver/Lung), Branch (You/Chicken, Lung/Kidney, 5PM-6:59PM, Mao/Rabbit, Liver/Large Intestine, 5AM-6:59AM)

Ban Lan Gen, Bei Ban Lan Gen (Radix Isatidis, Isatis Root)
Clear Heat Clean Toxin
Bitter
Cold
Heart, **Stomach**, Lung[471]

Da Qing Ye (Folium Isatidis, Woad Leaf, Indigo Leaf)
Clear Heat Clean Toxin
Bitter, Salty[472]
Very Cold
Heart, Lung, **Stomach**, Liver[473]
Clock Neighbor (Liver/Lung) + Heart, Stomach

Nan Ban Lan Ye, Ma Lian Ye (Folium Baphicacanthis)
Clear Heat Clean Toxin
Bitter, Salty
Cold
Lung, **Stomach**, Heart, Liver
Clock Neighbor (Liver/Lung) + Stomach, Heart

Long Kui, Ku Kui (Herba Solanum Nigrum, Black Nightshade)
Clear Heat Clean Toxin
Slightly Bitter, slightly Sweet[474]
Cold, non-Toxic[475] to slightly Toxic*
Lung, Urinary Bladder, **Stomach**[476]
Bie Jing (Tai Yin/Tai Yang, Lung/Urinary Bladder), Clock Opposite (Lung/Urinary Bladder), Qian/Hou (Front/Back, Stomach/Urinary Bladder)

Qing Dai (Indigo Naturalis)
Clear Heat Clean Toxin
Salty
Cold to very Cold[477]
Liver, Lung, **Stomach**
Clock Neighbor (Liver/Lung) + Stomach

Bai Tou Weng (Radix Pulsatillae, Chinese Anemone Root, Pulsatilla)
Clear Heat Clean Toxin
Bitter
Cold
Large Intestine, **Stomach**[478]
Name (Yang Ming, Large Intestine/Stomach), Clock Neighbor (Large Intestine/Stomach)

Lou Lu (Radix Rhapontici, Rhaponticum Root)
Clear Heat Clean Toxin
Bitter, Salty[479]
Cold
Stomach, Large Intestine[480]
Name (Yang Ming, Large Intestine/Stomach), Clock Neighbor (Large Intestine/Stomach)

Bai Hua She She Cao (Herba Oldenlandia, Heydyotis)
Clear Heat Clean Toxin
Slightly Bitter, Sweet
Cold
Stomach, Large Intestine, Small Intestine, Liver[481]
Name (Yang Ming, Large Intestine/Stomach), Bie Jing (Jue Yin/Yang Ming, Liver/Large Intestine), Clock Opposite (Liver/Small Intestine), Clock Neighbor (Large Intestine/Stomach), Branch (Mao/Rabbit, Liver/Large Intestine, 5AM-6:59AM)

Qin Pi (Cortex Fraxini, Bark of Korean Ash Branch)
Clear Heat Dry Dampness/Clear Heat Clean Toxin
Bitter, Acrid,[482] Astringent[483]
Cold
Gall Bladder, Liver, Large Intestine, **Stomach**[484]
Name (Yang Ming, Large Intestine/Stomach), Bie Jing (Jue Yin/Yang Ming, Liver/Large Intestine), Biao/Li (Gall Bladder/Liver), Clock Neighbor (Large Intestine/Stomach), Branch (Mao/Rabbit, Liver/Large Intestine, 5AM-6:59AM)

Bai Jiang Cao (Herba cum Radice Patriniae, Patrinia, Thlaspi)
Clear Heat Clean Toxin
Acrid, Bitter, Salty[485]
Cool to slightly Cold
Stomach, Large Intestine, Liver
Name (Yang Ming, Large Intestine/Stomach), Bie Jing (Yang Ming/Jue Yin, Large Intestine/Liver), Clock Neighbor (Large Intestine/Stomach), Branch (Mao/Rabbit, Liver/Large Intestine, 5AM-6:59AM)

Quan Shen (Rhizoma Bistortae)
Clear Heat Clean Toxin
Bitter, Astringent
Cool, slightly Toxic*
Liver, **Stomach**, Large Intestine
Name (Yang Ming, Large Intestine/Stomach), Bie Jing (Jue Yin/Yang Ming, Liver/Large Intestine), Clock Neighbor (Large Intestine/Stomach), Branch (Mao/Rabbit, Liver/Large Intestine, 5AM-6:59AM)

Bai Xian Pi, Bai Tian (Cortex Dictamni, Dictamnus Root Bark)
Clear Heat Clean Toxin
Bitter
Cold
Spleen, **Stomach**
Biao/Li (Stomach/Spleen)

He Ye Geng, Lian Geng (Nelumbinis Petiolus, Lotus Leafstalk)
Clear Heat Clean Toxin/Astringe, Stabilize and Bind
Bitter
Neutral
Spleen, **Stomach**
Biao/Li (Stomach/Spleen)

Bai Lian, Bai Cao, Tu He, Kun Lun, Mao Er Luan (Radix Ampelopsis)
Clear Heat Clean Toxin
Bitter, Acrid, Sweet[486]
Neutral to Cool to Cold[487]
Heart, **Stomach**, Liver, Spleen[488]
Biao/Li (Stomach/Spleen), Clock Neighbor (Spleen/Heart), Branch (Chou/Ox, Spleen/Liver, 1AM-2:59AM)

Guan Zhong, Mian Ma Guan Zhong (Rhizoma Dryopteridis, Dryopteris Root, Shield-Fern Root)
Clear Heat Clean Toxin/Expel Parasites
Bitter
Cool to Cold,[489] slightly Toxic*
Liver, Spleen, **Stomach**[490]
Biao/Li (Stomach/Spleen), Branch (Chou/Ox, Spleen/Liver, 1AM-2:59AM)

Dong Ling Cao (Herba Rabdosiae, Rabdosia)
Clear Heat Clean Toxin
Bitter, Sweet
Cool
Liver, Spleen, **Stomach**
Biao/Li (Stomach/Spleen), Branch (Chou/Ox, Spleen/Liver, 1AM-2:59AM)

Lu Dou Yi (Pericarpium Phaseoli Radiati, Mung Bean Skin)
Clear Heat Clean Toxin
Sweet
Cold
Heart, **Stomach**

Lu Dou (Semen Phaseoli Radiati, Mung Bean)
Clear Heat Clean Toxin
Sweet
Cold
Heart, **Stomach**

Zi Hua Di Ding, Jian Tou Cao, Di Ding Cao (Herba Violae, Yedeon's Violet)
Clear Heat Clean Toxin
Bitter, Acrid
Cold
Heart, Liver, **Stomach**,[491] Pericardium[492]
Name (Jue Yin, Pericardium/Liver), Bie Jing (Jue Yin/Yang Ming, Pericardium/Stomach), Clock Opposite (Pericardium/Stomach), Branch (Shu/Dog, Stomach/Pericardium, 7PM-8:59PM) + Heart

Nan Ban Lan Gen (Rhizoma et Radix Baphicacathis)
Clear Heat Clean Toxin
Bitter
Cold
Heart, Liver, **Stomach**

Pu Gong Ying, Huang Hua Di Ding (Herba Taraxaci, Dandelion)
Clear Heat Clean Toxin
Bitter, Sweet
Cold
Liver, **Stomach**

Shan Ci Gu, Mao Ci Gu, Guang Ci Gu (Psuedobulbus Cremastrae/Pleiones, Cremastra)
Clear Heat Clean Toxin
Sweet, Bland,[493] slightly Acrid
Cold, slightly Toxic*
Liver, **Stomach**

Clear Deficient Heat

Bai Wei (Radix Cynanchi Atrati, Black Swallow-Wort Root)
Clear Deficient Heat
Bitter, Salty
Cold
Stomach, Liver, Kidney,[494] Lung,[495] Ren and Chong[496]
Clock Neighbor (Liver/Lung), Branch (You/Chicken, Lung/Kidney, 5PM-6:59PM) + Stomach, Ren, Chong

Hu Huang Lian, Hu Lian (Rhizoma Picrorhizae, Picrorhiza, Figwort Rhizome)
Clear Deficient Heat
Bitter, Astringing[497]
Cold
Heart, Liver, **Stomach**, Large Intestine
Name (Yang Ming, Large Intestine, Stomach), Bie Jing (Jue Yin/Yang Ming, Liver/Large Intestine), Clock Neighbor (Large Intestine, Stomach), Branch (Mao/Rabbit, Liver/Large Intestine, 5AM-6:59AM) + Heart

Qing Hao (Herba Artemesiae Annuae, Sweet Wormwood)
Clear Deficient Heat
Bitter, Acrid, Aromatic
Cold
Liver, Gall Bladder, **Stomach**,[498] Kidney[499]
Biao/Li (Gall Bladder/Liver), Branch (Zi/Rat, Kidney/Gall Bladder, 11PM-12:59AM) + Stomach

Yin Chai Hu, Niu Dan Gen (Radix Stellariae, Stellaria Root, Starwort Root)
Clear Deficient Heat
Sweet, Bitter[500]
Cool to slightly Cold
Liver, **Stomach**

Purgative

Mang Xiao (Natri Sulfas, Mirabilite, Glauber's Salt, Epsom Salts)
Purgative
Salty, Bitter, Acrid[501]
Cold
Lung,[502] **Stomach**, Large Intestine
Name (Yang Ming, Large Intestine/Stomach), Biao/Li (Large Intestine/Lung), Clock Neighbor (Large Intestine/Stomach)

Ba Dou (Fructus Crotonis, Croton)
Purgative/Cathartic
Acrid
Hot, extremely Toxic*
Stomach, Large Intestine, Lung[503]
Name (Yang Ming, Large Intestine/Stomach), Biao/Li (Large Intestine/Lung), Clock Neighbor (Large Intestine/Stomach)

Da Huang (Radix et Rhizoma Rhei, Rhubarb Root and Rhizome)
Purgative
Bitter to very Bitter[504] to purely Bitter,[505] Aromatic[506]
Cold to very Cold[507]
Spleen, **Stomach**, Large Intestine, Liver, Heart, Du[508]
Name (Yang Ming, Large Intestine/Stomach), Bie Jing (Jue Yin/Yang Ming, Liver/Large Intestine), Biao/Li (Stomach/Spleen), Clock Neighbor (Spleen/Heart, Large Intestine/Stomach), Branch (Chou/Ox, Spleen/Liver, 1AM-2:59AM and Mao/Rabbit, Liver/Large Intestine, 5AM-6:59AM) + Du

Lu Hui, Xiang Dan (Aloe, Dried Aloe Leaf Juice)
Purgative
Very Bitter
Very Cold
Liver, Large Intestine, **Stomach**[509]
Name (Yang Ming, Large Intestine/Stomach), Bie Jing (Jue Yin/Yang Ming, Liver/Large Intestine), Clock Neighbor (Large Intestine/Stomach), Branch (Mao/Rabbit, Liver/Large Intestine, 5AM-6:59AM)

Moist Laxative

Huo Ma Ren (Semen Cannabis, Hemp Seeds)
Moist Laxative
Sweet
Neutral, slightly Toxic*
Spleen, **Stomach**, Large Intestine
Name (Yang Ming, Large Intestine/Stomach), Biao/Li (Stomach/Spleen), Clock Neighbor (Large Intestine/Stomach)

Cathartic

Ba Dou (Fructus Crotonis, Croton)
Purgative/Cathartic
Acrid
Hot, extremely Toxic*
Stomach, Large Intestine, Lung[510]
Name (Yang Ming, Large Intestine/Stomach), Biao/Li (Large Intestine/Lung), Clock Neighbor (Large Intestine/Stomach)

Dispel Wind Dampness, Open Channels and Luo-Network Vessels and Relieve Pain

Hong Gu She (Radix Kadsura Japonicae, Kadsura)
Dispel Wind Dampness, Open Channels and Luo-Network Vessels and Relieve Pain
Acrid, Bitter
Cool
Lung, Liver, **Stomach**
Clock Neighbor (Liver/Lung) + Stomach

Qin Jiao (Radix Gentianae Macrophyllae, Gentiana)
Dispel Wind Dampness, Open Channels and Luo-Network Vessels and Relieve Pain
Bitter, Acrid, Aromatic[511]
Neutral[512] to Cool to slightly Cold
Stomach, Liver, Gall Bladder, Spleen[513]
Biao/Li (Gall Bladder/Liver, Stomach/Spleen), Branch (Chou/Ox, Spleen/Liver, 1AM-2:59AM)

Can Sha, Can Shi (Excrementum Bombycis Mori, Silkworm Feces)
Dispel Wind Dampness, Open Channels and Luo-Network Vessels and Relieve Pain
Sweet,[514] Acrid
Warm
Liver, Spleen, **Stomach**
Biao/Li (Stomach/Spleen), Branch (Chou/Ox, Spleen/Liver, 1AM-2:59AM)

Xu Chang Qing, Liao Diao Zhu (Radix Cynanchi Paniculati, Paniculate Swallow-Wort Root)
Dispel Wind Dampness, Open Channels and Luo-Network Vessels and Relieve Pain
Acrid, Aromatic
Warm
Liver, **Stomach**

Dispel Wind-Dampness Strengthen Sinew/Tendon and Bone

Zou Ma Tai (Rhizoma Ardisiae, Ardisia Root, Giant Leaf Ardisia Rhizome)
Dispel Wind-Dampness Strengthen Sinew/Tendon and Bone
Acrid
Neutral
Lung, **Stomach**, Spleen, Large Intestine
Name (Tai Yin, Lung/Spleen, Yang Ming, Large Intestine/Stomach), Biao/Li (Large Intestine/Lung, Stomach/Spleen), Clock Neighbor (Large Intestine/Stomach)

Aromatic Dissolve Dampness

Hou Po, Chuan Po, Lie Po (Cortex Magnoliae Officinalis, Officinal Magnolia Bark)
Aromatic Dissolve Dampness
Bitter, Acrid, Aromatic
Warm
Large Intestine, Lung, Spleen, **Stomach**
Name (Tai Yin, Lung/Spleen and Yang Ming, Large Intestine/Stomach), Biao/Li (Large Intestine/Lung, Stomach/Spleen), Clock Neighbor (Large Intestine/Stomach)

Huo Xiang (Herba Agastache *or* Herba Pogostemonis, Patchouli)
Aromatic Dissolve Dampness
Acrid, Sweet,[515] Aromatic
Slightly Warm
Spleen, **Stomach**, Lung
Name (Tai Yin, Spleen/Lung), Biao/Li (Stomach/Spleen)

Pei Lan (Herba Eupatorii, Fortune Eupatorium)
Aromatic Dissolve Dampness
Acrid, Aromatic
Neutral
Spleen, **Stomach**, Lung
Name (Tai Yin, Spleen/Lung), Biao/Li (Stomach/Spleen)

Hong Dou Kou (Fructus Galangae, Galanga Seed)
Aromatic Dissolve Dampness/Warm Interior
Acrid, Aromatic
Warm
Spleen, **Stomach**,[516] Lung
Name (Tai Yin, Spleen/Lung), Biao/Li (Stomach/Spleen)

Bai Dou Kou (Fructus Amomi Rotundus, Round Cardamom Fruit)
Aromatic Dissolve Dampness
Intensely[517] Acrid, not Astringent,[518] Aromatic
Warm
Lung, Spleen, **Stomach** and possibly San Jiao[519]
Name (Tai Yin, Lung/Spleen), Biao/Li (Stomach/Spleen) and possibly Clock Opposite (Spleen/San Jiao)

Sha Ren (Fructus Amomi, Amomum Fruit)
Aromatic Dissolve Dampness
Acrid, Aromatic
Warm
Spleen, **Stomach**
Biao/Li (Stomach/Spleen)

Cao Guo (Fructus Tsaoko)
Aromatic Dissolve Dampness
Acrid to intensely Acrid,[520] Aromatic
Warm
Spleen, **Stomach**
Biao/Li (Stomach/Spleen)

Cao Dou Kou (Semen Alpiniae Katsumadai, Katsumada's Galangal Seed)
Aromatic Dissolve Dampness
Acrid, Aromatic
Warm
Spleen, **Stomach**
Biao/Li (Stomach/Spleen)

Cang Zhu (Rhizoma Atractylodis, Atractylodis)
Aromatic Dissolve Dampness
Acrid, Bitter, Sweet,[521] Aromatic
Warm
Spleen, **Stomach**, Yang Qiao[522]
Biao/Li (Stomach/Spleen) + Yang Qiao

Regulate Water Resolve Dampness

Dong Gua Zi (Semen Benincasae, White Gourd Seed, Winter Melon Seed)
Regulate Water Resolve Dampness
Sweet
Cool to Cold[523]
Lung, **Stomach**, Small Intestine, Large Intestine
Name (Yang Ming, Large Intestine/Stomach), Biao/Li (Large Intestine/Lung), Clock Neighbor (Large Intestine/Stomach) + Small Intestine

Tong Cao (Medulla Tetrapanacis, Rice Paper Pith)
Regulate Water Resolve Dampness
Sweet, Bland
Cool to slightly Cold[524]
Lung, **Stomach**

Yi Yi Ren (Semen Coicis, Job's Tears)
Regulate Water Resolve Dampness
Sweet, Bland
Cool to slightly Cold
Spleen, **Stomach**, Lung, Kidney[525]
Name (Tai Yin, Spleen/Lung), Biao/Li (Stomach/Spleen), Branch (You/Chicken, Lung/Kidney, 5PM-6:59PM)

Cha Ye (Folium Theae, Tea Leaves)
Regulate Water Resolve Dampness
Bitter, Sweet
Cool
Heart, Lung, **Stomach**

Dong Kui Guo (Fructus Malvae, Mallow Fruit, Cluster Mallow Fruit)
Regulate Water Resolve Dampness
Sweet
Cold
Urinary Bladder, Small Intestine, **Stomach**,[526] Large Intestine[527]
Name (Tai Yang, Small Intestine/Urinary Bladder, Yang Ming, Large Intestine/Stomach), Clock Neighbor (Large Intestine/Stomach, Small Intestine/Urinary Bladder), Qian/Hou (Front/Back, Stomach/Urinary Bladder), Branch (Shen/Monkey, Large Intestine/Urinary Bladder, 3PM-4:59PM)

Yin Chen Hao, Yin Chen (Herba Artemesia Scopariae, Virgate Wormwood, Capillary Wormwood)
Regulate Water Resolve Dampness
Bitter, Aromatic
Cool to Cold[528]
Liver, Spleen, Gall Bladder, **Stomach**
Biao/Li (Gall Bladder/Liver, Stomach/Spleen), Branch (Chou/Ox, Spleen/Liver, 1AM-2:59AM)

Hua Shi, Fei Hua Shi (Talcum)
Regulate Water Resolve Dampness
Sweet, Bland
Cold
Stomach, Urinary Bladder
Qian/Hou (Front/Back, Stomach/Urinary Bladder)

Bi Xie (Rhizoma Dioscoriae Hypoglaucae, Fish Poison Yam, Tokoro)
Regulate Water Resolve Dampness
Bitter
Neutral
Urinary Bladder, Liver, **Stomach**
Qian/Hou (Front/Back, Stomach/Urinary Bladder) + Liver

Warm Interior

Hong Dou Kou (Fructus Galangae, Galanga Seed)
Aromatic Dissolve Dampness/Warm Interior
Acrid, Aromatic
Warm
Spleen, **Stomach**,[529] Lung
Name (Tai Yin, Spleen/Lung), Biao/Li (Stomach/Spleen)

Gan Jiang (Rhizoma Zingiberis, Dried Ginger Root)
Warm Interior
Acrid, Aromatic
Hot
Heart, Lung, Spleen, **Stomach**
Name (Tai Yin, Lung/Spleen), Biao/Li (Stomach/Spleen), Clock Neighbor (Spleen/Heart)

Hu Jiao, Bai Hu Jiao, Hei Hu Jiao (Fructus Piper, Black Pepper, White Pepper)
Warm Interior
Acrid, Aromatic
Hot
Stomach, Large Intestine
Name (Yang Ming, Large Intestine/Stomach), Clock Neighbor (Large Intestine/Stomach)

Bi Ba, Bi Bo (Fructus Piperis Longi, Long Pepper)
Warm Interior
Acrid, Aromatic
Hot
Stomach, Large Intestine, Spleen[530]
Name (Yang Ming, Large Intestine/Stomach), Biao/Li (Stomach/Spleen), Clock Neighbor (Large Intestine/Stomach)

Gao Liang Jiang (Rhizoma Alpiniae Officinarium, Galanga, Alpinia, Lesser Galangal Rhizome)
Warm Interior
Acrid, Aromatic
Hot
Spleen, **Stomach**
Biao/Li (Stomach/Spleen)

Bi Cheng Qie, Cheng Qie Zi (Fructus Litseae, Cubeb Fruit)
Warm Interior
Acrid, Aromatic[531]
Warm
Spleen, **Stomach**, Kidney, Urinary Bladder
Biao/Li (Stomach/Spleen, Urinary Bladder/Kidney), Qian/Hou (Front/Back, Stomach/Urinary Bladder)

Ding Xiang (Flos Caryophylli, Clove Flower Bud)
Warm Interior
Acrid, Aromatic
Warm
Kidney, Spleen, **Stomach**
Biao/Li (Stomach/Spleen) + Kidney

Hua Jiao, Chuan Jiao (Pericarpium Zanthoxyli, Sichuan Peppercorn)
Warm Interior
Acrid, Aromatic
Warm[532] to Hot, slightly Toxic*
Kidney, Spleen, **Stomach**
Biao/Li (Stomach/Spleen) + Kidney

Wu Zhu Yu, Wu Yu (Fructus Evodiae, Evodia Fruit)
Warm Interior
Acrid, Bitter, Aromatic
Hot, slightly Toxic*
Liver, Spleen, **Stomach**, Kidney[533]
Biao/Li (Stomach/Spleen), Branch (Chou/Ox, Spleen/Liver, 1AM-2:59AM) + Kidney

Xiao Hui Xiang, Gui Hui Xiang (Fructus Foeniculi, Fennel Seed)
Warm Interior
Acrid, Aromatic
Warm
Liver, Kidney, Spleen, **Stomach**
Biao/Li (Stomach/Spleen), Branch (Chou/Ox, Spleen/Liver, 1AM-2:59AM) + Kidney

Regulate and Rectify Qi

Xie Bai, Xiao Suan, Ye Suan (Bulbus Alli Macrostemonis, Chive Bulb)
Regulate and Rectify Qi
Acrid, Bitter, Aromatic
Warm
Large Intestine, **Stomach**, Lung
Name (Yang Ming, Large Intestine/Stomach), Biao/Li (Large Intestine/Lung), Clock Neighbor (Large Intestine/Stomach)

Ju Hong, Yun Pi, Yun Hong (Exocarpium Citri Rubrum, Tangerine Flavedo)
Regulate and Rectify Qi
Bitter, Acrid, Aromatic
Warm
Lung, **Stomach**

Shi Di, Shi Ding, Shi Zi Ba (Calyx Kaki, Persimmon Calyx)
Regulate and Rectify Qi
Bitter, Astringent[534]
Neutral
Lung,[535] **Stomach**

Hua Ju Hong, Hua Pi, You Pi Ju Hong (Exocarpium Citri Grandis, Pumelo Peel)
Regulate and Rectify Qi
Bitter, Acrid, Aromatic
Warm
Lung, Spleen, **Stomach**
Name (Tai Yin, Lung/Spleen), Biao/Li (Stomach/Spleen)

Chen Pi, Ju Pi, Hong Pi (Pericarpium Citri Reticulatae, Aged Tangerine Peel)
Regulate and Rectify Qi
Acrid, Bitter, Aromatic
Warm
Lung, Spleen, **Stomach**[536]
Name (Tai Yin, Lung/Spleen), Biao/Li (Stomach/Spleen)

Zi Su Geng (Caulis Perillae, Perilla Stem)
Acrid Warm Exterior Releasing/Regulate and Rectify Qi
Acrid, Sweet, Aromatic
Slightly Warm
Lung, Spleen, **Stomach**
Name (Tai Yin, Lung/Spleen), Biao/Li (Stomach/Spleen)

Tan Xiang (Lignum Santali Albi, Sandalwood)
Regulate and Rectify Qi
Acrid, Aromatic
Warm
Spleen, **Stomach**, Lung
Name (Tai Yin, Spleen/Lung), Biao/Li (Stomach/Spleen)

Fo Shou (Fructus Citri Sarcodactylis, Finger Citron Fruit, Buddha's Hand Citron)
Regulate and Rectify Qi
Acrid, Bitter, Aromatic
Warm
Liver, Lung, **Stomach**, Spleen
Name (Tai Yin, Lung/Spleen), Biao/Li (Stomach/Spleen), Clock Neighbor (Liver/Lung), Branch (Chou/Ox, Spleen/Liver, 1AM-2:59AM)

Zhi Ke, Zhi Qiao (Fructus Aurantii, Ripened Bitter Orange)
Regulate and Rectify Qi
Bitter, Acrid, Aromatic
Cool to slightly Cold[537]
Large Intestine, Spleen, **Stomach**
Name (Yang Ming, Large Intestine/Stomach), Biao/Li (Stomach/Spleen), Clock Neighbor (Large Intestine/Stomach)

Zhi Shi (Fructus Aurantii Immaturus, Immature Bitter Orange)
Regulate and Rectify Qi
Bitter, Acrid, Aromatic
Warm[538] to Cool to slightly Cold[539]
Large Intestine, Spleen, **Stomach**
Name (Yang Ming, Large Intestine/Stomach), Biao/Li (Stomach/Spleen) Clock Neighbor (Large Intestine/Stomach)

Da Fu Pi (Pericarpium Arecae, Areca Peel, Betel Husk)
Regulate and Rectify Qi
Acrid
Slightly Warm
Large Intestine, Small Intestine, Spleen, **Stomach**
Name (Yang Ming, Large Intestine/Stomach), Bie Jing (Tai Yin/Tai Yang, Spleen/Small Intestine), Biao/Li (Stomach/Spleen), Clock Neighbor (Large Intestine/Stomach), Branch (Si/Snake, Small Intestine/Spleen, 9AM-10:59AM, Wei/Sheep, Spleen/Small Intestine, 1PM-2:59PM)

Dao Dou (Semen Canavaliae, Sword Bean)
Regulate and Rectify Qi
Sweet
Warm
Stomach, Spleen,[540] Kidney, Large Intestine[541]
Name (Yang Ming, Large Intestine/Stomach), Biao/Li (Stomach/Spleen), Clock Opposite (Kidney/Large Intestine), Clock Neighbor (Large Intestine/Stomach)

Mu Xiang (Radix Aucklandiae, Costus Root)
Regulate and Rectify Qi
Acrid, Bitter, slightly Astringent,[542] Aromatic
Warm
Gall Bladder, Large Intestine, Spleen, **Stomach**, San Jiao[543]
Name (Yang Ming, Large Intestine/Stomach, Shao Yang, Gall Bladder/San Jiao), Biao/Li (Stomach/Spleen), Clock Opposite (Spleen/San Jiao), Clock Neighbor (Large Intestine/Stomach, San Jiao/Gall Bladder)

Gan Song (Radix seu Rhizoma Nardostachys, Spoon-Leaf Nardostachys Rhizome)
Regulate and Rectify Qi
Acrid, Sweet, Aromatic
Warm
Spleen, **Stomach**
Biao/Li (Stomach/Spleen)

Chen Xiang (Lignum Aquilariae Resinatum, Aloeswood)
Regulate and Rectify Qi
Acrid, Bitter, Aromatic
Warm
Kidney, Spleen, **Stomach**
Biao/Li (Stomach/Spleen) + Kidney

Chuan Lian Zi, Jin Ling Zi (Fructus Toosendan, Sichuan Pagoda Tree Fruit, Sichuan Chinaberry)
Regulate and Rectify Qi
Bitter, slightly Sour[544]
Cold, slightly Toxic*
Liver, Small Intestine, **Stomach**, Urinary Bladder
Name (Tai Yang, Small Intestine/Urinary Bladder), Clock Opposite (Liver/Small Intestine), Clock Neighbor (Small Intestine/Urinary Bladder), Qian/Hou (Front/Back, Stomach/Urinary Bladder)

Po Bu Zi Ye (Folium Cordia Dichotoma, Sebastan Plum Cordia Leaf)
Regulate and Rectify Qi
Bitter, slightly Astringent
Cool
Liver, Kidney, **Stomach**

Jiu Ceng Ta (Herba Ocimi Basilici, Basil)
Regulate and Rectify Qi
Acrid
Warm
Stomach, Liver, Kidney

Qing Pi, Qing Ju Pi (Pericarpium Citri Reticulatae Viride, Green or Unripened Tangerine Peel)
Regulate and Rectify Qi
Acrid, Bitter, slightly Sour,[545] Aromatic
Warm
Liver, Gall Bladder, **Stomach**, San Jiao[546]
Name (Shao Yang, San Jiao/Gall Bladder), Biao/Li (Gall Bladder/Liver), Clock Neighbor (San Jiao/Gall Bladder) + Stomach

Ba Yue Zha, Yu Zhi Zi (Fructus Akebiae, Akebia Fruit)
Regulate and Rectify Qi
Bitter, Sweet[547]
Neutral to slightly Cool[548]
Liver, **Stomach**

Li Zhi He, Li He, Li Ren (Semen Litchi, Litchee Nut)
Regulate and Rectify Qi
Acrid,[549] slightly Bitter,[550] Sweet, Astringent
Warm
Liver, **Stomach**

Qing Mu Xiang, Ma Dou Ling Gen (Radix Aristolochiae, Aristolochia Root, Slender Dutchman's Pipe Root)
Regulate and Rectify Qi
Acrid, Bitter
Cool to Cold, Toxic*
Liver, **Stomach**

Suo Luo Zi, Kai Xin Guo (Semen Aesculi, Horse Chestnut, Chinese Buckeye Seed, Wilson's Buckeye Seed)
Regulate and Rectify Qi
Sweet
Warm
Liver, **Stomach**

Digestive

Lai Fu Zi (Semen Raphani, Radish/Daikon/Turnip Seeds)
Digestive
Acrid, Sweet
Neutral
Spleen, **Stomach**, Lung
Name (Tai Yin, Spleen/Lung), Biao/Li (Stomach/Spleen)

Su Ya (Fructus Setariae Germinatus, Millet Sprouts)
Digestive
Sweet, Bitter[551]
Warm
Spleen, **Stomach**
Biao/Li (Stomach/Spleen)

Gu Ya, Xiao Gu Ya, Dao Ya (Fructus Setariae Germinatus, Rice Sprout)
Digestive
Sweet
Neutral
Spleen, **Stomach**
Biao/Li (Stomach/Spleen)

Dao Ya (Fructus Oryzae germinatus, Rice Sprouts)
Digestive
Sweet
Neutral
Spleen, **Stomach**
Biao/Li (Stomach/Spleen)

Liu Shen Qu, Shen Qu (Massa Fermentata, Medicated Leaven)
Digestive
Sweet, Acrid
Warm
Spleen, **Stomach**
Biao/Li (Stomach/Spleen)

Ji Nei Jin (Endothelium Corneum Gigerae Galli, Chicken Gizzard Lining)
Digestive
Sweet
Neutral
Urinary Bladder, Small Intestine, Spleen, **Stomach**
Name (Tai Yang, Small Intestine/Urinary Bladder), Biao/Li (Stomach/Spleen), Bie Jing (Tai Yin/Tai Yang, Spleen/Small Intestine), Clock Neighbor (Small Intestine/Urinary Bladder), Qian/Hou (Front/Back, Stomach/Urinary Bladder), Branch (Si/Snake, Small Intestine/Spleen, 9AM-10:59AM and Wei/Sheep, Spleen/Small Intestine, 1PM-2:59PM)

Shan Zha (Fructus Crategi, Crategus, Hawthorn Fruit)
Digestive
Sweet, Sour
Neutral[552] to slightly Warm
Liver, Spleen, **Stomach**
Biao/Li (Stomach/Spleen), Branch (Chou/Ox, Spleen/Liver, 1AM-2:59AM)

Mai Ya, Da Mai Ya (Fructus Hordei Germinatus, Barley Sprout, Malt)
Digestive
Sweet, Salty[553]
Neutral
Liver, Spleen, **Stomach**
Biao/Li (Stomach/Spleen), Branch (Chou/Ox, Spleen/Liver, 1AM-2:59AM)

Expel Parasites

Fei Zi (Semen Torreyae, Torreya Seeds)
Expel Parasites
Sweet, Astringent[554]
Neutral, relatively Non-Toxic[555]
Lung, Large Intestine, **Stomach**[556]
Name (Yang Ming, Large Intestine/Stomach), Biao/Li (Large Intestine/Lung), Clock Neighbor (Large Intestine/Stomach)

Da Suan (Bulbus Alli Sativi, Garlic)
Expel Parasites/External Application
Acrid, Sweet[557]
Neutral to Warm
Spleen, **Stomach**, Lung, Large Intestine[558]
Name (Tai Yin, Spleen/Lung, Yang Ming, Large Intestine/Stomach), Biao/Li (Stomach/Spleen, Large Intestine/Lung), Clock Neighbor (Large Intestine/Stomach)

Lei Wan (Omphalia, Fruiting Body of Omphalia)
Expel Parasites
Bitter
Cold, slightly Toxic*[559]
Stomach, Large Intestine
Name (Yang Ming, Large Intestine/Stomach), Clock Neighbor (Large Intestine/Stomach)

Bing Lang, Hai Nan Zi, Bing Men (Semen Arecae, Betel Nut, Areca Seeds)
Expel Parasites
Acrid, Bitter
Warm
Large Intestine, **Stomach**
Name (Yang Ming, Large Intestine/Stomach), Clock Neighbor (Large Intestine/Stomach)

Nan Gua Zi, Nan Gua Ren (Semen Cucurbitae Moschatae, Pumpkin Seed)
Expel Parasites
Sweet
Neutral
Stomach, Large Intestine
Name (Yang Ming, Large Intestine/Stomach), Clock Neighbor (Large Intestine/Stomach)

Wu Yi, Chou Wu Yi, Bai Wu Yi (Fructus Ulmi Praeparatus, Ulmus, Paste of Stinking Elm Cake)
Expel Parasites
Acrid, Bitter, Sour[560]
Neutral[561] to Warm
Spleen, **Stomach**
Biao/Li (Stomach/Spleen)

Nan He Shi, Shan Luo Bo Zi (Fructus Carotae, Daucus Fruit, Wild Carrot Seed)
Expel Parasites
Bitter, Acrid
Neutral, slightly Toxic*
Spleen, **Stomach**
Biao/Li (Stomach/Spleen)

Shi Jun Zi (Fructus Quisqualis, Rangoon Creeper Fruit and Seeds)
Expel Parasites
Sweet, Aromatic
Warm, relatively non-Toxic[562] to slightly Toxic*
Spleen, **Stomach**
Biao/Li (Stomach/Spleen)

Ku Lian Pi, Ku Lian Gen Pi (Cortex Meliae, Chinaberry Bark)
Expel Parasites
Bitter
Cold, Toxic*
Liver, Spleen, **Stomach**
Biao/Li (Stomach/Spleen), Branch (Chou/Ox, Spleen/Liver, 1AM-2:59AM)

Guan Zhong, Mian Ma Guan Zhong (Rhizoma Dryopteridis, Dryopteris Root, Shield-Fern Root)
Clear Heat Clean Toxin/Expel Parasites
Bitter
Cool to Cold,[563] slightly Toxic*
Liver, Spleen, **Stomach**[564]
Biao/Li (Stomach/Spleen), Branch (Chou/Ox, Spleen/Liver, 1AM-2:59AM)

He Shi, Bei He Shi (Fructus Carpesii, Carpesium Fruit)
Expel Parasites
Bitter, Acrid
Neutral, slightly Toxic*
Spleen, **Stomach**, Liver[565]
Biao/Li (Stomach/Spleen), Branch (Chou/Ox, Spleen/Liver, 1AM-2:59AM)

Stop Bleeding

Bai Mao Gen (Rhizoma Imperatae, Wolly Grass Rhizome, Cogon Rhizome)
Stop Bleeding
Sweet
Cold
Lung, **Stomach**, Urinary Bladder, Small Intestine[566]
Name (Tai Yang, Small Intestine/Urinary Bladder), Bie Jing (Tai Yin/Tai Yang, Lung/Urinary Bladder), Clock Opposite (Lung/Urinary Bladder), Clock Neighbor (Small Intestine/Urinary Bladder), Qian/Hou (Front/Back, Stomach/Urinary Bladder)

Zhu Fan Hua Tou, Su Xiang (Rhizoma Mirabilidis, Mirabilis)
Stop Bleeding
Sweet, Bitter, Astringent
Neutral
Lung, **Stomach**, Urinary Bladder
Bie Jing (Tai Yin/Tai Yang, Lung/Urinary Bladder), Clock Opposite (Lung/Urinary Bladder), Qian/Hou (Front/Back, Stomach/Urinary Bladder)

Bai Ji, Bai Gen, Gan Gen (Rhizoma Bletillae, Bletilla Rhizome)
Stop Bleeding
Bitter, Sweet, Astringent
Cool to slightly Cold[567]
Lung, **Stomach**, Liver
Clock Neighbor (Liver/Lung) + Stomach

Zi Zhu, Zi Zhu Cao (Folium Callicarpae, Callicarpa Leaf, Beauty-Berry Leaf)
Stop Bleeding
Bitter, Astringent
Cool
Liver, Lung, **Stomach**
Clock Neighbor (Liver/Lung) + Stomach

Ou Jie (Nodus Nelumbinis Rhizomatis, Lotus Rhizome Nodes)
Stop Bleeding/Astringe, Stabilize and Bind
Sweet, Astringent
Neutral
Lung, **Stomach**, Liver
Clock Neighbor (Liver/Lung) + Stomach

San Qi, Tian Qi (Radix Notoginseng, Pseudoginseng Root)
Stop Bleeding
Sweet, slightly Bitter
Warm
Liver, **Stomach**,[568] Spleen,[569] Large Intestine,[570] Pericardium[571]
Name (Yang Ming, Large Intestine/Stomach and Jue Yin, Liver/Pericardium), Bie Jing (Jue Yin/Yang Ming, Pericardium/Stomach and Liver/Large Intestine), Biao/Li (Stomach/Spleen), Clock Opposite (Pericardium/Stomach), Clock Neighbor (Large Intestine/Stomach), Branch (Chou/Ox, Spleen/Liver, 1AM-2:59AM, Mao/Rabbit, Liver/Large Intestine, 5AM-6:59AM and Shu/Dog, Stomach/Pericardium, 7PM-8:59PM)

Di Yu (Radix Sanguisorbae, Bloodwort Root, Burnet Root)
Stop Bleeding
Bitter, Sour, Astringent[572]
Cool to Cold[573]
Liver, Large Intestine, **Stomach**
Name (Yang Ming, Large Intestine/Stomach), Bie Jing (Jue Yin/Yang Ming, Liver/Large Intestine), Clock Neighbor (Large Intestine/Stomach), Branch (Mao/Rabbit, Liver/Large Intestine, 5AM-6:59AM)

Fu Long Gan, Zao Xin Tu (Terra Flava Usta, Oven Clay, Fire Pit Ash)
Stop Bleeding
Acrid, Bitter
Warm
Spleen, **Stomach**
Biao/Li (Stomach/Spleen)

Xue Yu Tan (Crinis Carbonitsatus, Charred Human Hair)
Stop Bleeding
Bitter, Astringent[574]
Neutral
Liver, **Stomach**, Heart,[575] Kidney[576]
Name (Shao Yin, Heart/Kidney) + Liver, Stomach

Vitalize Blood Transform Stasis

Wa Leng Zi (Concha Arcae, Cockle Shell, Ark Shell)
Vitalize Blood Transform Stasis/Transform Phlegm/External Application
Salty
Neutral
Liver, **Stomach**, Lung, Spleen[577]
Name (Tai Yin, Lung/Spleen), Biao/Li (Stomach/Spleen), Clock Neighbor (Liver/Lung), Branch (Chou/Ox, Spleen/Liver, 1AM-2:59AM)

Yan Hu Suo (Rhizoma Corydalis, Corydalis Rhizome)
Vitalize Blood Transform Stasis
Acrid, Bitter, Aromatic
Warm
Heart, Liver, Spleen, **Stomach**[578]
Biao/Li (Stomach/Spleen), Clock Neighbor (Spleen/Heart), Branch (Chou/Ox, Spleen/Liver, 1AM-2:59AM)

Jiang Xiang (Lignum Dalbergiae Odoriferae, Dalbergia Heartwood, Rosewood)
Vitalize Blood Transform Stasis
Acrid, Aromatic
Warm
Liver, Spleen, Heart, **Stomach**[579]
Biao/Li (Stomach/Spleen), Clock Neighbor (Spleen/Heart), Branch (Chou/Ox, Spleen/Liver, 1AM-2:59AM)

Jiang Huang (Rhizoma Curcumae Longae, Turmeric Rhizome)
Vitalize Blood Transform Stasis
Acrid, Bitter, Aromatic
Warm
Spleen, Liver, **Stomach**[580]
Biao/Li (Stomach/Spleen), Branch (Chou/Ox, Spleen/Liver, 1AM-2:59AM)

Wang Bu Liu Xing (Semen Vaccariae, Vaccaria Seeds, Cow Soapwort Seed)
Vitalize Blood Transform Stasis
Acrid,[581] Bitter
Neutral
Liver, **Stomach**, Urinary Bladder[582]
Qian/Hou (Front/Back, Stomach/Urinary Bladder) + Liver

Lu Lu Tong, Feng Guo, Jiu Kong Zi (Fructus Liquidambaris, Sweetgum Fruit)
Vitalize Blood Transform Stasis
Bitter
Neutral
Liver, **Stomach**

Gan Qi (Resina Toxicodendri, Lacquer)
Vitalize Blood Transform Stasis
Acrid, Bitter
Warm, slightly Toxic
Liver, **Stomach**

Chuan Shan Jia (Squama Manis, Pangolin Scales)
Vitalize Blood Transform Stasis
Salty
Cool to slightly Cold[583]
Liver, **Stomach**, some sources say that it enters and affects every channel and Luo-Network vessel.[584]

Transform Phlegm

Gua Lou Shi, Quan Gua Lou, Gua Lou (Fructus Trichosanthis, Snake Gourd Fruit)
Transform Phlegm
Sweet, slightly Bitter[585]
Cold
Large Intestine, Lung, **Stomach**
Name (Yang Ming, Large Intestine/Stomach), Biao/Li (Large Intestine/Lung), Clock Neighbor (Large Intestine/Stomach)

Gua Lou Pi (Pericarpium Trichosanthis, Trichosanthis Peel, Snake Gourd Peel)
Transform Phlegm
Sweet
Cold
Large Intestine, Lung, **Stomach**
Name (Yang Ming, Large Intestine/Stomach), Biao/Li (Large Intestine/Lung), Clock Neighbor (Large Intestine/Stomach)

Gua Lou Ren (Semen Trichosanthis, Trichosanthes Seed, Snake Gourd Seed)
Transform Phlegm
Sweet
Cold
Large Intestine, Lung, **Stomach**
Name (Yang Ming, Large Intestine/Stomach), Biao/Li (Large Intestine/Lung), Clock Neighbor (Large Intestine/Stomach)

Xuan Fu Hua, Jin Fei Hua, Jin Fu Hua (Flos Inulae, Inula Flower)
Transform Phlegm
Bitter, Acrid, Salty
Slightly Warm
Large Intestine, Lung, **Stomach**, Spleen, Liver[586]
Name (Yang Ming, Large Intestine/Stomach, Tai Yin, Lung/Spleen), Bie Jing (Jue Yin/Yang Ming, Liver/Large Intestine), Biao/Li (Large Intestine/Lung, Stomach/Spleen), Clock Neighbor (Large Intestine/Stomach, Liver/Lung), Branch (Chou/Ox, Spleen/Liver, 1AM-2:59AM and Mao/Rabbit, Liver/Large Intestine, 5AM-6:59AM)

Bi Qi, Di Li, Wu Yu, Ma Ti (Rhizoma Eleocharitis, Water Chestnut)
Transform Phlegm
Sweet
Slightly Cold
Lung, Liver,[587] **Stomach**, Large Intestine
Name (Yang Ming, Large Intestine/Stomach), Bie Jing (Jue Yin/Yang Ming, Liver/Large Intestine), Biao/Li (Large Intestine/Lung), Clock Neighbor (Large Intestine/Stomach, Liver/Lung), Branch (Mao/Rabbit, Liver/Large Intestine, 5AM-6:59AM)

Ge Qiao, Ge Ke, Hai Ge Ke Fen (Concha Meretricis seu Cyclinae, Clam Shell)
Transform Phlegm
Bitter,[588] Salty
Neutral[589] to Cold
Lung, **Stomach**

Zhi Ban Xia, Ban Xia (Rhizoma Pinelliae preparatum)
Transform Phlegm
Acrid
Warm, Toxic* if unprocessed
Spleen, **Stomach**, Lung
Name (Tai Yin, Spleen/Lung), Biao/Li (Stomach/Spleen)

Bai Jie Zi, Huang Jie Zi, Jie Cai Zi (Semen Sinapis, White Mustard Seed)
Transform Phlegm
Acrid
Warm
Lung, **Stomach**,[590] Spleen[591]
Name (Tai Yin, Lung/Spleen), Biao/Li (Stomach/Spleen)

Zhi Bai Fu Zi, Bai Fu Zi (Rhizoma Typhonii preparatum, Typhonium)
Transform Phlegm
Acrid, Sweet
Warm, Toxic*
Spleen, **Stomach**, Lung,[592] Liver[593]
Name (Tai Yin, Spleen/Lung), Biao/Li (Stomach/Spleen), Clock Neighbor (Liver/Lung), Branch (Chou/Ox, Spleen/Liver, 1AM-2:59AM)

Wa Leng Zi (Concha Arcae, Cockle Shell, Ark Shell)
Vitalize Blood Transform Stasis/Transform Phlegm/External Application
Salty
Neutral
Liver, **Stomach**, Lung, Spleen[594]
Name (Tai Yin, Lung/Spleen), Biao/Li (Stomach/Spleen), Clock Neighbor (Liver/Lung), Branch (Chou/Ox, Spleen/Liver, 1AM-2:59AM)

Zhu Li (Succus Bambusae, Dried Bamboo Sap)
Transform Phlegm
Sweet, Bitter[595]
Cold
Heart, Lung, **Stomach**, Liver[596]
Clock Neighbor (Liver/Lung) + Heart, Stomach

Hai Zao (Sargassum, Seaweed, Gulfweed)
Transform Phlegm
Bitter,[597] Salty
Cold
Liver, Kidney, **Stomach**,[598] Lung[599]
Clock Neighbor (Liver/Lung), Branch (You/Chicken, Lung/Kidney, 5PM-6:59PM) + Stomach

Zhu Ru (Caulis Bambusae in Taenia, Bamboo Shavings)
Transform Phlegm
Sweet, Bitter[600]
Cool to slightly Cold[601]
Lung, **Stomach**, Gall Bladder
Branch (Yin/Tiger, Gall Bladder/Lung, 3AM-4:59AM) + Stomach

Si Gua Luo (Retinervus Luffae Fructus, Dried Vegetable Sponge)
Transform Phlegm/External Application
Sweet
Neutral to Cold[602]
Lung, **Stomach**, Liver
Clock Neighbor (Liver/Lung) + Stomach

Jin Meng Shi (Micae Lapis Aureus, Vermiculite Schist)
Transform Phlegm
Sweet, Salty
Neutral
Liver, Lung, **Stomach**
Clock Neighbor (Liver/Lung) + Stomach

Zao Jiao Ci, Tian Ding, Zao Ci, Zao Ding (Spina Gleditsiae, Spine of Honeylocust Plant)
Transform Phlegm
Acrid
Warm
Liver, **Stomach**, Lung[603]
Clock Neighbor (Liver/Lung) + Stomach

Kun Bu (Thallus Laminariae seu Eckloniae, Kelp)
Transform Phlegm
Salty
Cold
Liver, **Stomach**, Kidney

Relieve Cough and Wheezing/Panting

Pi Pa Ye, Liu Jie Ye (Folium Eriobotryae, Eriobotrya Leaf, Loquat Leaf)
Relieve Cough and Wheezing/Panting
Bitter
Neutral[604] to Cool to slightly Cold[605]
Lung, **Stomach**

Zhong Ru Shi (Stalactitum, Stalactite Tip)
Relieve Cough and Wheezing/Panting/Tonify Yang
Sweet, Acrid[606]
Warm
Lung, Kidney, **Stomach**
Branch (You/Chicken, Lung/Kidney, 5PM-6:59PM) + Stomach

Li Lu (Radix et Rhizoma Veratri, Lack False Hellebore, Vanity Grass)
Relieve Cough and Wheezing/Panting/Emetic
Acrid, Bitter
Cold, extremely Toxic*
Lung, Liver, **Stomach**
Clock Neighbor (Liver/Lung) + Stomach

Gua Di (Pedicellus Cucumeris, Melon Pedicle)
Relieve Cough and Wheezing/Panting/Emetic
Bitter
Cold, Toxic*
Stomach
Branch (Chen/Dragon, Stomach/Stomach, 7AM-8:59AM)

Nourish and Calm Shen

He Huan Hua, Ye He Hua, Ye He Mi (Flos Albiziae, Mimosa Flower)
Nourish and Calm Shen
Sweet
Neutral
Liver, **Stomach**, Spleen,[607] Heart,[608] Lung[609]
Name (Tai Yin, Lung/Spleen), Biao/Li (Stomach/Spleen), Clock Neighbor (Spleen/Heart, Liver/Lung), Branch (Chou/Ox, Spleen/Liver, 1AM-2:59AM)

Open Orifices

Shui Chang Pu, Bai Chang Pu (Rhizoma Acori Calami, Calamus, Sweetflag Rhizome)
Open Orifices
Bitter, Acrid
Warm, slightly Toxic*
Heart, Liver, **Stomach**, Spleen,[610] Large Intestine[611]
Name (Yang Ming, Large Intestine/Stomach), Bie Jing (Jue Yin/Yang Ming, Liver/Large Intestine), Biao/Li (Stomach/Spleen), Clock Neighbor (Spleen/Heart, Large Intestine/Stomach), Branch (Chou/Ox, Spleen/Liver, 1AM-2:59AM and Mao/Rabbit, Liver/Large Intestine, 5AM-6:59AM)

Shi Chang Pu (Rhizoma Acori Tatarinowii, Grassleaf Sweetflag Rhizome, Acorus)
Open Orifices
Bitter,[612] Acrid, Aromatic
Warm, slightly Toxic*
Heart, **Stomach**

Tonify Qi

Sha Ji, Cu Liu Guo (Fructus Hippophae, Sea Buckthorn Fruit, Swallow Thorn Fruit)
Tonify Qi
Sour, slightly Sweet, Astringent
Warm
Lung, Spleen, **Stomach**, Large Intestine, Liver, Small Intestine[613]
Name (Tai Yin, Lung/Spleen, Yang Ming, Large Intestine/Stomach), Bie Jing (Jue Yin/Yang Ming, Liver/Large Intestine, Tai Yin/Tai Yang, Spleen/Small Intestine), Biao/Li (Large Intestine/Lung, Stomach/Spleen), Clock Opposite (Liver/Small Intestine), Clock Neighbor (Liver/Lung, Large Intestine/Stomach), Branch (Chou/Ox, Spleen/Liver, 1AM-2:59AM, Mao/Rabbit, Liver/Large Intestine, 5AM-6:59AM, Si/Snake, Small Intestine/Spleen, 9AM-10:59AM, Wei/Sheep, Spleen/Small Intestine, 1PM-2:59PM)

Yi Tang (Saccharum Granorum, Maltosum, Malt Sugar, Maltose)
Tonify Qi
Sweet
Slightly Warm[614] to Warm
Spleen, **Stomach**, Lung
Name (Tai Yin, Spleen/Lung), Biao/Li (Stomach/Spleen)

Gan Cao (Radix Glycyrrhizae, Licorice Root)
Tonify Qi
Sweet
Neutral
Spleen, **Stomach**, Lung, Heart, Dai,[615] some sources indicate that it enters all channels
Name (Tai Yin, Spleen/Lung), Biao/Li (Stomach/Spleen), Clock Neighbor (Spleen/Heart) + Dai, some sources indicate that Gan Cao enters all channels and therefore creates every relationship.

Bai Zhu (Rhizoma Atractylodis Macrocephalae, White Atractylodes Rhizome)
Tonify Qi
Bitter, Sweet, Aromatic
Warm to very Warm[616]
Spleen, **Stomach**
Biao/Li (Stomach/Spleen)

Geng Mi, Jing Mi (Semen Oryzae)
Tonify Qi
Sweet
Neutral[617] to Cool
Spleen, **Stomach**
Biao/Li (Stomach/Spleen)

Da Zao (Fructus Jujubae, Chinese Date, Jujube)
Tonify Qi
Sweet
Warm
Spleen, **Stomach**
Biao/Li (Stomach/Spleen)

Bian Dou, Bai Bian Dou (Semen Lablab Album, Hyacinth Bean)
Tonify Qi
Sweet, Bland[618]
Neutral[619] to slightly Warm
Spleen, **Stomach**
Biao/Li (Stomach/Spleen)

Tonify Yang

Zhong Ru Shi (Stalactitum, Stalactite Tip)
Relieve Cough and Wheezing/Panting/Tonify Yang
Sweet, Acrid[620]
Warm
Lung, Kidney, **Stomach**
Branch (You/Chicken, Lung/Kidney, 5PM-6:59PM) + Stomach

Yin Yang Huo, Xian Ling Pi (Herba Epimedii, Arial Parts of Epimedium, Horny Goat Weed)
Tonify Yang
Acrid, Sweet, Aromatic[621]
Warm
Kidney, Liver, and possibly Large Intestine, **Stomach** and San Jiao[622]
Possibly Name (Yang Ming, Large Intestine/Stomach), Bie Jing (Jue Yin/Yang Ming, Liver/Large Intestine, Shao Yin/Shao Yang, Kidney/San Jiao), Clock Opposite (Kidney/Large Intestine), Clock Neighbor (Large Intestine/Stomach), Branch (Mao/Rabbit, Liver/Large Intestine, 5AM-6:59AM)

Tonify Yin

Bei Sha Shen (Radix Glehniae, Glehniae)
Tonify Yin
Sweet, slightly Bitter[623]
Cool to slightly Cold[624]
Lung, **Stomach**

Nan Sha Shen (Radix Adenophorae, Adenophora, Four Leaf Lady Bell Root)
Tonify Yin
Sweet, slightly Bitter, Bland[625]
Cool
Lung, **Stomach**

Yu Zhu (Rhizoma Polygonati Odorati, Polygonatum, Solomon's Seal Rhizome)
Tonify Yin
Sweet
Neutral to slightly Cold[626]
Lung, **Stomach**

Bai Mu Er, Yin Er (Fructifactio Tremellae Fuciformis, Tremella, White Wood Ear)
Tonify Yin
Sweet, Bland
Neutral
Lung, **Stomach**

Mai Men Dong, Mai Dong (Radix Ophiopogonis, Ophiopogon Tuber)
Tonify Yin
Sweet, slightly Bitter
Cool to slightly Cold[627]
Spleen,[628] Lung,[629] **Stomach**, Heart
Name (Tai Yin, Spleen/Lung), Biao/Li (Stomach/Spleen), Clock Neighbor (Spleen/Heart)

Tian Men Dong, Tian Dong (Radix Asparagi, Asparagus Tuber)
Tonify Yin
Sweet, Bitter
Cold to very Cold
Lung, Kidney, **Stomach**[630]
Branch (You/Chicken, Lung/Kidney, 5PM-6:59PM) + Stomach

Zhi Ju Zi (Fructus Hoveniae, Hovenia)
Tonify Yin
Sweet
Neutral
Stomach
Branch (Chen/Dragon, Stomach/Stomach, 7AM-8:59AM)

Shi Hu (Herba Dendrobii, Dendrobium Stem)
Tonify Yin
Sweet, slightly Salty,[631] Bland[632]
Slightly Cold
Kidney, **Stomach**

Astringe, Stabilize and Bind

He Zi, Ke Zi, He Li, He Li Le (Fructus Chebulae, Black Myrobalan Fruit, Terminalia, Chebula)
Astringe, Stabilize and Bind
Sour, Bitter, Astringent
Neutral
Lung, **Stomach**,[633] Large Intestine
Name (Yang Ming, Large Intestine/Stomach), Biao/Li (Large Intestine/Lung), Clock Neighbor (Large Intestine/Stomach)

Chun Gen Pi, Chun Pi (Cortex Ailanthi, Ailanthus Bark, Tree of Heaven Bark, Chinese Sumac Bark)
Astringe, Stabilize and Bind
Bitter, Astringent
Cold
Large Intestine, **Stomach**,[634] Liver, Lung[635]
Name (Yang Ming, Large Intestine/Stomach), Bie Jing (Jue Yin/Yang Ming, Liver/Large Intestine), Biao/Li (Large Intestine/Lung), Clock Neighbor (Large Intestine/Stomach, Liver/Lung), Branch (Mao/Rabbit, Liver/Large Intestine, 5AM-6:59AM)

Ou Jie (Nodus Nelumbinis Rhizomatis, Lotus Rhizome Nodes)
Stop Bleeding/Astringe, Stabilize and Bind
Sweet, Astringent
Neutral
Lung, **Stomach**, Liver
Clock Neighbor (Liver/Lung) + Stomach

Shi Liu Pi, Shi Liu Ke, An Shi Liu (Pericarpium Granati, Pomegranate Husk)
Astringe, Stabilize and Bind
Sour, Sweet,[636] Astringent
Slightly Cooling[637] to Warm, slightly Toxic*
Stomach,[638] Large Intestine
Name (Yang Ming, Large Intestine/Stomach), Clock Neighbor (Large Intestine/Stomach)

Yu Yu Liang (Limonitum)
Astringe, Stabilize and Bind
Sweet, slightly Salty,[639] Bland,[640] Astringent
Neutral
Large Intestine, **Stomach**
Name (Yang Ming, Large Intestine/Stomach), Clock Neighbor (Large Intestine/Stomach)

Chi Shi Zhi (Halloysitum Rubrum, Red Halloysite)
Astringe, Stabilize and Bind
Sweet, Sour, Astringent[641]
Warm
Stomach, Large Intestine, Spleen[642]
Name (Yang Ming, Large Intestine/Stomach), Biao/Li (Stomach/Spleen), Clock Neighbor (Large Intestine/Stomach)

Rou Dou Kou (Semen Mystericae, Nutmeg Seeds)
Astringe, Stabilize and Bind
Acrid, Astringent, Aromatic
Warm
Large Intestine, Spleen, **Stomach**
Name (Yang Ming, Large Intestine/Stomach), Biao/Li (Stomach/Spleen), Clock Neighbor (Large Intestine/Stomach)

Chun Gen (Radix Ailanthus, Ailanthus Root, Tree of Heaven Root, Chinese Sumac Root)
Astringe, Stabilize and Bind
Bitter, Astringent
Cold
Stomach
Branch (Chen/Dragon, Stomach/Stomach, 7AM-8:59AM)

He Ye Geng, Lian Geng (Nelumbinis Petiolus, Lotus Leafstalk)
Clear Heat Clean Toxin/Astringe, Stabilize and Bind
Bitter
Neutral
Spleen, **Stomach**
Biao/Li (Stomach/Spleen)

Hai Piao Xiao, Wu Zei Gu (Endoconcha Sepiae, Cuttlefish Bone)
Astringe, Stabilize and Bind
Salty, Astringent
Slightly Warm
Liver, Kidney, **Stomach**[643]

Emetic

Li Lu (Radix et Rhizoma Veratri, Lack False Hellebore, Vanity Grass)
Relieve Cough and Wheezing/Panting/Emetic
Acrid, Bitter
Cold, extremely Toxic*
Lung, Liver, **Stomach**
Clock Neighbor (Liver/Lung) + Stomach

Gua Di (Pedicellus Cucumeris, Melon Pedicle)
Relieve Cough and Wheezing/Panting/Emetic
Bitter
Cold, Toxic*
Stomach
Branch (Chen/Dragon, Stomach/Stomach, 7AM-8:59AM)

External Application

Da Suan (Bulbus Alli Sativi, Garlic)
Expel Parasites/External Application
Acrid, Sweet[644]
Neutral to Warm
Spleen, **Stomach**, Lung, Large Intestine[645]
Name (Tai Yin, Spleen/Lung, Yang Ming, Large Intestine/Stomach), Biao/Li (Stomach/Spleen, Large Intestine/Lung), Clock Neighbor (Large Intestine/Stomach)

Ming Fan, Bai Fan, Ku Fan (Alumen, Alum)
External Application
Sour, Bitter,[646] Astringent
Cold, Toxic*
Lung, Liver, Spleen, **Stomach**,[647] Large Intestine[648]
Name (Tai Yin, Spleen/Lung, Yang Ming, Large Intestine/Stomach), Bie Jing (Jue Yin/Yang Ming, Liver/Large Intestine), Clock Neighbor (Liver/Lung, Large Intestine/Stomach), Biao/Li (Stomach/Spleen, Large Intestine/Lung), Branch (Chou/Ox, Spleen/Liver, 1AM-2:59AM, Mao/Rabbit, Liver/Large Intestine,[649] 5AM-6:59AM)

Xiong Huang (Realgar)
External Application
Acrid, Bitter
Neutral to Warm, Toxic*
Heart, Liver, Kidney,[650] **Stomach**,[651] Lung,[652] Large Intestine[653]
Name (Shao Yin, Heart/Kidney, Yang Ming, Large Intestine/Stomach), Bie Jing (Jue Yin/Yang Ming, Liver/Large Intestine), Biao/Li (Large Intestine/Lung), Clock Opposite (Kidney/Large Intestine), Clock Neighbor (Large Intestine/Stomach, Liver/Lung), Branch (Mao/Rabbit, Liver/Large Intestine, 5AM-6:59AM, You/Chicken, Lung, Kidney, 5PM-6:59PM)

Peng Sha, Yue Shi (Borax)
External Application
Sweet, Salty, Bitter[654]
Cool to slightly Cold,[655] Toxic*
Lung, **Stomach**

Wa Leng Zi (Concha Arcae, Cockle Shell, Ark Shell)
Vitalize Blood Transform Stasis/Transform Phlegm/External Application
Salty
Neutral
Liver, **Stomach**, Lung, Spleen[656]
Name (Tai Yin, Lung/Spleen), Biao/Li (Stomach/Spleen), Clock Neighbor (Liver/Lung), Branch (Chou/Ox, Spleen/Liver, 1AM-2:59AM)

Si Gua Luo (Retinervus Luffae Fructus, Dried Vegetable Sponge)
Transform Phlegm/External Application
Sweet
Neutral to Cold[657]
Lung, **Stomach**, Liver
Clock Neighbor (Liver/Lung) + Stomach

Lu Feng Fang, Feng Fang (Nidus Vespae, Wasp Nest)
External Application
Sweet
Neutral, Toxic*
Stomach, Lung,[658] Liver[659]
Clock Neighbor (Liver/Lung) + Stomach

Mu Bie Zi (Semen Momordicae, Momordica Seed)
External Application
Bitter, slightly Sweet
Warm, Toxic*
Large Intestine, Liver, **Stomach**
Name (Yang Ming, Large Intestine/Stomach), Bie Jing (Jue Yin/Yang Ming, Liver/Large Intestine), Clock Neighbor (Large Intestine/Stomach), Branch (Mao/Rabbit, Liver/Large Intestine, 5AM-6:59AM)

Chan Su (Venenum Bufonis, Poison Toad Venom)
External Application
Acrid, Sweet
Warm, Toxic*
Heart, **Stomach**[660]

Lu Gan Shi (Galamina, Calomine, Hydrozincite, Smithsonite)
External Application
Sweet
Neutral, Non-toxic[661] to Toxic*
Liver, **Stomach**

Foot Tai Yin Spleen Herbs

Acrid Warm Exterior Releasing

Bai Zhi (Radix Angelicae Dahuricae, Angelica Root)
Acrid Warm Exterior Releasing
Acrid, Aromatic
Warm
Lung, Stomach, **Spleen**,[662] Large Intestine[663]
Name (Tai Yin, Lung/Spleen, Yang Ming, Large Intestine/Stomach), Biao/Li (Stomach/Spleen, Large Intestine/Lung), Clock Neighbor (Large Intestine/Stomach)

Zi Su Geng (Caulis Perillae, Perilla Stem)
Acrid Warm Exterior Releasing/Regulate and Rectify Qi
Acrid, Sweet, Aromatic
Slightly Warm
Lung, **Spleen**, Stomach
Name (Tai Yin, Lung/Spleen), Biao/Li (Stomach/Spleen)

Sheng Jiang (Rhizoma Zingiberis Recens, Fresh Ginger Rhizome)
Acrid Warm Exterior Releasing
Acrid
Slightly Warm
Lung, **Spleen**, Stomach
Name (Tai Yin, Lung/Spleen), Biao/Li (Stomach/Spleen)

Xiang Ru, Hua Qi Ning, Shi Xiang Rou (Herba Elsholtziae seu Moslae, Aromatic Madder)
Acrid Warm Exterior Releasing
Acrid, Aromatic
Slightly Warm
Lung, **Spleen**,[664] Heart,[665] Stomach
Name (Tai Yin, Lung/Spleen), Biao/Li (Stomach/Spleen), Clock Neighbor (Spleen/Heart)

Zi Su Ye (Folium Perillae, Perilla Leaf)
Acrid Warm Exterior Releasing
Acrid, Aromatic
Warm
Lung, **Spleen**
Name (Tai Yin, Lung/Spleen)

Fang Feng, Pang Feng (Radix Saposhnikoviae, and sometimes Ledebouriella Root as a substitute)
Acrid Warm Exterior Releasing
Acrid, Sweet, Aromatic
Slightly Warm
Urinary Bladder, Liver, **Spleen**, Du,[666] Yang Qiao[667]
Branch (Chou/Ox, Spleen/Liver,1AM-2:59AM) + Urinary Bladder, Du, Yang Qiao

Acrid Cool Exterior Releasing

Sheng Ma (Radix Cimicifugae, Black Cohosh Rhizome, Bugbane Rhizome)
Acrid Cool Exterior Releasing
Acrid, Sweet
Cool to slightly Cold[668]
Lung, **Spleen**, Stomach, Large Intestine
Name (Tai Yin, Lung/Spleen, Yang Ming, Large Intestine/Stomach), Biao/Li (Large Intestine/Lung, Stomach/Spleen), Clock Neighbor (Large Intestine/Stomach)

Mao Zi Dun Tou (Herba Abutilon Indicum, Indian Abutilon)
Acrid Cool Exterior Releasing
Sweet
Neutral, slightly Toxic*
Lung, Liver, Gall Bladder, **Spleen**
Name (Tai Yin, Lung/Spleen), Biao/Li (Gall Bladder, Liver), Clock Neighbor (Liver/Lung), Branch (Yin/Tiger, Gall Bladder/Lung, 3AM-4:59AM, and Chou/Ox, Spleen/Liver, 1AM-2:59AM)

Ge Gen (Radix Puerariae, Kudzu Root, Pueraria)
Acrid Cool Exterior Releasing
Sweet, Acrid, slightly Bitter[669]
Cool
Spleen, Stomach, Tai Yang,[670] Yang Ming[671]
Biao/Li (Stomach/Spleen), possibly Name (Yang Ming Large Intestine/Stomach) and Clock Neighbor (Large Intestine/Stomach) if Yang Ming[672] really means the entire Yang Ming Jing-channel, and possibly Name (Tai Yang, Small Intestine/Urinary Bladder), Bie Jing (Spleen, Small Intestine), Clock Neighbor (Small Intestine/Urinary Bladder) and Qian/Hou (Front/Back, Stomach/Urinary Bladder) if Tai Yang[673] really means the entire Tai Yang Jing-channel.

Da Dou Juan, Dou Juan, Da Dou Huang Juan (Sojae Semen Germinatum, Dried Soybean Sprout)
Acrid Cool Exterior Releasing
Sweet, Bland
Neutral
Spleen, Stomach
Biao/Li (Stomach/Spleen)

Clear Heat Purge Fire

Qing Guo (Fructus Canarii, Chinese White Olive)
Clear Heat Purge Fire
Sweet, Sour, Astringent[674]
Neutral
Lung, Stomach, **Spleen**
Name (Tai Yin, Lung/Spleen), Biao/Li (Stomach, Spleen)

Clear Heat Dry Dampness

Ji Xue Cao, Beng Da Wan (Herba Centellae, Gotu Kola, Pennywort)
Clear Heat Dry Dampness/Clear Heat Clean Toxin
Acrid, Bitter
Cold
Liver, **Spleen**, Kidney, Small Intestine, Large Intestine
Bie Jing (Jue Yin/Yang Ming, Liver/Large Intestine, Tai Yin/Tai Yang, Spleen/Small Intestine), Clock Opposite (Liver/Small Intestine, Kidney/Large Intestine), Branch (Chou/Ox, Spleen/Liver, 1AM-2:59AM, Si/Snake, Small Intestine/Spleen, 9AM-10:59AM, Wei/Sheep, Spleen/Small Intestine, 1PM-2:59PM, Mao/Rabbit, Liver/Large Intestine, 5AM-6:59AM)

Clear Heat Cool Blood

Chi Shao (Radix Paeoniae Rubrae, Red Peony Root)
Clear Heat Cool Blood/Vitalize Blood Transform Stasis
Bitter, Sour[675]
Cool to slightly Cold
Liver, **Spleen**[676]
Branch (Chou/Ox, Spleen/Liver, 1AM-2:59AM)

Clear Heat Clean Toxin

Ren Dong Teng (Caulis Lonicerae, Honeysuckle Vine)
Clear Heat Clean Toxin
Sweet
Neutral to slightly Cold[677] to Cold
Lung, Stomach, Large Intestine,[678] **Spleen**[679]
Name (Yang Ming, Large Intestine/Stomach, Tai Yin, Lung/Spleen), Biao/Li (Large Intestine/Lung, Stomach/Spleen) Clock Neighbor (Large Intestine/Stomach)

Ji Xue Cao, Beng Da Wan (Herba Centellae, Gotu Kola, Pennywort)
Clear Heat Dry Dampness/Clear Heat Clean Toxin
Acrid, Bitter
Cold
Liver, **Spleen**, Kidney, Small Intestine, Large Intestine
Bie Jing (Jue Yin/Yang Ming, Liver/Large Intestine, Tai Yin/Tai Yang, Spleen/Small Intestine), Clock Opposite (Liver/Small Intestine, Kidney/Large Intestine), Branch (Chou/Ox, Spleen/Liver, 1AM-2:59AM, Si/Snake, Small Intestine/Spleen, 9AM-10:59AM, Wei/Sheep, Spleen/Small Intestine, 1PM-2:59PM, Mao/Rabbit, Liver/Large Intestine, 5AM-6:59AM)

Bai Xian Pi, Bai Tian (Cortex Dictamni, Dictamnus Root Bark)
Clear Heat Clean Toxin
Bitter
Cold
Spleen, Stomach
Biao/Li (Stomach/Spleen)

He Ye Geng, Lian Geng (Nelumbinis Petiolus, Lotus Leafstalk)
Clear Heat Clean Toxin/Astringe, Stabilize and Bind
Bitter
Neutral
Spleen, Stomach
Biao/Li (Stomach/Spleen)

Bai Lian, Bai Cao, Tu He, Kun Lun, Mao Er Luan (Radix Ampelopsis)
Clear Heat Clean Toxin
Bitter, Acrid, Sweet[680]
Neutral to Cool to Cold[681]
Heart, Stomach, Liver, **Spleen**[682]
Biao/Li (Stomach/Spleen), Clock Neighbor (Spleen/Heart), Branch (Chou/Ox, Spleen/Liver, 1AM-2:59AM)

Guan Zhong, Mian Ma Guan Zhong (Rhizoma Dryopteridis, Dryopteris Root, Shield-Fern Root)
Clear Heat Clean Toxin/Expel Parasites
Bitter
Cool to Cold,[683] slightly Toxic*
Liver, **Spleen**, Stomach[684]
Biao/Li (Stomach/Spleen), Branch (Chou/Ox, Spleen/Liver, 1AM-2:59AM)

Dong Ling Cao (Herba Rabdosiae, Rabdosia)
Clear Heat Clean Toxin
Bitter, Sweet
Cool
Liver, **Spleen**, Stomach
Biao/Li (Stomach/Spleen), Branch (Chou/Ox, Spleen/Liver, 1AM-2:59AM)

He Ye (Folium Nelumbinis, Lotus Leaf)
Clear Heat Clean Toxin/Astringe, Stabilize and Bind
Bitter, slightly Sweet,[685] Astringent, Aromatic
Neutral
Heart, Liver, **Spleen**
Clock Neighbor (Spleen/Heart), Branch (Chou/Ox, Spleen/Liver, 1AM-2:59AM)

Tian Kui Zi, Tian Kui, Zi Bei Tian Kui (Radix Semiaquilegiae, Muskroot-like Semiaquilegia Root)
Clear Heat Clean Toxin
Sweet, Bitter
Cold
Liver, **Spleen**, Urinary Bladder
Branch (Chou/Ox, Spleen/Liver, 1AM-2:59AM) + Urinary Bladder

Su Bai Jiang, Xi Ming (Herba Thlaspi, Thlaspi)
Clear Heat Clean Toxin
Bitter, Sweet
Slightly Cold
Liver, **Spleen**
Branch (Chou/Ox, Spleen/Liver, 1AM-2:59AM)

Purgative

Da Huang (Radix et Rhizoma Rhei, Rhubarb Root and Rhizome)
Purgative
Bitter to very Bitter[686] to purely Bitter,[687] Aromatic[688]
Cold to very Cold[689]
Spleen, Stomach, Large Intestine, Liver, Heart, Du[690]
Name (Yang Ming, Large Intestine/Stomach), Bie Jing (Jue Yin/Yang Ming, Liver/Large Intestine), Biao/Li (Stomach/Spleen), Clock Neighbor (Spleen/Heart, Large Intestine/Stomach), Branch (Chou/Ox, Spleen/Liver, 1AM-2:59AM and Mao/Rabbit, Liver/Large Intestine, 5AM-6:59AM) + Du

Moist Laxative

Huo Ma Ren (Semen Cannabis, Hemp Seeds)
Moist Laxative
Sweet
Neutral, slightly Toxic*
Spleen, Stomach, Large Intestine
Name (Yang Ming, Large Intestine/Stomach), Biao/Li (Stomach/Spleen), Clock Neighbor (Large Intestine/Stomach)

Yu Li Ren (Semen Pruni, Bush Cherry Kernel, Dwarf Flowering Cherry Kernel)
Moist Laxative
Acrid, Bitter, Sweet
Neutral
Spleen, Large Intestine, Small Intestine
Bie Jing (Tai Yin/Tai Yang, Spleen/Small Intestine), Branch (Si/Snake, Small Intestine/Spleen, 9AM-10:59AM and Wei/Sheep, Spleen/Small Intestine, 1PM-2:59PM) + Large Intestine

Cathartic

Shang Lu (Radix Phytolaccae, Poke Root)
Cathartic
Bitter
Cold, highly Toxic*
Lung, **Spleen**,[691] Kidney, Large Intestine, Urinary Bladder[692]
Name (Tai Yin, Lung/Spleen), Bie Jing (Tai Yin/Tai Yang, Lung/Urinary Bladder), Biao/Li (Large Intestine/Lung, Urinary Bladder/Kidney), Clock Opposite (Kidney/Large Intestine, Lung/Urinary Bladder), Branch (You/Chicken, Lung/Kidney, 5PM-6:59PM, Shen/Monkey, Large Intestine/Urinary Bladder, 3PM-4:59PM)

Da Ji (Radix Euphorbiae seu Knoxiae)
Cathartic
Bitter, Acrid
Cold, extremely Toxic*
Spleen,[693] Lung,[694] Kidney, Large Intestine, Liver,[695] Gall Bladder[696]
Name (Tai Yin, Lung/Spleen), Bie Jing (Jue Yin/Yang Ming, Liver/Large Intestine), Biao/Li (Large Intestine/Lung, Gall Bladder/Liver), Clock Opposite (Kidney/Large Intestine), Clock Neighbor (Liver/Lung), Branch (Zi/Rat, Kidney/Gall Bladder, 11PM-12:59AM, Chou/Ox, Spleen/Liver, 1AM-2:59AM, Mao/Rabbit, Liver/Large Intestine, 5AM-6:59AM, and You/Chicken, Lung/Kidney, 5PM-6:59PM)

Dispel Wind Dampness, Open Channels and Luo-Network Vessels and Relieve Pain

Han Fang Ji/Fen Fang Ji (Radix Stephaniae Tetandrae, Stephania Root)
Dispel Wind Dampness, Open Channels and Luo-Network Vessels and Relieve Pain
Acrid, Bitter to very Bitter[697]
Cold to very Cold[698]
Urinary Bladder, Lung,[699] **Spleen**,[700] Kidney, Yang Qiao,[701] and possibly San Jiao[702]
Name (Tai Yin, Spleen/Lung), Bie Jing (Tai Yin/Tai Yang, Lung/Urinary Bladder), Biao/Li (Urinary Bladder/Kidney), Clock Opposite (Lung/Urinary Bladder), Branch (You/Chicken, Lung/Kidney, 5PM-6:59PM) and possibly Bie Jing (Shao Yin/Shao Yang, Kidney/San Jiao), Clock Opposite (San Jiao/Spleen), Branch (Hai/Pig, Urinary Bladder/San Jiao, 9PM-10:59PM) + Yang Qiao

Mu Gua (Fructus Chaenomelis, Japanese Quince)
Dispel Wind Dampness, Open Channels and Luo-Network Vessels and Relieve Pain
Sour, not Astringent,[703] Aromatic[704]
Warm
Liver, **Spleen**, Lung[705]
Name (Tai Yin, Spleen/Lung), Clock Neighbor (Liver/Lung), Branch (Chou/Ox, Spleen/Liver, 1AM-2:59AM)

Lao Guan Cao (Herba Erodi seu Geranii, Geranium, Common Heron's Bill Herb)
Dispel Wind Dampness, Open Channels and Luo-Network Vessels and Relieve Pain
Acrid, Bitter
Neutral
Liver, Large Intestine, Kidney,[706] **Spleen**[707]
Bie Jing (Jue Yin/Yang Ming, Liver/Large Intestine), Clock Opposite (Kidney/Large Intestine), Branch (Mao/Rabbit, Liver/Large Intestine, 5AM-6:59AM, Chou/Ox, Spleen/Liver, 1AM-2:59AM)

Qin Jiao (Radix Gentianae Macrophyllae, Gentiana)
Dispel Wind Dampness, Open Channels and Luo-Network Vessels and Relieve Pain
Bitter, Acrid, Aromatic[708]
Neutral[709] to Cool to slightly Cold
Stomach, Liver, Gall Bladder, **Spleen**[710]
Biao/Li (Gall Bladder/Liver, Stomach/Spleen), Branch (Chou/Ox, Spleen/Liver, 1AM-2:59AM)

Can Sha, Can Shi (Excrementum Bombycis Mori, Silkworm Feces)
Dispel Wind Dampness, Open Channels and Luo-Network Vessels and Relieve Pain
Sweet,[711] Acrid
Warm
Liver, **Spleen**, Stomach
Biao/Li (Stomach/Spleen), Branch (Chou/Ox, Spleen/Liver, 1AM-2:59AM)

Mu Fang Ji (Radix Cocculi, Cocculus Root)
Dispel Wind Dampness, Open Channels and Luo-Network Vessels and Relieve Pain
Bitter, Acrid
Cold
Urinary Bladder, Kidney, **Spleen**
Biao/Li (Urinary Bladder/Kidney) + Spleen

Tou Gu Cao (Caulis Impatientis, Garden Balsam)
Dispel Wind Dampness, Open Channels and Luo-Network Vessels and Relieve Pain
Bitter, slightly Sweet, Acrid
Cool
Liver, **Spleen**, Kidney
Branch (Chou/Ox, Spleen/Liver, 1AM-2:59AM) + Kidney

Hai Tong Pi (Cortex Erythrinae, Coral Bean Bark)
Dispel Wind Dampness, Open Channels and Luo-Network Vessels and Relieve Pain
Bitter, Acrid
Neutral
Liver, **Spleen**,[712] Kidney[713]
Branch (Chou/Ox, Spleen/Liver, 1AM-2:59AM) + Kidney

Shen Jin Cao, Shi Song, Shi Wu Gong (Herba Lycopodii, Ground Pine, Staghorn Moss, Wolf's Claw Club Moss)
Dispel Wind Dampness, Open Channels and Luo-Network Vessels and Relieve Pain
Bitter, Acrid
Warm
Liver, **Spleen**,[714] Kidney[715]
Branch (Chou/Ox, Spleen/Liver, 1AM-2:59AM) + Kidney

Zhe Tong Pi (Cortex Zanthoxyli, Zanthoxylum Bark)
Dispel Wind Dampness, Open Channels and Luo-Network Vessels and Relieve Pain
Acrid, slightly Bitter
Neutral, slightly Toxic*
Liver, **Spleen**
Branch (Chou/Ox, Spleen/Liver, 1AM-2:59AM)

Qing Feng Teng (Caulis Sinomenii, Orient Vine)
Dispel Wind Dampness, Open Channels and Luo-Network Vessels and Relieve Pain
Bitter, Acrid
Neutral, Toxic*[716]
Liver, **Spleen**
Branch (Chou/Ox, Spleen/Liver, 1AM-2:59AM)

Wu Shao She (Zaocys, Black Striped Snake)
Dispel Wind Dampness, Open Channels and Luo-Network Vessels and Relieve Pain
Sweet, Salty
Neutral
Spleen,[717] Liver
Branch (Chou/Ox, Spleen/Liver, 1AM-2:59AM)

Dispel Wind-Dampness Strengthen Sinew/Tendon and Bone

Zou Ma Tai (Rhizoma Ardisiae, Ardisia Root, Giant Leaf Ardisia Rhizome)
Dispel Wind-Dampness Strengthen Sinew/Tendon and Bone
Acrid
Neutral
Lung, Stomach, **Spleen**, Large Intestine
Name (Tai Yin, Lung/Spleen, Yang Ming, Large Intestine/Stomach), Biao/Li (Large Intestine/Lung, Stomach/Spleen), Clock Neighbor (Large Intestine/Stomach)

Aromatic Dissolve Dampness

Hou Po, Chuan Po, Lie Po (Cortex Magnoliae Officinalis, Officinal Magnolia Bark)
Aromatic Dissolve Dampness
Bitter, Acrid, Aromatic
Warm
Large Intestine, Lung, **Spleen**, Stomach
Name (Tai Yin, Lung/Spleen and Yang Ming, Large Intestine/Stomach), Biao/Li (Large Intestine/Lung, Stomach/Spleen), Clock Neighbor (Large Intestine/Stomach)

Huo Xiang (Herba Agastache *or* Herba Pogostemonis, Patchouli)
Aromatic Dissolve Dampness
Acrid, Sweet,[718] Aromatic
Slightly Warm
Spleen, Stomach, Lung
Name (Tai Yin, Spleen/Lung), Biao/Li (Stomach/Spleen)

Pei Lan (Herba Eupatorii, Fortune Eupatorium)
Aromatic Dissolve Dampness
Acrid, Aromatic
Neutral
Spleen, Stomach, Lung
Name (Tai Yin, Spleen/Lung), Biao/Li (Stomach/Spleen)

Hong Dou Kou (Fructus Galangae, Galanga Seed)
Aromatic Dissolve Dampness/Warm Interior
Acrid, Aromatic
Warm
Spleen, Stomach,[719] Lung
Name (Tai Yin, Spleen/Lung), Biao/Li (Stomach/Spleen)

Bai Dou Kou (Fructus Amomi Rotundus, Round Cardamom Fruit)
Aromatic Dissolve Dampness
Acrid, not Astringent,[720] Aromatic
Warm
Lung, **Spleen**, Stomach and possibly San Jiao[721]
Name (Tai Yin, Lung/Spleen), Biao/Li (Stomach/Spleen) and possibly Clock Opposite (Spleen/San Jiao)

Sha Ren (Fructus Amomi, Amomum Fruit)
Aromatic Dissolve Dampness
Acrid, Aromatic
Warm
Spleen, Stomach
Biao/Li (Stomach/Spleen)

Cao Guo (Fructus Tsaoko)
Aromatic Dissolve Dampness
Acrid to intensely Acrid,[722] Aromatic
Warm
Spleen, Stomach
Biao/Li (Stomach/Spleen)

Cao Dou Kou (Semen Alpiniae Katsumadai, Katsumada's Galangal Seed)
Aromatic Dissolve Dampness
Acrid, Aromatic
Warm
Spleen, Stomach
Biao/Li (Stomach/Spleen)

Cang Zhu (Rhizoma Atractylodis, Atractylodis)
Aromatic Dissolve Dampness
Acrid, Bitter, Sweet,[723] Aromatic
Warm
Spleen, Stomach, Yang Qiao[724]
Biao/Li (Stomach/Spleen) + Yang Qiao

Regulate Water Resolve Dampness

Yi Yi Ren (Semen Coicis, Job's Tears)
Regulate Water Resolve Dampness
Sweet, Bland
Cool to slightly Cold
Spleen, Stomach, Lung, Kidney[725]
Name (Tai Yin, Spleen/Lung), Biao/Li (Stomach/Spleen), Branch (You/Chicken, Lung/Kidney, 5PM-6:59PM)

Fu Ling, Yun Ling (Poria, Hoelen, China Root)
Regulate Water Resolve Dampness
Sweet, Bland
Neutral
Heart, **Spleen**, Kidney, Lung[726]
Name (Shao Yin, Heart/Kidney, Tai Yin, Spleen/Lung), Clock Neighbor (Spleen/Heart)

Yin Chen Hao, Yin Chen (Herba Artemesia Scopariae, Virgate Wormwood, Capillary Wormwood)
Regulate Water Resolve Dampness
Bitter, Aromatic
Cool to Cold[727]
Liver, **Spleen**, Gall Bladder, Stomach
Biao/Li (Gall Bladder/Liver, Stomach/Spleen), Branch (Chou/Ox, Spleen/Liver, 1AM-2:59AM)

Warm Interior

Hong Dou Kou (Fructus Galangae, Galanga Seed)
Aromatic Dissolve Dampness/Warm Interior
Acrid, Aromatic
Warm
Spleen, Stomach,[728] Lung
Name (Tai Yin, Spleen/Lung), Biao/Li (Stomach/Spleen)

Gan Jiang (Rhizoma Zingiberis, Dried Ginger Root)
Warm Interior
Acrid, Aromatic
Hot
Heart, Lung, **Spleen**, Stomach
Name (Tai Yin, Lung/Spleen), Biao/Li (Stomach/Spleen), Clock Neighbor (Spleen/Heart)

Jiao Mu (Semen Zanthoxyli, Zanthoxylum Seed, Sichuan Peppercorn Seed)
Warm Interior
Bitter
Cold, Toxic*
Spleen, Urinary Bladder, Lung, Kidney
Name (Tai Yin, Spleen/Lung), Bie Jing (Tai Yin/Tai Yang, Lung/Urinary Bladder), Biao/Li (Urinary Bladder/Kidney), Clock Opposite (Lung/Urinary Bladder), Branch (You/Chicken, Lung/Kidney, 5PM-6:59PM)

Bi Ba, Bi Bo (Fructus Piperis Longi, Long Pepper)
Warm Interior
Acrid, Aromatic
Hot
Stomach, Large Intestine, **Spleen**[729]
Name (Yang Ming, Large Intestine/Stomach), Biao/Li (Stomach/Spleen), Clock Neighbor (Large Intestine/Stomach)

Gao Liang Jiang (Rhizoma Alpiniae Officinarium, Galanga, Alpinia, Lesser Galangal Rhizome)
Warm Interior
Acrid, Aromatic
Hot
Spleen, Stomach
Biao/Li (Stomach/Spleen)

Bi Cheng Qie, Cheng Qie Zi (Fructus Litseae, Cubeb Fruit)
Warm Interior
Acrid, Aromatic[730]
Warm
Spleen, Stomach, Kidney, Urinary Bladder
Biao/Li (Stomach/Spleen, Urinary Bladder/Kidney), Qian/Hou (Front/Back, Stomach/Urinary Bladder)

Ding Xiang (Flos Caryophylli, Clove Flower Bud)
Warm Interior
Acrid, Aromatic
Warm
Kidney, **Spleen**, Stomach
Biao/Li (Stomach/Spleen) + Kidney

Hua Jiao, Chuan Jiao (Pericarpium Zanthoxyli, Sichuan Peppercorn)
Warm Interior
Acrid
Warm[731] to Hot, slightly Toxic*
Kidney, **Spleen**, Stomach
Biao/Li (Stomach/Spleen) + Kidney

Wu Zhu Yu, Wu Yu (Fructus Evodiae, Evodia Fruit)
Warm Interior
Acrid, Bitter, Aromatic
Hot, slightly Toxic*
Liver, **Spleen**, Stomach, Kidney[732]
Biao/Li (Stomach/Spleen), Branch (Chou/Ox, Spleen/Liver, 1AM-2:59AM) + Kidney

Xiao Hui Xiang, Gui Hui Xiang (Fructus Foeniculi, Fennel Seed)
Warm Interior
Acrid, Aromatic
Warm
Liver, Kidney, **Spleen**, Stomach
Biao/Li (Stomach/Spleen), Branch (Chou/Ox, Spleen/Liver, 1AM-2:59AM) + Kidney

Zhi Cao Wu (Radix Aconiti Kusnezoffii, Wild Aconite Root)
Warm Interior
Acrid, Bitter
Hot, extremely Toxic**
Heart, Liver, **Spleen**, Kidney[733]
Name (Shao Yin, Kidney/Heart), Clock Neighbor (Spleen/Heart), Branch (Chou/Ox, Spleen/Liver, 1AM-2:59AM)

Rou Gui (Cortex Cinnamomi, Cinnamon Bark, Cassia Bark)
Warm Interior
Acrid to highly Acrid,[734] Sweet, Aromatic
Greatly Warming[735] to Hot
Heart, Kidney, Liver, **Spleen**
Name (Shao Yin, Heart/Kidney), Clock Neighbor (Spleen/Heart), Branch (Chou/Ox, Spleen/Liver, 1AM-2:59AM)

Zhi Fu Zi, Tian Xiong (Radix Aconiti Lateralis Praeparata, Aconite, Prepared/Processed Aconite Accessory Root)
Warm Interior
Acrid to extremely Acrid,[736] Sweet[737]
Hot to very Hot,[738] Toxic*
Heart, Kidney, **Spleen**, Du[739]
Name (Shao Yin, Heart/Kidney), Clock Neighbor (Spleen/Heart) + Du

Zhi Chuan Wu (Radix Aconiti Preparata, Prepared Aconite Main Root, Mother Root of Common Monk's Hood)
Warm Interior
Acrid, Bitter
Hot, extremely Toxic**
Heart, Liver, **Spleen**, Du[740]
Clock Neighbor (Spleen/Heart), Branch (Chou/Ox, Spleen/Liver, 1AM-2:59AM) + Du

Da Hui Xiang, Ba Jiao Huí, Ba Jiao Hui Xiang (Fructus Anisi Stellati, Star Anis)
Warm Interior
Acrid, Sweet, Aromatic
Warm
Liver, Kidney, **Spleen**
Branch (Chou/Ox, Spleen/Liver, 1AM-2:59AM) + Kidney

Regulate and Rectify Qi

Hua Ju Hong, Hua Pi, You Pi Ju Hong (Exocarpium Citri Grandis, Pumelo Peel)
Regulate and Rectify Qi
Bitter, Acrid, Aromatic
Warm
Lung, **Spleen**, Stomach
Name (Tai Yin, Lung/Spleen), Biao/Li (Stomach/Spleen)

Chen Pi, Ju Pi, Hong Pi (Pericarpium Citri Reticulatae, Aged Tangerine Peel)
Regulate and Rectify Qi
Acrid, Bitter, Aromatic
Warm
Lung, **Spleen**, Stomach[741]
Name (Tai Yin, Lung/Spleen), Biao/Li (Stomach/Spleen)

Zi Su Geng (Caulis Perillae, Perilla Stem)
Acrid Warm Exterior Releasing/Regulate and Rectify Qi
Acrid, Sweet, Aromatic
Slightly Warm
Lung, **Spleen**, Stomach
Name (Tai Yin, Lung/Spleen), Biao/Li (Stomach/Spleen)

Tan Xiang (Lignum Santali Albi, Sandalwood)
Regulate and Rectify Qi
Acrid, Aromatic
Warm
Spleen, Stomach, Lung
Name (Tai Yin, Spleen/Lung), Biao/Li (Stomach/Spleen)

Fo Shou (Fructus Citri Sarcodactylis, Finger Citron Fruit, Buddha's Hand Citron)
Regulate and Rectify Qi
Acrid, Bitter, Aromatic
Warm
Liver, Lung, Stomach, **Spleen**
Name (Tai Yin, Lung/Spleen), Biao/Li (Stomach/Spleen), Clock Neighbor (Liver/Lung), Branch (Chou/Ox, Spleen/Liver, 1AM-2:59AM)

Tian Xian Teng, Ma Dou Ling Teng (Herba Aristolochiae, Aristolochia, Dutchman's Pipe)
Regulate and Rectify Qi
Bitter
Warm, Toxic*
Heart, Lung, **Spleen**, Kidney
Name (Shao Yin, Heart/Kidney, Tai Yin, Spleen/Lung)
Clock Neighbor (Spleen/Heart), Branch (You/Chicken, Lung/Kidney, 5PM-6:59PM)

Wu Yao, Tai Wu Yao, Tai Wu (Radix Linderae, Lindera Root)
Regulate and Rectify Qi
Acrid, Aromatic[742]
Warm
Urinary Bladder, Kidney, Lung, **Spleen**
Name (Tai Yin, Lung/Spleen), Bie Jing (Tai Yin/Tai Yang, Lung/Urinary Bladder), Biao/Li (Urinary Bladder/Kidney), Clock Opposite (Lung/Urinary Bladder), Branch (You/Chicken, Lung/Kidney, 5PM-6:59PM)

Xiang Yuan (Fructus Citri, Citron)
Regulate and Rectify Qi
Acrid, slightly Bitter, Sour, Aromatic
Warm
Liver, **Spleen**, Lung
Name (Tai Yin, Spleen/Lung), Clock Neighbor (Liver/Lung), Branch (Chou/Ox, Spleen/Liver, 1AM-2:59AM)

Tu Mu Xiang, Qi Mu Xiang (Radix Inulae)
Regulate and Rectify Qi
Acrid, Bitter
Warm
Lung, Liver, **Spleen**
Name (Tai Yin, Lung/Spleen), Clock Neighbor (Liver/Lung) Branch (Chou/Ox, Spleen/Liver, 1AM-2:59AM)

Zhi Ke, Zhi Qiao (Fructus Aurantii, Ripened Bitter Orange)
Regulate and Rectify Qi
Bitter, Acrid, Aromatic
Cool to slightly Cold[743]
Large Intestine, **Spleen**, Stomach
Name (Yang Ming, Large Intestine/Stomach), Biao/Li (Stomach/Spleen), Clock Neighbor (Large Intestine/Stomach)

Zhi Shi (Fructus Aurantii Immaturus, Immature Bitter Orange)
Regulate and Rectify Qi
Bitter, Acrid, Aromatic
Warm[744] to Cool to slightly Cold[745]
Large Intestine, **Spleen**, Stomach
Name (Yang Ming, Large Intestine/Stomach), Biao/Li (Stomach/Spleen) Clock Neighbor (Large Intestine/Stomach)

Da Fu Pi (Pericarpium Arecae, Areca Peel, Betel Husk)
Regulate and Rectify Qi
Acrid
Slightly Warm
Large Intestine, Small Intestine, **Spleen**, Stomach
Name (Yang Ming, Large Intestine/Stomach), Bie Jing (Tai Yin/Tai Yang, Spleen/Small Intestine), Biao/Li (Stomach/Spleen), Clock Neighbor (Large Intestine/Stomach), Branch (Si/Snake, Small Intestine/Spleen, 9AM-10:59AM, Wei/Sheep, Spleen/Small Intestine, 1PM-2:59PM)

Dao Dou (Semen Canavaliae, Sword Bean)
Regulate and Rectify Qi
Sweet
Warm
Stomach, **Spleen**,[746] Kidney, Large Intestine[747]
Name (Yang Ming, Large Intestine/Stomach), Biao/Li (Stomach/Spleen), Clock Opposite (Kidney/Large Intestine), Clock Neighbor (Large Intestine/Stomach)

Mu Xiang (Radix Aucklandiae, Costus Root)
Regulate and Rectify Qi
Acrid, Bitter, slightly Astringent,[748] Aromatic
Warm
Gall Bladder, Large Intestine, **Spleen**, Stomach, San Jiao[749]
Name (Yang Ming, Large Intestine/Stomach, Shao Yang, Gall Bladder/San Jiao), Biao/Li (Stomach/Spleen), Clock Opposite (Spleen/San Jiao), Clock Neighbor (Large Intestine/Stomach, San Jiao/Gall Bladder)

Gan Song (Radix seu Rhizoma Nardostachys, Spoon-Leaf Nardostachys Rhizome)
Regulate and Rectify Qi
Acrid, Sweet, Aromatic
Warm
Spleen, Stomach
Biao/Li (Stomach/Spleen)

Chen Xiang (Lignum Aquilariae Resinatum, Aloeswood)
Regulate and Rectify Qi
Acrid, Bitter, Aromatic
Warm
Kidney, **Spleen**, Stomach
Biao/Li (Stomach/Spleen) + Kidney

Jiu Xiang Chong, Da Pi Chong (Aspongopus, Stinkbug)
Regulate and Rectify Qi
Salty
Warm
Spleen, Liver, Kidney
Branch (Chou/Ox, Spleen/Liver, 1AM-2:59AM) + Kidney

Xiang Fu (Rhizoma Cyperi, Cyperus Rhizome, Nut Grass Rhizome)
Regulate and Rectify Qi
Acrid to intensely Acrid,[750] slightly Bitter, slightly Sweet, Aromatic
Neutral
Liver, **Spleen**,[751] San Jiao, Gall Bladder,[752] some sources indicate that it enters all channels.
Name (Shao Yang, San Jiao/Gall Bladder), Biao/Li (Gall Bladder/Liver), Clock Opposite (Spleen/San Jiao), Clock Neighbor (San Jiao/Gall Bladder), Branch (Chou/Ox, Spleen/Liver, 1AM-2:59AM)

Mei Gui Hua (Rosa Rugosae Flos, Young Flower of Chinese Rose, Rosebud)
Regulate and Rectify Qi
Sweet, slightly Bitter, Aromatic
Warm
Liver, **Spleen**
Branch (Chou/Ox, Spleen/Liver, 1AM-2:59AM)

Digestive

Lai Fu Zi (Semen Raphani, Radish/Daikon/Turnip Seeds)
Digestive
Acrid, Sweet
Neutral
Spleen, Stomach, Lung
Name (Tai Yin, Spleen/Lung), Biao/Li (Stomach/Spleen)

Hong Qu (Monascus, Red Yeast Rice)
Digestive
Sweet, Acrid
Warm
Spleen, Liver, Large Intestine
Bie Jing (Jue Yin/Yang Ming, Liver/Large Intestine), Branch (Chou/Ox, Spleen/Liver, 1AM-2:59AM and Mao/Rabbit, Liver/Large Intestine, 5AM-6:59AM)

Su Ya (Fructus Setariae Germinatus, Millet Sprouts)
Digestive
Sweet, Bitter[753]
Warm
Spleen, Stomach
Biao/Li (Stomach/Spleen)

Gu Ya, Xiao Gu Ya, Dao Ya (Fructus Setariae Germinatus, Rice Sprout)
Digestive
Sweet
Neutral
Spleen, Stomach
Biao/Li (Stomach/Spleen)

Dao Ya (Fructus Oryzae germinatus, Rice Sprout)
Digestive
Sweet
Neutral
Spleen, Stomach
Biao/Li (Stomach/Spleen)

Liu Shen Qu, Shen Qu (Massa Fermentata, Medicated Leaven)
Digestive
Sweet, Acrid
Warm
Spleen, Stomach
Biao/Li (Stomach/Spleen)

Ji Nei Jin (Endothelium Corneum Gigerae Galli, Chicken Gizzard Lining)
Digestive
Sweet
Neutral
Urinary Bladder, Small Intestine, **Spleen**, Stomach
Name (Tai Yang, Small Intestine/Urinary Bladder), Biao/Li (Stomach/Spleen), Bie Jing (Tai Yin/Tai Yang, Spleen/Small Intestine), Clock Neighbor (Small Intestine/Urinary Bladder), Qian/Hou (Front/Back, Stomach/Urinary Bladder), Branch (Si/Snake, Small Intestine/Spleen, 9AM-10:59AM and Wei/Sheep, Spleen/Small Intestine, 1PM-2:59PM)

Shan Zha (Fructus Crategi, Crategus, Hawthorn Fruit)
Digestive
Sweet, Sour
Neutral[754] to slightly Warm
Liver, **Spleen**, Stomach
Biao/Li (Stomach/Spleen), Branch (Chou/Ox, Spleen/Liver, 1AM-2:59AM)

Mai Ya, Da Mai Ya (Fructus Hordei Germinatus, Barley Sprout, Malt)
Digestive
Sweet, Salty[755]
Neutral
Liver, **Spleen**, Stomach
Biao/Li (Stomach/Spleen), Branch (Chou/Ox, Spleen/Liver, 1AM-2:59AM)

Expel Parasites

Da Suan (Bulbus Alli Sativi, Garlic)
Expel Parasites/External Application
Acrid, Sweet[756]
Neutral to Warm
Spleen, Stomach, Lung, Large Intestine[757]
Name (Tai Yin, Spleen/Lung, Yang Ming, Large Intestine/Stomach), Biao/Li (Stomach/Spleen, Large Intestine/Lung), Clock Neighbor (Large Intestine/Stomach)

Wu Yi, Chou Wu Yi, Bai Wu Yi (Fructus Ulmi Praeparatus, Ulmus, Paste of Stinking Elm Cake)
Expel Parasites
Acrid, Bitter, Sour[758]
Neutral[759] to Warm
Spleen, Stomach
Biao/Li (Stomach/Spleen)

Nan He Shi, Shan Luo Bo Zi (Fructus Carotae, Daucus Fruit, Wild Carrot Seed)
Expel Parasites
Bitter, Acrid
Neutral, slightly Toxic*
Spleen, Stomach
Biao/Li (Stomach/Spleen)

Shi Jun Zi (Fructus Quisqualis, Rangoon Creeper Fruit and Seeds)
Expel Parasites
Sweet, Aromatic
Warm, relatively non-Toxic[760] to slightly Toxic*
Spleen, Stomach
Biao/Li (Stomach/Spleen)

Ku Lian Pi, Ku Lian Gen Pi (Cortex Meliae, Chinaberry Bark)
Expel Parasites
Bitter
Cold, Toxic*
Liver, **Spleen**, Stomach
Biao/Li (Stomach/Spleen), Branch (Chou/Ox, Spleen/Liver, 1AM-2:59AM)

Guan Zhong, Mian Ma Guan Zhong (Rhizoma Dryopteridis, Dryopteris Root, Shield-Fern Root)
Clear Heat Clean Toxin/Expel Parasites
Bitter
Cool to Cold,[761] slightly Toxic*
Liver, **Spleen**, Stomach[762]
Biao/Li (Stomach/Spleen), Branch (Chou/Ox, Spleen/Liver, 1AM-2:59AM)

He Shi, Bei He Shi (Fructus Carpesii, Carpesium Fruit)
Expel Parasites
Bitter, Acrid
Neutral, slightly Toxic*
Spleen, Stomach, Liver[763]
Biao/Li (Stomach/Spleen), Branch (Chou/Ox, Spleen/Liver, 1AM-2:59AM)

Stop Bleeding

Zong Lu Tan (Trachycarpi Petiolus Carbonisatus, Charred Trachycarpus Petiole)
Stop Bleeding
Bitter, Astringent
Neutral
Lung, Liver, Large Intestine, **Spleen**[764]
Name (Tai Yin, Lung/Spleen), Bie Jing (Jue Yin/Yang Ming, Liver/Large Intestine), Biao/Li (Large Intestine/Lung), Clock Neighbor (Liver/Lung), Branch (Mao/Rabbit, Liver/Large Intestine, 5AM-6:59AM)

Xian He Cao, Tuo Li Cao, Lang Ya Cao (Herba Agrimoniae, Agrimony Grass)
Stop Bleeding
Bitter, Astringent
Neutral
Lung, Liver, **Spleen**
Name (Tai Yin, Lung/Spleen), Clock Neighbor (Liver/Lung), Branch (Chou/Ox, Spleen/Liver, 1AM-2:59AM)

San Qi, Tian Qi (Radix Notoginseng, Pseudoginseng Root)
Stop Bleeding
Sweet, slightly Bitter
Warm
Liver, Stomach,[765] **Spleen**,[766] Large Intestine,[767] Pericardium[768]
Name (Yang Ming, Large Intestine/Stomach and Jue Yin, Liver/Pericardium), Bie Jing (Jue Yin/Yang Ming, Pericardium/Stomach and Liver/Large Intestine), Biao/Li (Stomach/Spleen), Clock Opposite (Pericardium/Stomach), Clock Neighbor (Large Intestine/Stomach), Branch (Chou/Ox, Spleen/Liver, 1AM-2:59AM, Mao/Rabbit, Liver/Large Intestine, 5AM-6:59AM and Shu/Dog, Stomach/Pericardium, 7PM-8:59PM)

Fu Long Gan, Zao Xin Tu (Terra Flava Usta, Oven Clay, Fire Pit Ash)
Stop Bleeding
Acrid, Bitter
Warm
Spleen, Stomach
Biao/Li (Stomach/Spleen)

Pu Huang (Pollen Typhae, Cattail Pollen, Bulrush Pollen)
Stop Bleeding
Sweet, Acrid,[769] Astringent,[770] Aromatic[771]
Neutral
Liver, Pericardium,[772] Heart,[773] **Spleen**[774]
Name (Jue Yin, Liver/Pericardium), Clock Neighbor (Spleen/Heart), Branch (Chou/Ox, Spleen/Liver, 1AM-2:59AM)

Da Ji, Da Xiao Ji (Herba seu Radix Cirsii Japonici, Japanese Thistle)
Stop Bleeding
Sweet, Bitter, slightly Acrid[775]
Cool
Liver, Heart, **Spleen**[776]
Clock Neighbor (Spleen/Heart), Branch (Chou/Ox, Spleen/Liver, 1AM-2:59AM)

Lian Fang (Receptaculum Nelumbinis, Lotus Peduncle)
Stop Bleeding
Bitter, Astringent
Warm
Liver, **Spleen**, Kidney
Branch (Chou/Ox, Spleen/Liver, 1AM-2:59AM) + Kidney

Ai Ye (Folium Artemisiae Argyi, Mugwort Leaf, Moxa)
Stop Bleeding
Bitter, Acrid, Aromatic
Warm
Spleen, Liver, Kidney, Dai[777]
Branch (Chou/Ox, Spleen/Liver, 1AM-2:59AM) + Kidney, Dai

Pao Jiang (Zingiberis Rhizoma Praeparatum, Blast-Fried Ginger)
Stop Bleeding
Bitter, slightly Acrid, Astringent
Warm
Liver, **Spleen**
Branch (Chou/Ox, Spleen/Liver, 1AM-2:59AM)

Vitalize Blood Transform Stasis

Wa Leng Zi (Concha Arcae, Cockle Shell, Ark Shell)
Vitalize Blood Transform Stasis/Transform Phlegm/External Application
Salty
Neutral
Liver, Stomach, Lung, **Spleen**[778]
Name (Tai Yin, Lung/Spleen), Biao/Li (Stomach/Spleen), Clock Neighbor (Liver/Lung), Branch (Chou/Ox, Spleen/Liver, 1AM-2:59AM)

Yan Hu Suo (Rhizoma Corydalis, Corydalis Rhizome)
Vitalize Blood Transform Stasis
Acrid, Bitter, Aromatic
Warm
Heart, Liver, **Spleen**, Stomach[779]
Biao/Li (Stomach/Spleen), Clock Neighbor (Spleen/Heart), Branch (Chou/Ox, Spleen/Liver, 1AM-2:59AM)

Jiang Xiang (Lignum Dalbergiae Odoriferae, Dalbergia Heartwood, Rosewood)
Vitalize Blood Transform Stasis
Acrid, Aromatic
Warm
Liver, **Spleen**, Heart, Stomach[780]
Biao/Li (Stomach/Spleen), Clock Neighbor (Spleen/Heart), Branch (Chou/Ox, Spleen/Liver, 1AM-2:59AM)

Jiang Huang (Rhizoma Curcumae Longae, Turmeric Rhizome)
Vitalize Blood Transform Stasis
Acrid, Bitter, Aromatic
Warm
Spleen, Liver, Stomach[781]
Biao/Li (Stomach/Spleen), Branch (Chou/Ox, Spleen/Liver, 1AM-2:59AM)

Liu Ji Nu, Hua Shi Dan (Herba Artemisiae Anomalae, Artemesia)
Vitalize Blood Transform Stasis
Bitter, Aromatic
Warm
Heart, **Spleen**
Clock Neighbor (Spleen/Heart)

Mao Dong Qing (Radix Ilicis Pubescentis, Hairy Holly Root)
Vitalize Blood Transform Stasis
Bitter, Acrid,[782] Astringent
Neutral to slightly Cold[783]
Heart, **Spleen**
Clock Neighbor (Spleen, Heart)

Ji Xue Teng, Da Xue Teng (Caulis Spatholobi, Spatholobus, Millettia Vine)
Vitalize Blood Transform Stasis
Bitter, slightly Sweet, Acrid[784]
Warm
Heart,[785] Liver, **Spleen**[786]
Clock Neighbor (Spleen/Heart), Branch (Chou/Ox, Spleen/Liver, 1AM-2:59AM)

Mo Yao (Commiphora Myrrha, Myrrh)
Vitalize Blood Transform Stasis
Acrid,[787] Bitter, Aromatic
Neutral
Heart, Liver, **Spleen**
Clock Neighbor (Spleen/Heart), Branch (Chou/Ox, Spleen/Liver, 1AM-2:59AM)

Ru Xiang (Boswelia Carterii, Gummi Olibanum, Frankincense)
Vitalize Blood Transform Stasis
Acrid, Bitter, Aromatic
Warm
Heart, Liver, **Spleen**
Clock Neighbor (Spleen/Heart), Branch (Chou/Ox, Spleen/Liver, 1AM-2:59AM)

Su Mu (Lignum Sappan, Sappan Wood, Brazilwood)
Vitalize Blood Transform Stasis
Sweet, Salty, slightly Acrid to Acrid[788]
Neutral to slightly Cooling[789]
Heart, Liver, **Spleen**[790]
Clock Neighbor (Spleen/Heart), Branch (Chou/Ox, Spleen/Liver, 1AM-2:59AM)

Di Bie Chong, Tu Bie Chong, Zhe Chong (Eupolyphagia, Wingless Cockroach, Ground Beetle)
Vitalize Blood Transform Stasis
Salty
Cold, slightly Toxic*
Liver, Heart, **Spleen**
Clock Neighbor (Spleen/Heart), Branch (Chou/Ox, Spleen/Liver, 1AM-2:59AM)

Chi Shao (Radix Paeoniae Rubrae, Red Peony Root)
Clear Heat Cool Blood/Vitalize Blood Transform Stasis
Bitter, Sour[791]
Cool to slightly Cold
Liver, **Spleen**[792]
Branch (Chou/Ox, Spleen/Liver, 1AM-2:59AM)

Ma Bian Cao, Tie Ma Bian, Feng Jing Cao (Herba Verbena, Verbena, Iron Herb)
Vitalize Blood Transform Stasis
Bitter
Cool to slightly Cold[793]
Liver, **Spleen**
Branch (Chou/Ox, Spleen/Liver, 1AM-2:59AM)

Mei Gui Hua (Flos Rugosae)
Vitalize Blood Transform Stasis
Sweet, slightly Bitter
Warm
Liver, **Spleen**
Branch (Chou/Ox, Spleen/Liver,1AM-2:59AM)

San Leng (Rhizoma Sparganii, Scirpus Rhizome, Burr Reed Rhizome)
Vitalize Blood Transform Stasis
Bitter, Acrid[794]
Neutral to Warm[795]
Liver, **Spleen**
Branch (Chou/Ox, Spleen/Liver, 1AM-2:59AM)

Ze Lan (Herba Lycopi, Bugleweed, Water Horehound)
Vitalize Blood Transform Stasis
Bitter, Acrid, Aromatic
Slightly Warm
Liver, **Spleen**
Branch (Chou/Ox, Spleen/Liver, 1AM-2:59AM)

E Zhu (Rhizoma Curcumae, Zedoaria Rhizome)
Vitalize Blood Transform Stasis
Bitter, Acrid, Aromatic
Warm
Spleen, Liver
Branch (Chou/Ox, Spleen/Liver, 1AM-2:59AM)

Chong Wei Zi (Fructus Leonuri, Leonurus Fruit)
Vitalize Blood Transform Stasis
Sweet
Cool[796] to slightly Cold
Liver, **Spleen**
Branch (Chou/Ox, Spleen/Liver, 1AM-2:59AM)

Transform Phlegm

Xuan Fu Hua, Jin Fei Hua, Jin Fu Hua (Flos Inulae, Inula Flower)
Transform Phlegm
Bitter, Acrid, Salty
Slightly Warm
Large Intestine, Lung, Stomach, **Spleen**, Liver[797]
Name (Yang Ming, Large Intestine/Stomach, Tai Yin, Lung/Spleen), Bie Jing (Jue Yin/Yang Ming, Liver/Large Intestine), Biao/Li (Large Intestine/Lung, Stomach/Spleen), Clock Neighbor (Large Intestine/Stomach, Liver/Lung), Branch (Chou/Ox, Spleen/Liver, 1AM-2:59AM and Mao/Rabbit, Liver/Large Intestine, 5AM-6:59AM)

Luo Han Guo (Fructus Momordicae, Momordica Fruit)
Transform Phlegm/Relieve Cough and Wheezing/Panting
Sweet
Cool
Lung, Large Intestine, **Spleen**[798]
Name (Tai Yin, Lung/Spleen), Biao/Li (Large Intestine, Lung)

Zhi Ban Xia, Ban Xia (Rhizoma Pinelliae preparatum)
Transform Phlegm
Acrid
Warm, Toxic* if unprocessed
Spleen, Stomach, Lung
Name (Tai Yin, Spleen/Lung), Biao/Li (Stomach/Spleen)

Bai Jie Zi, Huang Jie Zi, Jie Cai Zi (Semen Sinapis, White Mustard Seed)
Transform Phlegm
Acrid
Warm
Lung, Stomach,[799] **Spleen**[800]
Name (Tai Yin, Lung/Spleen), Biao/Li (Stomach/Spleen)

Zhi Bai Fu Zi, Bai Fu Zi (Rhizoma Typhonii preparatum, Typhonium)
Transform Phlegm
Acrid, Sweet
Warm, Toxic*
Spleen, Stomach, Lung,[801] Liver[802]
Name (Tai Yin, Spleen/Lung), Biao/Li (Stomach/Spleen), Clock Neighbor (Liver/Lung), Branch (Chou/Ox, Spleen/Liver, 1AM-2:59AM)

Wa Leng Zi (Concha Arcae, Cockle Shell, Ark Shell)
Vitalize Blood Transform Stasis/Transform Phlegm/External Application
Salty
Neutral
Liver, Stomach, Lung, **Spleen**[803]
Name (Tai Yin, Lung/Spleen), Biao/Li (Stomach/Spleen), Clock Neighbor (Liver/Lung), Branch (Chou/Ox, Spleen/Liver, 1AM-2:59AM)

Dan Nan Xing, Dan Xing (Arisaema cum Bile)
Transform Phlegm
Bitter, slightly Acrid[804]
Cool, slightly Toxic*
Liver, Lung,[805] **Spleen**,[806] Gall Bladder[807]
Name (Tai Yin, Spleen/Lung), Biao/Li (Gall Bladder/Liver), Clock Neighbor (Liver/Lung), Branch (Chou/Ox, Spleen/Liver, 1AM-2:59AM and Yin/Tiger, Gall Bladder/Lung, 3AM-4:59AM)

Zhi Tian Nan Xing, Tian Nan Xing (Rhizoma Arisaematis preparatum, prepared Arisaema, Jack in the Pulpit)
Transform Phlegm
Bitter, very Acrid
Warm, Toxic*
Liver, Lung, **Spleen**
Name (Tai Yin, Spleen/Lung), Clock Neighbor (Liver/Lung), Branch (Chou/Ox, Spleen/Liver, 1AM-2:59AM)

Relieve Cough and Wheezing/Panting

Luo Han Guo (Fructus Momordicae, Momordica Fruit)
Transform Phlegm/Relieve Cough and Wheezing/Panting
Sweet
Cool
Lung, Large Intestine, **Spleen**[808]
Name (Tai Yin, Lung/Spleen), Biao/Li (Large Intestine, Lung)

Yang Jin Hua (Flos Daturae, Datura Flower)
Relieve Cough and Wheezing/Panting
Acrid
Warm, Toxic*
Lung, Liver, Heart, **Spleen**
Name (Tai Yin, Lung/Spleen), Clock Neighbor (Liver/Lung, Spleen/Heart), Branch (Chou/Ox, Spleen/Liver, 1AM-2:59AM)

Nourish and Calm Shen

He Huan Hua, Ye He Hua, Ye He Mi (Flos Albiziae, Mimosa Flower)
Nourish and Calm Shen
Sweet
Neutral
Liver, Stomach, **Spleen**,[809] Heart,[810] Lung[811]
Name (Tai Yin, Lung/Spleen), Biao/Li (Stomach/Spleen), Clock Neighbor (Spleen/Heart, Liver/Lung), Branch (Chou/Ox, Spleen/Liver, 1AM-2:59AM)

Suan Zao Ren, Dong Zao (Semen Zizyphi Spinosae, Sour Jujube Seed)
Nourish and Calm Shen
Sweet, Sour[812]
Neutral
Heart, Liver, Gall Bladder,[813] **Spleen**[814]
Bie Jing (Shao Yin/Shao Yang, Heart/Gall Bladder), Biao/Li (Gall Bladder/Liver), Clock Opposite (Heart/Gall Bladder), Clock Neighbor (Spleen/Heart), Branch (Chou/Ox, Spleen/Liver, 1AM-2:59AM)

Calm Shen Sedative

Zi Bei Chi, Bei Zi, Zi Bei, Bao Bei (Concha Mauritiae/Cypraeae, Cowry Shell)
Calm Shen Sedative
Salty
Neutral
Spleen, Liver
Branch (Chou/Ox, Spleen/Liver, 1AM-2:59AM)

Calm Liver Extinguish Wind

Di Long, Qiu Yin (Pheretima, Earthworm)
Calm Liver Extinguish Wind
Salty
Cold
Liver, **Spleen**, Kidney,[815] Urinary Bladder, Lung[816]
Name (Tai Yin, Spleen/Lung), Bie Jing (Tai Yin/Tai Yang, Lung/Urinary Bladder), Biao/Li (Urinary Bladder/Kidney), Clock Opposite (Lung/Urinary Bladder), Clock Neighbor (Liver/Lung), Branch (Chou/Ox, Spleen/Liver, 1AM-2:59AM)

Hei Dou (Semen Glycinis, Black Soybean)
Calm Liver Extinguish Wind
Sweet
Neutral
Spleen, Kidney

Open Orifices

Bing Pian, Long Nao Bing Pian (Borneolum, Borneolum Syntheticum, Borneol)
Open Orifices
Acrid, Bitter, Aromatic
Slightly Cold[817] to Hot[818]
Heart, **Spleen**, Lung
Name (Tai Yin, Spleen/Lung), Clock Neighbor (Spleen/Heart)

Shui Chang Pu, Bai Chang Pu (Rhizoma Acori Calami, Calamus, Sweetflag Rhizome)
Open Orifices
Bitter, Acrid, slightly Toxic*
Warm
Heart, Liver, Stomach, **Spleen**,[819] Large Intestine[820]
Name (Yang Ming, Large Intestine/Stomach), Bie Jing (Jue Yin/Yang Ming, Liver/Large Intestine), Biao/Li (Stomach/Spleen), Clock Neighbor (Spleen/Heart, Large Intestine/Stomach), Branch (Chou/Ox, Spleen/Liver, 1AM-2:59AM and Mao/Rabbit, Liver/Large Intestine, 5AM-6:59AM)

Su He Xiang (Styrax, Resin of Rose Maloes, Styrax)
Open Orifices
Acrid, Sweet,[821] Aromatic
Warm
Heart, **Spleen**
Clock Neighbor (Spleen/Heart)

An Xi Xiang (Benzoinum, Benzoin)
Open Orifices
Acrid, Bitter, Aromatic
Neutral
Heart, Liver, **Spleen**
Clock Neighbor (Spleen/Heart), Branch (Chou/Ox, Spleen/Liver, 1AM-2:59AM)

Jiu Jie Chang Pu, Jing Chang Pu (Rhizoma Anemones Altaicae)
Open Orifices
Acrid
Warm, slightly Toxic*
Heart, Liver, **Spleen**
Clock Neighbor (Spleen/Heart), Branch (Chou/Ox, Spleen/Liver, 1AM-2:59AM)

She Xiang (Moschus, Musk, Navel Gland Secretions of Musk Deer)
Open Orifices
Acrid, Aromatic
Warm
Heart, Liver, **Spleen**, some sources say all channels.
Clock Neighbor (Spleen/Heart), Branch (Chou/Ox, Spleen/Liver, 1AM-2:59AM)

Tonify Qi

Sha Ji, Cu Liu Guo (Fructus Hippophae, Sea Buckthorn Fruit, Swallow Thorn Fruit)
Tonify Qi
Sour, slightly Sweet, Astringent
Warm
Lung, **Spleen**, Stomach, Large Intestine, Liver, Small Intestine[822]
Name (Tai Yin, Lung/Spleen, Yang Ming, Large Intestine/Stomach), Bie Jing (Jue Yin/Yang Ming, Liver/Large Intestine, Tai Yin/Tai Yang, Spleen/Small Intestine), Biao/Li (Large Intestine/Lung, Stomach/Spleen), Clock Opposite (Liver/Small Intestine), Clock Neighbor (Liver/Lung, Large Intestine/Stomach), Branch (Chou/Ox, Spleen/Liver, 1AM-2:59AM, Mao/Rabbit, Liver/Large Intestine, 5AM-6:59AM, Si/Snake, Small Intestine/Spleen, 9AM-10:59AM, Wei/Sheep, Spleen/Small Intestine, 1PM-2:59PM)

Feng Mi (Mel, Honey)
Tonify Qi
Sweet
Neutral
Spleen, Lung, Large Intestine
Name (Tai Yin, Spleen/Lung), Biao/Li (Large Intestine/Lung)

Yi Tang (Saccharum Granorum, Maltosum, Malt Sugar, Maltose)
Tonify Qi
Sweet
Slightly Warm[823] to Warm
Spleen, Stomach, Lung
Name (Tai Yin, Spleen/Lung), Biao/Li (Stomach/Spleen)

Gan Cao (Radix Glycyrrhizae, Licorice Root)
Tonify Qi
Sweet
Neutral
Spleen, Stomach, Lung, Heart, Dai,[824] some sources indicate that it enters all channels.
Name (Tai Yin, Spleen/Lung), Biao/Li (Stomach/Spleen), Clock Neighbor (Spleen/Heart) + Dai, some sources indicate that Gan Cao enters all channels and therefore creates every relationship.

Tai Zi Shen (Radix Psuedostellariae, Pseudostellaria)
Tonify Qi
Sweet, slightly Bitter
Neutral to slightly Cold[825]
Lung, **Spleen**
Name (Tai Yin, Spleen/Lung)

Dong Yang Shen (Radix Ginseng Japonica, Japanese Ginseng)
Tonify Qi
Sweet, slightly Bitter
Cool
Spleen, Lung
Name (Tai Yin, Spleen/Lung)

Dang Shen (Radix Codonopsis, Codonopsis Root)
Tonify Qi
Sweet
Neutral
Spleen, Lung
Name (Tai Yin, Spleen/Lung)

Hong Qi (Radix Hedysari, Many Inflorescenced Sweetvetch)
Tonify Qi
Sweet
Warm
Lung, **Spleen**
Name (Tai Yin, Lung/Spleen)

Hong Jing Tian, Qi Ye Dan (Herba Rhodiolae, Rhodiola)
Tonify Qi
Sweet, Astringent[826]
Cold
Spleen, Lung
Name (Tai Yin, Spleen/Lung)

Jiao Gu Lan, Qi Dan Ye, Long Xu Teng (Rhizoma seu Herba Gynostemmatis)
Tonify Qi
Sweet,[827] slightly Bitter
Cold
Spleen,[828] Lung, Heart[829]
Name (Tai Yin, Spleen/Lung), Clock Neighbor (Spleen/Heart)

Xi Yang Shen, Hua Qi Shen (Radix Panacis Quinquefoli, American Ginseng Root)
Tonify Qi/Tonify Yin
Sweet, slightly Bitter[830] to Bitter to very Bitter[831]
Cold
Kidney, Heart, Lung, **Spleen**[832]
Name (Shao Yin, Kidney/Heart, Tai Yin, Spleen/Lung), Clock Neighbor (Spleen/Heart), Branch (You/Chicken, Lung/Kidney, 5PM-6:59PM)

Ren Shen (Radix Ginseng, Ginseng Root)
Tonify Qi
Sweet, slightly Bitter
Slightly Warm
Lung, **Spleen**, Heart,[833] Kidney[834]
Name (Tai Yin, Lung/Spleen, Shao Yin, Kidney/Heart), Clock Neighbor (Spleen/Heart), Branch (You/Chicken, Lung/Kidney, 5PM-6:59PM)

Ci Wu Jia, Wu Jia Shen (Radix et Caulis Acanthopanacis Senticosi, Siberian Ginseng, Eleutherococcus Ginseng)
Tonify Qi
Acrid, slightly Bitter
Warm
Spleen, Kidney, Heart, Lung[835]
Name (Tai Yin, Spleen/Lung, Shao Yin, Kidney/Heart), Clock Neighbor (Spleen/Heart), Branch (You/Chicken, Lung/Kidney, 5PM-6:59PM)

Shan Yao, Huai Shan Yao, Huai Shan, Shan Shu (Rhizoma Dioscoriae, Chinese Yam)
Tonify Qi
Sweet, Sour,[836] slightly Astringent
Neutral
Kidney, Lung, **Spleen**, Dai[837]
Name (Tai Yin, Lung/Spleen), Branch (You/Chicken, Lung/Kidney, 5PM-6:59PM) + Dai

Huang Qi (Radix Astragali, Astragalus Root, Milk Vetch Root)
Tonify Qi
Sweet
Slightly Warm
Spleen, Lung, San Jiao[838]
Name (Tai Yin, Spleen/Lung), Clock Opposite (Spleen/San Jiao)

Bai Zhu (Rhizoma Atractylodis Macrocephalae, White Atractylodes Rhizome)
Tonify Qi
Bitter, Sweet, Aromatic[839]
Warm to very Warm[840]
Spleen, Stomach
Biao/Li (Stomach/Spleen)

Geng Mi, Jing Mi (Semen Oryzae)
Tonify Qi
Sweet
Neutral[841] to Cool
Spleen, Stomach
Biao/Li (Stomach/Spleen)

Da Zao (Fructus Jujubae, Chinese Date, Jujube)
Tonify Qi
Sweet
Warm
Spleen, Stomach
Biao/Li (Stomach/Spleen)

Bian Dou, Bai Bian Dou (Semen Lablab Album, Hyacinth Bean)
Tonify Qi
Sweet, Bland[842]
Neutral[843] to slightly Warm
Spleen, Stomach
Biao/Li (Stomach/Spleen)

Tonify Yang

Bu Gu Zhi, Gu Zi, Po Gu Zhi (Fructus Psoraleae, Psoralea Fruit)
Tonify Yang
Bitter, Acrid, Astringent[844]
Very Warm to Hot
Kidney, **Spleen**

Yi Zhi Ren, Yi Zhi, Yi Zhi Zi (Fructus Alpiniae Oxyphyllae, Black Cardamon)
Tonify Yang
Acrid, Astringent,[845] Aromatic
Warm
Kidney, **Spleen**

Xian Mao (Rhizoma Curculiginis, Golden Eye Grass Rhizome)
Tonify Yang
Acrid
Warm[846] to Hot, Toxic*
Kidney, Liver,[847] **Spleen**[848] and possibly San Jiao[849]
Branch (Chou/Ox, Spleen/Liver, 1AM-2:59AM) + Kidney
and possibly Bie Jing (Shao Yin/Shao Yang, Kidney/San Jiao), Clock Opposite (Spleen/San Jiao)

Tu Si Zi (Semen Cuscutae, Chinese Dodder Seeds)
Tonify Yang
Acrid, Sweet, Astringent[850]
Neutral to Warm[851]
Liver, Kidney, **Spleen**[852]
Branch (Chou/Ox, Spleen/Liver, 1AM-2:59AM) + Kidney

Tonify Blood

Long Yan Rou (Arillus Longan, Longan Fruit Flesh)
Tonify Blood
Sweet, not Astringent[853]
Warm
Heart, **Spleen**
Clock Neighbor (Spleen/Heart)

Dang Gui (Radix Angelica Sinensis, Chinese Angelica Root)
Tonify Blood
Sweet, Acrid, Bitter,[854] Aromatic
Warm
Heart, Liver, **Spleen**, Dai[855]
Clock Neighbor (Spleen/Heart), Branch (Chou/Ox, Spleen/Liver, 1AM-2:59AM) + Dai

Bai Shao (Radix Paeoniae Alba, White Peony Root)
Tonify Blood
Bitter, Sour, Sweet,[856] slightly Astringent
Cool to slightly Cold[857]
Liver, **Spleen**, Dai[858]
Branch (Chou/Ox, Spleen/Liver, 1AM-2:59AM) + Dai

Tonify Yin

Mai Men Dong, Mai Dong (Radix Ophiopogonis, Ophiopogon Tuber)
Tonify Yin
Sweet, slightly Bitter
Cool to slightly Cold[859]
Spleen,[860] Lung,[861] Stomach, Heart
Name (Tai Yin, Spleen/Lung), Biao/Li (Stomach/Spleen), Clock Neighbor (Spleen/Heart)

Xi Yang Shen, Hua Qi Shen (Radix Panacis Quinquefoli, American Ginseng Root)
Tonify Qi/Tonify Yin
Sweet, slightly Bitter[862] to Bitter to very Bitter[863]
Cold
Kidney, Heart, Lung, **Spleen**[864]
Name (Shao Yin, Kidney/Heart, Tai Yin, Spleen/Lung), Clock Neighbor (Spleen/Heart), Branch (You/Chicken, Lung/Kidney, 5PM-6:59PM)

Huang Jing, Mi Pu (Rhizoma Polygonati, Siberian Solomon Seal Rhizome)
Tonify Yin
Sweet
Neutral
Spleen, Lung, Kidney
Name (Tai Yin, Spleen/Lung), Branch (You/Chicken, Lung/Kidney, 5PM-6:59PM)

Chu Shi Zi, Chu Shi, Chu Shi Mi (Fructus Broussonetiae, Paper Mulberry Fruit)
Tonify Yin
Sweet
Cold
Kidney, Liver, **Spleen**[865]
Branch (Chou/Ox, Spleen/Liver, 1AM-2:59AM) + Kidney

Bie Jia (Carapax Trionycis, Chinese Soft Shell Turtle Shell)
Tonify Yin
Salty
Slightly Cold[866] to Cold
Liver, Kidney,[867] **Spleen**,[868] Chong[869]
Branch (Chou/Ox, Spleen/Liver, 1AM-2:59AM) + Kidney, Chong

Astringe, Stabilize and Bind

Wu Mei (Fructus Mume, Mume Fruit, Smoked Plum)
Astringe, Stabilize and Bind
Sour, Astringent
Neutral to Warm[870]
Liver, **Spleen**, Lung, Large Intestine
Name (Tai Yin, Spleen/Lung), Bie Jing (Jue Yin/Yang Ming, Liver/Large Intestine), Biao/Li (Large Intestine/Lung), Clock Neighbor (Liver/Lung), Branch (Chou/Ox, Spleen/Liver, 1AM-2:59AM, Mao/Rabbit, Liver/Large Intestine, 5AM-6:59AM)

Chi Shi Zhi (Halloysitum Rubrum, Red Halloysite)
Astringe, Stabilize and Bind
Sweet, Sour, Astringent[871]
Warm
Stomach, Large Intestine, **Spleen**[872]
Name (Yang Ming, Large Intestine/Stomach), Biao/Li (Stomach/Spleen), Clock Neighbor (Large Intestine/Stomach)

Rou Dou Kou (Semen Mystericae, Nutmeg Seeds)
Astringe, Stabilize and Bind
Acrid, Aromatic
Warm
Large Intestine, **Spleen**, Stomach
Name (Yang Ming, Large Intestine/Stomach), Biao/Li (Stomach/Spleen), Clock Neighbor (Large Intestine/Stomach)

He Ye Geng, Lian Geng (Nelumbinis Petiolus, Lotus Leafstalk)
Clear Heat Clean Toxin/Astringe, Stabilize and Bind
Bitter
Neutral
Spleen, Stomach
Biao/Li (Stomach/Spleen)

Lian Zi, Ou Shi, Lian Shi, Pi Guo (Semen Nelumbinis, Lotus Seed)
Astringe, Stabilize and Bind
Sweet, Astringent
Neutral
Heart, Kidney, **Spleen**
Name (Shao Yin, Heart/Kidney), Clock Neighbor (Spleen/Heart)

He Ye (Folium Nelumbinis, Lotus Leaf)
Clear Heat Clean Toxin/Astringe, Stabilize and Bind
Bitter, slightly Sweet,[873] Astringent, Aromatic[874]
Neutral
Heart, Liver, **Spleen**
Clock Neighbor (Spleen/Heart), Branch (Chou/Ox, Spleen/Liver, 1AM-2:59AM)

Qian Shi (Semen Euryales, Euryale Seed)
Astringe, Stabilize and Bind
Sweet, Astringent
Neutral
Kidney, **Spleen**, Dai[875]

External Application

Da Suan (Bulbus Alli Sativi, Garlic)
Expel Parasites/External Application
Acrid, Sweet[876]
Neutral to Warm
Spleen, Stomach, Lung, Large Intestine[877]
Name (Tai Yin, Spleen/Lung, Yang Ming, Large Intestine/Stomach), Biao/Li (Stomach/Spleen, Large Intestine/Lung), Clock Neighbor (Large Intestine/Stomach)

Ming Fan, Bai Fan, Ku Fan (Alumen, Alum)
External Application
Sour, Bitter,[878] Astringent
Cold, Toxic*
Lung, Liver, **Spleen**, Stomach,[879] Large Intestine[880]
Name (Tai Yin, Spleen/Lung, Yang Ming, Large Intestine/Stomach), Bie Jing (Jue Yin/Yang Ming, Liver/Large Intestine), Clock Neighbor (Liver/Lung, Large Intestine/Stomach), Biao/Li (Stomach/Spleen, Large Intestine/Lung), Branch (Chou/Ox, Spleen/Liver, 1AM-2:59AM, Mao/Rabbit, Liver/Large Intestine,[881] 5AM-6:59AM)

Wa Leng Zi (Concha Arcae, Cockle Shell, Ark Shell)
Vitalize Blood Transform Stasis/Transform Phlegm/External Application
Salty
Neutral
Liver, Stomach, Lung, **Spleen**[882]
Name (Tai Yin, Lung/Spleen), Biao/Li (Stomach/Spleen), Clock Neighbor (Liver/Lung), Branch (Chou/Ox, Spleen/Liver, 1AM-2:59AM)

Tu Jing Pi, Tu Jin Pi (Cortex Psuedolaricis, Golden Larch Bark)
External Application
Acrid, Bitter[883]
Warm, Toxic
Lung, **Spleen**
Name (Tai Yin, Lung/Spleen)

Zhang Nao (Camphora, Camphor)
External Application
Acrid, Aromatic
Hot, Toxic*
Heart, **Spleen**
Clock Neighbor (Spleen/Heart)

Qian Dan, Huang Dan (Minium, Lead Oxide)
External Application
Bitter, Acrid[884]
Cool to slightly Cold,[885] Toxic*
Heart, Liver, **Spleen**[886]
Clock Neighbor (Spleen, Heart), Branch (Chou/Ox, Spleen/Liver, 1AM-2:59AM)

Da Feng Zi (Semen Hydnocarpi, Hydnocarpus Seed, Chaulmoogra Seed)
External Application
Acrid, Bitter[887]
Hot, extremely Toxic*
Liver, **Spleen**, Kidney
Branch (Chou/Ox, Spleen/Liver,1AM-2:59AM) + Kidney

Ma Qian Zi (Semen Strychni, Nux Vomica)
External Application
Bitter, Acrid[888]
Cold, extremely Toxic*
Liver, **Spleen**
Branch (Chou/Ox, Spleen/Liver, 1AM-2:59AM)

Mi Tuo Seng (Lithargyum)
External Application
Salty, Acrid
Neutral, Toxic*
Liver, **Spleen**
Branch (Chou/Ox, Spleen/Liver, 1AM-2:59AM)

Hand Shao Yin Heart Herbs

Acrid Warm Exterior Releasing

Xiang Ru, Hua Qi Ning, Shi Xiang Rou (Herba Elsholtziae seu Moslae, Aromatic Madder)
Acrid Warm Exterior Releasing
Acrid, Aromatic
Slightly Warm
Lung, Spleen,[889] **Heart**,[890] Stomach
Name (Tai Yin, Lung/Spleen), Biao/Li (Stomach/Spleen), Clock Neighbor (Spleen/Heart)

Xi He Liu, Guan Yin Liu (Cacumen Tamaricis, Tamarisk stems and leaves)
Acrid Warm Exterior Releasing
Acrid, Sweet, Salty[891]
Warm
Lung, Stomach, **Heart**

Gui Zhi, Liu Gui (Ramulus Cinnamomi, Cassia Twig)
Acrid Warm Exterior Releasing
Acrid, Sweet
Warm
Heart, Lung, Urinary Bladder
Bie Jing (Tai Yin/Tai Yang, Lung/Urinary Bladder), Clock Opposite (Lung/Urinary Bladder) + Heart

Xi Xin (Radix et Rhizoma Asari, Asarum, Chinese Wild Ginger)
Acrid Warm Exterior Releasing/Warm Interior
Acrid to extremely Acrid,[892] Aromatic
Warm, slightly Toxic*
Lung, **Heart**, Kidney, Du,[893] all channels[894]
Name (Shao Yin, Heart/Kidney), Branch (You/Chicken, Lung/Kidney, 5PM-6:59PM) + Du

Clear Heat Purge Fire

Zhu Ye (Herba Phyllostachys, Bamboo Leaves)
Clear Heat Purge Fire
Sweet, Bland
Cold
Heart, Stomach, Lung

Lu Gen (Rhizoma Phragmitis, Reed Rhizome)
Clear Heat Purge Fire
Sweet, Bland[895]
Cold
Lung, Stomach, **Heart**[896]

Wu Long Cha (Folium Camellia Sinensis Fermentata, 'Oolong' Tea)
Clear Heat Purge Fire
Bitter, Sweet
Cool
Heart, Lung, Stomach, Small Intestine
Biao/Li (Small Intestine/Heart) + Lung, Stomach

Xi Gua (Fructus Citrulli, Watermelon Fruit)
Clear Heat Purge Fire
Sweet
Cold
Heart, Stomach, Urinary Bladder, Lung[897]
Bie Jing (Tai Yin/Tai Yang, Lung/Urinary Bladder), Clock Opposite (Lung/Urinary Bladder), Qian/Hou (Front/Back, Stomach/Urinary Bladder) + Heart

Shan Zhi Zi, Zhi Zi (Fructus Gardeniae, Cape Jasmine Fruit, Gardenia Fruit)
Clear Heat Purge Fire
Bitter
Cold
Heart, Lung, Stomach, San Jiao, Liver[898]
Clock Neighbor (Liver/Lung) + Heart, Stomach, San Jiao

Dan Zhu Ye (Herba Lophatheri, Lophatherum)
Clear Heat Purge Fire
Sweet, Bland
Cold
Heart, Stomach, Small Intestine
Biao/Li (Small Intestine/Heart) + Stomach

Xi Gua Pi (Exocarpium Citrulli, Watermelon Rind)
Clear Heat Purge Fire
Sweet
Cold
Heart, Stomach, Urinary Bladder
Qian/Hou (Front/Back, Stomach/Urinary Bladder) + Heart

Lian Zi Xin (Plumula Nelumbinis, Lotus Plumule)
Clear Heat Purge Fire
Bitter, Astringent
Slightly Cold to Cold[899]
Heart, Pericardium

Clear Heat Dry Dampness

Ku Shen, Ku Shen Gen, Ku Gu (Radix Sophorae Flavescentis, Flavescent Sophora Root)
Clear Heat Dry Dampness
Bitter to extremely Bitter[900]
Cold
Heart, Liver, Stomach, Large Intestine, Urinary Bladder, Small Intestine[901]
Name (Yang Ming, Large Intestine/Stomach, Tai Yang, Small Intestine/Urinary Bladder), Bie Jing (Jue Yin/Yang Ming, Liver/Large Intestine), Biao/Li (Small Intestine/Heart), Clock Opposite (Liver/Small Intestine), Clock Neighbor (Large Intestine/Stomach, Small Intestine/Urinary Bladder), Branch (Shen/Monkey, Large Intestine/Urinary Bladder, 3PM-4:59PM and Mao/Rabbit, Liver/Large Intestine, 5AM-6:59AM), Qian/Hou (Front/Back, Stomach/Urinary Bladder)

Huang Lian (Rhizoma Coptidis, Goldthread Rhizome, Coptis Root)
Clear Heat Dry Dampness
Very Bitter, purely Bitter[902]
Very Cold
Heart, Liver, Stomach, Large Intestine, Du[903]
Name (Yang Ming, Large Intestine/Stomach), Bie Jing (Jue Yin/Yang Ming, Liver/Large Intestine), Clock Neighbor (Large Intestine/Stomach), Branch (Mao/Rabbit, Liver/Large Intestine, 5AM-6:59AM) + Heart, Du

Clear Heat Cool Blood

Dong Qing Ye (Folium Ilexis, Ilex)
Clear Heat Cool Blood
Bitter, Astringent
Cold
Lung, **Heart**

Shui Niu Jiao (Bubali Cornu, Water Buffalo Horn)
Clear Heat Cool Blood
Salty, Bitter[904]
Cold
Heart, Liver, Stomach

Mu Dan Pi, Mu Shao Yao (Cortex Moutan, Peony Tree Root Cortex)
Clear Heat Cool Blood/Vitalize Blood Transform Stasis
Bitter, Acrid, Aromatic
Cool to slightly Cold
Heart, Liver, Kidney, Pericardium[905]
Name (Shao Yin, Heart/Kidney, Jue Yin, Liver/Pericardium), Clock Neighbor (Kidney/Pericardium)

Sheng Di Huang (Radix Rehmanniae, Chinese Foxglove Root)
Clear Heat Cool Blood
Sweet, Bitter
Cold
Heart, Liver, Kidney
Name (Shao Yin, Heart/Kidney) + Liver

Zi Cao, Zi Cao Gen (Radix Lithospermi, Arnebia, Groomwell Root)
Clear Heat Cool Blood
Sweet, Salty,[906] Bitter[907]
Cold
Heart, Liver

Clear Heat Clean Toxin

Shan Dou Gen, Dou Gen, Nan Dou Gen (Radix Sophorae Tonkinensis, Subprostrate, Sophora Root)
Clear Heat Clean Toxin
Bitter to very Bitter[908]
Cold, slightly Toxic*
Lung, Stomach,[909] Large Intestine,[910] **Heart**[911]
Name (Yang Ming, Large Intestine/Stomach), Biao/Li (Large Intestine/Lung), Clock Neighbor (Large Intestine/Stomach) + Heart

Jin Yin Hua (Flos Lonicerae, Honeysuckle Flower, Lonicera Flower)
Clear Heat Clean Toxin
Sweet
Cold
Lung, Stomach, Large Intestine, **Heart**[912]
Name (Yang Ming, Large Intestine/Stomach), Biao/Li (Large Intestine/Lung), Clock Neighbor (Large Intestine/Stomach) + Heart

Ban Lan Gen, Bei Ban Lan Gen (Radix Isatidis, Isatis Root)
Clear Heat Clean Toxin
Bitter
Cold
Heart, Stomach, Lung[913]

Da Qing Ye (Folium Isatidis, Woad Leaf, Indigo Leaf)
Clear Heat Clean Toxin
Bitter, Salty[914]
Very Cold
Heart, Lung, Stomach, Liver[915]
Clock Neighbor (Liver/Lung) + Heart, Stomach

Nan Ban Lan Ye, Ma Lian Ye (Folium Baphicacanthis)
Clear Heat Clean Toxin
Bitter, Salty
Cold
Lung, Stomach, **Heart**, Liver
Clock Neighbor (Liver/Lung) + Stomach, Heart

Ban Bian Lian (Herba Lobeliae Chinensis)
Clear Heat Clean Toxin/Regulate Water Resolve Dampness
Acrid, Sweet,[916] Bland[917]
Slightly Cold[918] to Cold, Toxic*[919]
Heart, Lung, Small Intestine
Biao/Li (Small Intestine/Heart) + Lung

Lian Qiao (Fructus Forsythiae, Forsythia Fruit)
Clear Heat Clean Toxin
Bitter, slightly Acrid[920]
Cool to slightly Cold[921]
Lung, **Heart**, Gall Bladder
Bie Jing (Shao Yin/Shao Yang, Heart/Gall Bladder), Clock Opposite (Heart/Gall Bladder), Branch (Yin/Tiger, Gall Bladder/Lung, 3AM-4:59AM)

Shan Ma Ti (Radix Rauvolfiae, Devil Pepper Root)
Clear Heat Clean Toxin
Bitter
Cold, slightly Toxic*
Lung, Liver, **Heart**
Clock Neighbor (Liver/Lung) + Heart

Bai Lian, Bai Cao, Tu He, Kun Lun, Mao Er Luan (Radix Ampelopsis)
Clear Heat Clean Toxin
Bitter, Acrid, Sweet[922]
Neutral to Cool to Cold[923]
Heart, Stomach, Liver, Spleen[924]
Biao/Li (Stomach/Spleen), Clock Neighbor (Spleen/Heart), Branch (Chou/Ox, Spleen/Liver, 1AM-2:59AM)

Lu Dou Yi (Pericarpium Phaseoli Radiati, Mung Bean Skin)
Clear Heat Clean Toxin
Sweet
Cold
Heart, Stomach

Lu Dou (Semen Phaseoli Radiati, Mung Bean)
Clear Heat Clean Toxin
Sweet
Cold
Heart, Stomach

Zi Hua Di Ding, Jian Tou Cao, Di Ding Cao (Herba Violae, Yedeon's Violet)
Clear Heat Clean Toxin
Bitter, Acrid
Cold
Heart, Liver, Stomach,[925] Pericardium[926]
Name (Jue Yin, Pericardium/Liver), Bie Jing (Jue Yin/Yang Ming, Pericardium/Stomach), Clock Opposite (Pericardium/Stomach), Branch (Shu/Dog, Stomach/Pericardium, 7PM-8:59PM) + Heart

Nan Ban Lan Gen (Rhizoma et Radix Baphicacathis)
Clear Heat Clean Toxin
Bitter
Cold
Heart, Liver, Stomach

He Ye (Folium Nelumbinis, Lotus Leaf)
Clear Heat Clean Toxin/Astringe, Stabilize and Bind
Bitter, slightly Sweet,[927] Astringent, Aromatic
Neutral
Heart, Liver, Spleen
Clock Neighbor (Spleen/Heart), Branch (Chou/Ox, Spleen/Liver, 1AM-2:59AM)

Niu Huang (Calculus Bovis, Cattle Bezoar, Cattle Gallstone)
Clear Heat Clean Toxin/Open Orifices
Bitter, Aromatic
Cool to Cold[928]
Liver, **Heart**, Gall Bladder[929]
Bie Jing (Shao Yin/Shao Yang, Heart/Gall Bladder), Biao/Li (Gall Bladder/Liver), Clock Opposite (Heart/Gall Bladder)

Clear Deficient Heat

Hu Huang Lian, Hu Lian (Rhizoma Picrorhizae, Picrorhiza, Figwort Rhizome)
Clear Deficient Heat
Bitter, Astringing[930]
Cold
Heart, Liver, Stomach, Large Intestine
Name (Yang Ming, Large Intestine, Stomach), Bie Jing (Jue Yin/Yang Ming, Liver/Large Intestine), Clock Neighbor (Large Intestine, Stomach), Branch (Mao/Rabbit, Liver/Large Intestine, 5AM-6:59AM) + Heart

Purgative

Da Huang (Radix et Rhizoma Rhei, Rhubarb Root and Rhizome)
Purgative
Bitter to very Bitter[931] to purely Bitter,[932] Aromatic[933]
Cold to very Cold[934]
Spleen, Stomach, Large Intestine, Liver, **Heart**, Du[935]
Name (Yang Ming, Large Intestine/Stomach), Bie Jing (Jue Yin/Yang Ming, Liver/Large Intestine), Biao/Li (Stomach/Spleen), Clock Neighbor (Spleen/Heart, Large Intestine/Stomach), Branch (Chou/Ox, Spleen/Liver, 1AM-2:59AM and Mao/Rabbit, Liver/Large Intestine, 5AM-6:59AM) + Du

Dispel Wind Dampness, Open Channels and Luo-Network Vessels and Relieve Pain

Hai Feng Teng (Caulis Piperis Kadsurae, Kadsura Pepper Stem, Futokadsura Stem)
Dispel Wind Dampness, Open Channels and Luo-Network Vessels and Relieve Pain
Acrid, Bitter, Aromatic
Slightly Warm
Liver, **Heart**,[936] Kidney[937]
Name (Shao Yin, Heart/Kidney) + Liver

Luo Shi Teng, Luo Shi, Bai Hua Teng (Caulis Trachelospermi, Star Jasmine Stem)
Dispel Wind Dampness, Open Channels and Luo-Network Vessels and Relieve Pain
Bitter
Cool to slightly Cold[938]
Heart, Liver

Dispel Wind-Dampness Strengthen Sinew/Tendon and Bone

Xiang Jia Pi (Cortex Periplocae, Chinese Silkvine Root Bark)
Dispel Wind-Dampness Strengthen Sinew/Tendon and Bone
Acrid, Bitter
Warm, Toxic*
Liver, Kidney, **Heart**
Name (Shao Yin, Kidney/Heart) + Liver

Regulate Water Resolve Dampness

Cha Ye (Folium Theae, Tea Leaves)
Regulate Water Resolve Dampness
Bitter, Sweet
Cool
Heart, Lung, Stomach

Fu Ling, Yun Ling (Poria, Hoelen, China Root)
Regulate Water Resolve Dampness
Sweet, Bland
Neutral
Heart, Spleen, Kidney, Lung[939]
Name (Shao Yin, Heart/Kidney, Tai Yin, Spleen/Lung), Clock Neighbor (Spleen/Heart)

Deng Xin Cao (Medulla Junci, Juncus, Rush Pith)
Regulate Water Resolve Dampness
Sweet, Bland
Cool to slightly Cold[940]
Heart, Lung, Small Intestine
Biao/Li (Small Intestine/Heart) + Lung

Ban Bian Lian (Herba Lobeliae Chinensis)
Clear Heat Clean Toxin/Regulate Water Resolve Dampness
Acrid, Sweet,[941] Bland[942]
Slightly Cold[943] to Cold, Toxic*[944]
Heart, Lung, Small Intestine
Biao/Li (Small Intestine/Heart) + Lung

Chuan Mu Tong (Caulis Clematidis Armandii, Armand's Clematis)
Regulate Water Resolve Dampness
Bitter, Bland[945]
Cold
Urinary Bladder, **Heart**, Lung,[946] Small Intestine
Name (Tai Yang, Small Intestine/Urinary Bladder), Bie Jing (Tai Yin/Tai Yang, Lung/Urinary Bladder), Biao/Li (Small Intestine/Heart), Clock Opposite (Lung/Urinary Bladder), Clock Neighbor (Small Intestine/Urinary Bladder)

Chi Xiao Dou, Hong Dou (Semen Phaseoli, Phaseolus, Adzuki Bean, Rice Bean)
Regulate Water Resolve Dampness
Sweet, Sour
Neutral
Heart, Small Intestine
Biao/Li (Small Intestine/Heart)

Qu Mai (Herba Dianthi, Dianthus, Fringed Pink, Lilac Pink, Chinese Pink, Rainbow Pink)
Regulate Water Resolve Dampness
Bitter
Cold
Urinary Bladder, **Heart**, Small Intestine
Name (Tai Yang, Small Intestine/Urinary Bladder), Biao/Li (Small Intestine/Heart), Clock Neighbor (Small Intestine/Urinary Bladder)

Mu Tong (Caulis Akebiae, Akebia)
Regulate Water Resolve Dampness
Bitter
Slightly Cold
Urinary Bladder, **Heart**, Small Intestine
Name (Tai Yang, Small Intestine/Urinary Bladder), Biao/Li (Small Intestine/Heart), Clock Neighbor (Small Intestine/Urinary Bladder)

Warm Interior

Gan Jiang (Rhizoma Zingiberis, Dried Ginger Root)
Warm Interior
Acrid, Aromatic
Hot
Heart, Lung, Spleen, Stomach
Name (Tai Yin, Lung/Spleen), Biao/Li (Stomach/Spleen), Clock Neighbor (Spleen/Heart)

Xi Xin (Radix et Rhizoma Asari, Asarum, Chinese Wild Ginger)
Acrid Warm Exterior Releasing/Warm Interior
Acrid to extremely Acrid,[947] Aromatic
Warm, slightly Toxic*
Lung, **Heart**, Kidney, Du,[948] all channels[949]
Name (Shao Yin, Heart/Kidney), Branch (You/Chicken, Lung/Kidney, 5PM-6:59PM) + Du

Zhi Cao Wu (Radix Aconiti Kusnezoffii, Wild Aconite Root)
Warm Interior
Acrid, Bitter
Hot, extremely Toxic**
Heart, Liver, Spleen, Kidney[950]
Name (Shao Yin, Kidney/Heart), Clock Neighbor (Spleen/Heart), Branch (Chou/Ox, Spleen/Liver, 1AM-2:59AM)

Rou Gui (Cortex Cinnamomi, Cinnamon Bark, Cassia Bark)
Warm Interior
Acrid to highly Acrid,[951] Sweet, Aromatic
Greatly Warming[952] to Hot
Heart, Kidney, Liver, Spleen
Name (Shao Yin, Heart/Kidney), Clock Neighbor (Spleen/Heart), Branch (Chou/Ox, Spleen/Liver, 1AM-2:59AM)

Zhi Fu Zi, Tian Xiong (Radix Aconiti Lateralis Praeparata, Aconite, Prepared/Processed Aconite Accessory Root)
Warm Interior
Acrid to extremely Acrid,[953] Sweet[954]
Hot to very Hot,[955] Toxic*
Heart, Kidney, Spleen, Du[956]
Name (Shao Yin, Heart/Kidney), Clock Neighbor (Spleen/Heart) + Du

Zhi Chuan Wu (Radix Aconiti Preparata, Prepared Aconite Main Root, Mother Root of Common Monk's Hood)
Warm Interior
Acrid, Bitter
Hot, extremely Toxic**
Heart, Liver, Spleen, Du[957]
Clock Neighbor (Spleen/Heart), Branch (Chou/Ox, Spleen/Liver, 1AM-2:59AM) + Du

Regulate and Rectify Qi

Tian Xian Teng, Ma Dou Ling Teng (Herba Aristolochiae, Aristolochia, Dutchman's Pipe)
Regulate and Rectify Qi
Bitter
Warm, Toxic*
Heart, Lung, Spleen, Kidney
Name (Shao Yin, Heart/Kidney, Tai Yin, Spleen/Lung)
Clock Neighbor (Spleen/Heart), Branch (You/Chicken, Lung/Kidney, 5PM-6:59PM)

Expel Parasites

Chang Shan (Radix Dichroae, Dichroa Root)
Expel Parasites/Emetic
Acrid, Bitter
Cold, Toxic*
Lung, **Heart**, Liver
Clock Neighbor (Liver/Lung) + Heart

Stop Bleeding

Xue Yu Tan (Crinis Carbonitsatus, Charred Human Hair)
Stop Bleeding
Bitter, Astringent[958]
Neutral
Liver, Stomach, **Heart**,[959] Kidney[960]
Name (Shao Yin, Heart/Kidney) + Liver, Stomach

Pu Huang (Pollen Typhae, Cattail Pollen, Bulrush Pollen)
Stop Bleeding
Sweet, Acrid,[961] Astringent,[962] Aromatic[963]
Neutral
Liver, Pericardium,[964] **Heart**,[965] Spleen[966]
Name (Jue Yin, Liver/Pericardium), Clock Neighbor (Spleen/Heart), Branch (Chou/Ox, Spleen/Liver, 1AM-2:59AM)

Da Ji, Da Xiao Ji (Herba seu Radix Cirsii Japonici, Japanese Thistle)
Stop Bleeding
Sweet, Bitter, slightly Acrid[967]
Cool
Liver, **Heart**, Spleen[968]
Clock Neighbor (Spleen/Heart), Branch (Chou/Ox, Spleen/Liver, 1AM-2:59AM)

Xiao Ji, Da Xiao Ji (Herba Cirisii, Cirsium, Field Thistle)
Stop Bleeding
Bitter,[969] Sweet
Cool
Liver, **Heart**, Small Intestine,[970] Urinary Bladder[971]
Name (Tai Yang, Small Intestine/Urinary Bladder), Biao/Li (Small Intestine/Heart), Clock Opposite (Liver/Small Intestine), Clock Neighbor (Small Intestine/Urinary Bladder)

Qian Cao, Qian Cao Gen, Qian Gen (Radix Rubiae, Rubia Root)
Stop Bleeding
Bitter
Cold
Liver, **Heart**[972]

Zhu Ma Gen (Boemeriae Radix, Ramie Root)
Stop Bleeding
Sweet
Cold
Heart, Liver

Vitalize Blood Transform Stasis

Tao Ren (Semen Persicae, Peach Kernel)
Vitalize Blood Transform Stasis
Bitter, Sweet[973]
Neutral, slightly Toxic*
Heart, Large Intestine, Liver, Lung
Bie Jing (Jue Yin/Yang Ming, Liver/Large Intestine), Biao/Li (Large Intestine/Lung), Clock Neighbor (Liver/Lung), Branch (Mao/Rabbit, Liver/Large Intestine, 5AM-6:59AM) + Heart

Yu Jin (Radix Curcumae, Aromatic Tumeric Tuber)
Vitalize Blood Transform Stasis
Acrid, Bitter, Aromatic
Cold
Heart, Liver, Gall Bladder, Lung[974]
Bie Jing (Shao Yin/Shao Yang, Heart/Gall Bladder), Biao/Li (Gall Bladder/Liver), Clock Opposite (Heart/Gall Bladder), Clock Neighbor (Liver/Lung), Branch (Yin/Tiger, Gall Bladder/Lung, 3AM-4:59AM)

Yan Hu Suo (Rhizoma Corydalis, Corydalis Rhizome)
Vitalize Blood Transform Stasis
Acrid, Bitter, Aromatic
Warm
Heart, Liver, Spleen, Stomach[975]
Biao/Li (Stomach/Spleen), Clock Neighbor (Spleen/Heart), Branch (Chou/Ox, Spleen/Liver, 1AM-2:59AM)

Jiang Xiang (Lignum Dalbergiae Odoriferae, Dalbergia Heartwood, Rosewood)
Vitalize Blood Transform Stasis
Acrid, Aromatic
Warm
Liver, Spleen, **Heart**, Stomach[976]
Biao/Li (Stomach/Spleen), Clock Neighbor (Spleen/Heart), Branch (Chou/Ox, Spleen/Liver, 1AM-2:59AM)

Liu Ji Nu, Hua Shi Dan (Herba Artemisiae Anomalae, Artemesia)
Vitalize Blood Transform Stasis
Bitter, Aromatic
Warm
Heart, Spleen
Clock Neighbor (Spleen/Heart)

Mao Dong Qing (Radix Ilicis Pubescentis, Hairy Holly Root)
Vitalize Blood Transform Stasis
Bitter, Acrid,[977] Astringent
Neutral to slightly Cold[978]
Heart, Spleen
Clock Neighbor (Spleen, Heart)

Ji Xue Teng, Da Xue Teng (Caulis Spatholobi, Spatholobus, Millettia Vine)
Vitalize Blood Transform Stasis
Bitter, slightly Sweet, Acrid[979]
Warm
Heart,[980] Liver, Spleen[981]
Clock Neighbor (Spleen/Heart), Branch (Chou/Ox, Spleen/Liver, 1AM-2:59AM)

Mo Yao (Commiphora Myrrha, Myrrh)
Vitalize Blood Transform Stasis
Acrid,[982] Bitter, Aromatic
Neutral
Heart, Liver, Spleen
Clock Neighbor (Spleen/Heart), Branch (Chou/Ox, Spleen/Liver, 1AM-2:59AM)

Ru Xiang (Boswelia Carterii, Gummi Olibanum, Frankincense)
Vitalize Blood Transform Stasis
Acrid, Bitter, Aromatic
Warm
Heart, Liver, Spleen
Clock Neighbor (Spleen/Heart), Branch (Chou/Ox, Spleen/Liver, 1AM-2:59AM)

Su Mu (Lignum Sappan, Sappan Wood, Brazilwood)
Vitalize Blood Transform Stasis
Sweet, Salty, slightly Acrid to Acrid[983]
Neutral to slightly Cooling[984]
Heart, Liver, Spleen[985]
Clock Neighbor (Spleen/Heart), Branch (Chou/Ox, Spleen/Liver, 1AM-2:59AM)

Di Bie Chong, Tu Bie Chong, Zhe Chong (Eupolyphagia, Wingless Cockroach, Ground Beetle)
Vitalize Blood Transform Stasis
Salty
Cold, slightly Toxic*
Liver, **Heart**, Spleen
Clock Neighbor (Spleen/Heart), Branch (Chou/Ox, Spleen/Liver, 1AM-2:59AM)

Yi Mu Cao (Herba Leonuri, Chinese Motherwort)
Vitalize Blood Transform Stasis
Acrid, Bitter
Cool to slightly Cold[986]
Heart, Liver, Urinary Bladder

Mu Dan Pi, Mu Shao Yao (Cortex Moutan, Peony Tree Root Cortex)
Clear Heat Cool Blood/Vitalize Blood Transform Stasis
Bitter, Acrid, Aromatic
Cool to slightly Cold
Heart, Liver, Kidney, Pericardium[987]
Name (Shao Yin, Heart/Kidney, Jue Yin, Liver/Pericardium), Clock Neighbor (Kidney/Pericardium)

Dan Shen (Radix Salviae Miltiorrhizae, Salvia Root)
Vitalize Blood Transform Stasis
Bitter
Cool to slightly Cold[988] to Warm[989]
Heart, Pericardium,[990] Liver
Name (Jue Yin, Pericardium/Liver) + Heart

Hong Hua (Flos Carthami, Safflower Flower)
Vitalize Blood Transform Stasis
Acrid, Bitter,[991] Sweet[992]
Slightly Cool[993] to Warm
Heart, Liver

Xi Hong Hua, Fan Hong Hua, Zhang Hong Hua (Flos Crocus Sativus, Crocus Stigma, Saffron)
Vitalize Blood Transform Stasis
Sweet
Cool to slightly Cold[994] to Cold[995]
Heart, Liver

Xue Jie (Daemonoropis Resina, Sanguis Draconis, Dragon's Blood)
Vitalize Blood Transform Stasis/External Application
Sweet, Acrid,[996] Salty,[997] Aromatic
Neutral
Heart, Liver

Transform Phlegm

Zhu Li (Succus Bambusae, Dried Bamboo Sap)
Transform Phlegm
Sweet, Bitter[998]
Cold
Heart, Lung, Stomach, Liver[999]
Clock Neighbor (Liver/Lung) + Heart, Stomach

Zhe Bei Mu, Da Bei Mu (Bulbus Fritillariae Thunbergii, Thunbergy Fritillary Bulb)
Transform Phlegm
Bitter
Cold
Heart, Lung

Chuan Bei Mu (Bulbus Fritillarie Cirrhosae, Sichuan Fritillaria Bulb, Tendrilled Fritillaria Bulb)
Transform Phlegm
Bitter, Sweet
Cool to slightly Cold[1000]
Heart, Lung

Tian Zhu Huang (Concretio Silicea Bambusae, Siliceous Secretions of Bamboo, Bamboo Sugar, Tabasheer)
Transform Phlegm
Sweet, Bitter[1001]
Cold
Gall Bladder, **Heart**, Liver
Bie Jing (Shao Yin/Shao Yang, Heart/Gall Bladder), Biao/Li (Gall Bladder/Liver), Clock Opposite (Heart/Gall Bladder)

Relieve Cough and Wheezing/Panting

Yang Jin Hua (Flos Daturae, Datura Flower)
Relieve Cough and Wheezing/Panting
Acrid
Warm, Toxic*
Lung, Liver, **Heart**, Spleen
Name (Tai Yin, Lung/Spleen), Clock Neighbor (Liver/Lung, Spleen/Heart), Branch (Chou/Ox, Spleen/Liver, 1AM-2:59AM)

Kuan Dong Hua, Dong Hua, Jiu Jiu Hua (Flos Farfarae, Coltsfoot Flower)
Relieve Cough and Wheezing/Panting
Acrid, slightly Bitter,[1002] Sweet[1003]
Warm
Lung, **Heart**,[1004] Liver[1005]
Clock Neighbor (Liver/Lung) + Heart

Nourish and Calm Shen

He Huan Hua, Ye He Hua, Ye He Mi (Flos Albiziae, Mimosa Flower)
Nourish and Calm Shen
Sweet
Neutral
Liver, Stomach, Spleen,[1006] **Heart**,[1007] Lung[1008]
Name (Tai Yin, Lung/Spleen), Biao/Li (Stomach/Spleen), Clock Neighbor (Spleen/Heart, Liver/Lung), Branch (Chou/Ox, Spleen/Liver, 1AM-2:59AM)

Yuan Zhi (Radix Polygalae, Senega Root)
Nourish and Calm Shen
Acrid, Bitter
Slightly Warm
Lung, **Heart**, Kidney[1009]
Name (Shao Yin, Heart/Kidney), Branch (You/Chicken, Lung/Kidney, 5PM-6:59PM)

Ling Zhi, Zhi, Ling Zhi Cao (Ganoderma, Reishi Mushroom)
Nourish and Calm Shen
Sweet
Neutral
Heart, Liver, Lung
Clock Neighbor (Liver/Lung) + Heart

Bai Zi Ren (Semen Platycadi, Arbor-Vitae Seed, Biota)
Nourish and Calm Shen
Sweet, Acrid,[1010] Aromatic[1011]
Neutral to Cool[1012]
Heart, Kidney, Large Intestine
Name (Shao Yin, Kidney/Heart), Clock Opposite (Kidney/Large Intestine)

Suan Zao Ren, Dong Zao (Semen Zizyphi Spinosae, Sour Jujube Seed)
Nourish and Calm Shen
Sweet, Sour[1013]
Neutral
Heart, Liver, Gall Bladder,[1014] Spleen[1015]
Bie Jing (Shao Yin/Shao Yang, Heart/Gall Bladder), Biao/Li (Gall Bladder/Liver), Clock Opposite (Heart/Gall Bladder), Clock Neighbor (Spleen/Heart), Branch (Chou/Ox, Spleen/Liver, 1AM-2:59AM)

Xiao Mai, Jing Xiao Mai (Fructus Tritici, Wheat)
Nourish and Calm Shen
Sweet
Cool
Heart
Branch (Wu/Horse, Heart/Heart, 11AM-12:59PM)

Ye Jiao Teng, Shou Wu Teng (Caulis Polygoni Multiflori, Polygonum Vine, Fleeceflower Vine, Flowery Knotweed Stem)
Nourish and Calm Shen
Sweet, slightly Bitter
Neutral
Heart, Liver

Xie Cao, Jie Cao (Radix et Rhizoma Valerianae, Valerian Root)
Nourish and Calm Shen
Bitter, Sweet, Acrid[1016]
Neutral to Warm[1017]
Heart, Liver

He Huan Pi (Cortex Albiziae, Mimosa Tree Bark)
Nourish and Calm Shen
Sweet
Neutral
Heart, Liver

Ye He Hua (Flos Magnoliae Cocinis, Magnolia Flower)
Nourish and Calm Shen
Acrid, Aromatic[1018]
Warm
Liver, **Heart**

Calm Shen Sedative

Long Chi (Fossilia Mastodi Dentis, fossilized teeth)
Calm Shen Sedative
Sweet, Astringent
Cool
Heart, Liver, Lung[1019]
Clock Neighbor (Liver/Lung) + Heart

Hu Po (Succinum, Amber)
Calm Shen Sedative
Sweet, Bland[1020]
Neutral
Heart, Liver, Urinary Bladder[1021]

Ci Shi (Magnetitum, Magnetite, Loadstone)
Calm Shen Sedative
Acrid,[1022] Salty
Cold
Liver, Kidney, **Heart**
Name (Shao Yin, Kidney/Heart) + Liver

Long Gu (Os Draconis, Fossilia Mastodi Ossis, Fossilized Bones)
Calm Shen Sedative
Sweet, slightly Acrid,[1023] Astringent[1024]
Neutral[1025] to Cool to slightly Cold[1026]
Heart, Liver, Kidney,[1027] Dai[1028]
Name (Shao Yin, Heart/Kidney) + Liver, Dai

Zhen Zhu (Margarita, Pearl)
Calm Shen Sedative/Calm Liver Extinguish Wind
Sweet, Salty, Bland,[1029] Astringent[1030]
Cold
Heart, Liver

Zhen Zhu Mu (Concha Margaritaferae, Mother of Pearl)
Calm Shen Sedative/Calm Liver Extinguish Wind
Salty, Sweet[1031]
Cool[1032] to Cold
Heart, Liver

Sheng Tie Luo, Tie Luo (Frusta Ferri, Oxidized Iron Filings)
Calm Shen Sedative/Anchor, Settle and Calm the Spirit
Acrid
Cool
Heart, Liver

Zi Shi Ying (Floritum, Flourite)
Calm Shen Sedative/Calm Liver Extinguish Wind
Sweet, Acrid
Warm
Heart, Liver, Chong and Ren[1033]

Calm Liver Extinguish Wind

Dai Zhe Shi, Zhe Shi (Haematitum, Hematite)
Calm Liver Extinguish Wind
Bitter
Cold
Heart, Liver, Pericardium[1034]
Name (Jue Yin, Liver/Pericardium) + Heart

Gou Teng (Ramulus Uncariae cum Uncis, Gambir Vine Stems and Thorns)
Calm Liver Extinguish Wind
Sweet
Cool to slightly Cold[1035]
Liver, Pericardium, **Heart**[1036]
Name (Jue Yin, Liver/Pericardium) + Heart

Zhen Zhu (Margarita, Pearl)
Calm Shen Sedative/Calm Liver Extinguish Wind
Sweet, Salty, Bland,[1037] Astringent[1038]
Cold
Heart, Liver

Zhen Zhu Mu (Concha Margaritaferae, Mother of Pearl)
Calm Shen Sedative/Calm Liver Extinguish Wind
Salty, Sweet[1039]
Cool[1040] to Cold
Heart, Liver

Ling Yang Jiao (Cornu Saigae Tataricae, Antelope Horn)
Calm Liver Extinguish Wind
Salty
Cold
Liver, **Heart**

Zi Shi Ying (Floritum, Flourite)
Calm Shen Sedative/Calm Liver Extinguish Wind
Sweet, Acrid
Warm
Heart, Liver, Chong and Ren[1041]

Open Orifices

Bing Pian, Long Nao Bing Pian (Borneolum, Borneolum Syntheticum, Borneol)
Open Orifices
Acrid, Bitter, Aromatic
Slightly Cold[1042] to Hot[1043]
Heart, Spleen, Lung
Name (Tai Yin, Spleen/Lung), Clock Neighbor (Spleen/Heart)

Shui Chang Pu, Bai Chang Pu (Rhizoma Acori Calami, Calamus, Sweetflag Rhizome)
Open Orifices
Bitter, Acrid, slightly Toxic*
Warm
Heart, Liver, Stomach, Spleen,[1044] Large Intestine[1045]
Name (Yang Ming, Large Intestine/Stomach), Bie Jing (Jue Yin/Yang Ming, Liver/Large Intestine), Biao/Li (Stomach/Spleen), Clock Neighbor (Spleen/Heart, Large Intestine/Stomach), Branch (Chou/Ox, Spleen/Liver, 1AM-2:59AM and Mao/Rabbit, Liver/Large Intestine, 5AM-6:59AM)

Shi Chang Pu (Rhizoma Acori Tatarinowii, Grassleaf Sweetflag Rhizome, Acorus)
Open Orifices
Bitter,[1046] Acrid, Aromatic
Warm, slightly Toxic*
Heart, Stomach

Su He Xiang (Styrax, Resin of Rose Maloes, Styrax)
Open Orifices
Acrid, Sweet,[1047] Aromatic
Warm
Heart, Spleen
Clock Neighbor (Spleen/Heart)

An Xi Xiang (Benzoinum, Benzoin)
Open Orifices
Acrid, Bitter, Aromatic
Neutral
Heart, Liver, Spleen
Clock Neighbor (Spleen/Heart), Branch (Chou/Ox, Spleen/Liver, 1AM-2:59AM)

Jiu Jie Chang Pu, Jing Chang Pu (Rhizoma Anemones Altaicae)
Open Orifices
Acrid
Warm, slightly Toxic*
Heart, Liver, Spleen
Clock Neighbor (Spleen/Heart), Branch (Chou/Ox, Spleen/Liver, 1AM-2:59AM)

She Xiang (Moschus, Musk, Navel Gland Secretions of Musk Deer)
Open Orifices
Acrid, Aromatic
Warm
Heart, Liver, Spleen, some sources say all channels.
Clock Neighbor (Spleen/Heart), Branch (Chou/Ox, Spleen/Liver, 1AM-2:59AM)

Niu Huang (Calculus Bovis, Cattle Bezoar, Cattle Gallstone)
Clear Heat Clean Toxin/Open Orifices
Bitter, Aromatic
Cool to Cold[1048]
Liver, **Heart**, Gall Bladder[1049]
Bie Jing (Shao Yin/Shao Yang, Heart/Gall Bladder), Biao/Li (Gall Bladder/Liver), Clock Opposite (Heart/Gall Bladder)

Tonify Qi

Gan Cao (Radix Glycyrrhizae, Licorice Root)
Tonify Qi
Sweet
Neutral
Spleen, Stomach, Lung, **Heart**, Dai,[1050] some sources indicate that it enters all channels.
Name (Tai Yin, Spleen/Lung), Biao/Li (Stomach/Spleen), Clock Neighbor (Spleen/Heart) + Dai, some sources indicate that Gan Cao enters all channels and therefore creates every relationship.

Jiao Gu Lan, Qi Dan Ye, Long Xu Teng (Rhizoma seu Herba Gynostemmatis)
Tonify Qi
Sweet,[1051] slightly Bitter
Cold
Spleen,[1052] Lung, **Heart**[1053]
Name (Tai Yin, Spleen/Lung), Clock Neighbor (Spleen/Heart)

Xi Yang Shen, Hua Qi Shen (Radix Panacis Quinquefoli, American Ginseng Root)
Tonify Qi/Tonify Yin
Sweet, slightly Bitter[1054] to Bitter to very Bitter[1055]
Cold
Kidney, **Heart**, Lung, Spleen[1056]
Name (Shao Yin, Kidney/Heart, Tai Yin, Spleen/Lung), Clock Neighbor (Spleen/Heart), Branch (You/Chicken, Lung/Kidney, 5PM-6:59PM)

Ren Shen (Radix Ginseng, Ginseng Root)
Tonify Qi
Sweet, slightly Bitter
Slightly Warm
Lung, Spleen, **Heart**,[1057] Kidney[1058]
Name (Tai Yin, Lung/Spleen, Shao Yin, Kidney/Heart), Clock Neighbor (Spleen/Heart), Branch (You/Chicken, Lung/Kidney, 5PM-6:59PM)

Ci Wu Jia, Wu Jia Shen (Radix et Caulis Acanthopanacis Senticosi, Siberian Ginseng, Eleutherococcus Ginseng)
Tonify Qi
Acrid, slightly Bitter
Warm
Spleen, Kidney, **Heart**, Lung[1059]
Name (Tai Yin, Spleen/Lung, Shao Yin, Kidney/Heart), Clock Neighbor (Spleen/Heart), Branch (You/Chicken, Lung/Kidney, 5PM-6:59PM)

Tonify Yang

Hai Shen, Hai Shu, Ci Shen (Strichopus Japonicus, Sea Cucumber, Sea Slug, Trepang)
Tonify Yang
Sweet, Salty
Warm
Heart, Kidney
Name (Shao Yin, Heart/Kidney)

Lu Jiao Shuang (Cornu Cervi Degelatinatium)
Tonify Yang
Sweet, Salty, Astringent[1060]
Slightly Warm
Kidney, Liver, **Heart**, Pericardium
Name (Shao Yin, Kidney/Heart, Jue Yin, Liver/Pericardium), Clock Neighbor (Kidney/Pericardium)

Tonify Blood

Sheng He Shou Wu (Radix Polygoni Multiflori Recens, Fresh Fleeceflower Root)
Tonify Blood
Bitter, Sweet, Astringent, not Astringent[1061]
Neutral to Cold[1062]
Liver, **Heart**, Large Intestine
Bie Jing (Jue Yin/Yang Ming, Liver/Large Intestine), Branch (Mao/Rabbit, Liver/Large Intestine, 5AM-6:59AM) + Heart

Long Yan Rou (Arillus Longan, Longan Fruit Flesh)
Tonify Blood
Sweet, not Astringent[1063]
Warm
Heart, Spleen
Clock Neighbor (Spleen/Heart)

Dang Gui (Radix Angelica Sinensis, Chinese Angelica Root)
Tonify Blood
Sweet, Acrid, Bitter,[1064]Aromatic
Warm
Heart, Liver, Spleen, Dai[1065]
Clock Neighbor (Spleen/Heart), Branch (Chou/Ox, Spleen/Liver, 1AM-2:59AM) + Dai

Sang Shen Zi, Sang Shen, Sang Guo (Fructus Mori, Mulberry Fruit, White Mulberry Fruit)
Tonify Blood/Tonify Yin
Sweet
Cold
Heart,[1066] Liver, Kidney
Name (Shao Yin, Heart/Kidney) + Liver

Shu Di Huang (Radix Rehmanniae Preparata, Cooked and Cured Rehmannia, Cooked and Cured Chinese Foxglove Root)
Tonify Blood
Sweet
Slightly Warm
Liver, Kidney, **Heart**[1067]
Name (Shao Yin, Heart/Kidney) + Liver

Tonify Yin

Mai Men Dong, Mai Dong (Radix Ophiopogonis, Ophiopogon Tuber)
Tonify Yin
Sweet, slightly Bitter
Cool to slightly Cold[1068]
Spleen,[1069] Lung,[1070] Stomach, **Heart**
Name (Tai Yin, Spleen/Lung), Biao/Li (Stomach/Spleen), Clock Neighbor (Spleen/Heart)

Xi Yang Shen, Hua Qi Shen (Radix Panacis Quinquefoli, American Ginseng Root)
Tonify Qi/Tonify Yin
Sweet, slightly Bitter[1071] to Bitter to very Bitter[1072]
Cold
Kidney, **Heart**, Lung, Spleen[1073]
Name (Shao Yin, Kidney/Heart, Tai Yin, Spleen/Lung), Clock Neighbor (Spleen/Heart), Branch (You/Chicken, Lung/Kidney, 5PM-6:59PM)

Bai He (Bulbus Lilii, Lilly Bulb)
Tonify Yin
Sweet, slightly Bitter,[1074] Bland[1075]
Neutral[1076] to Cool to slightly Cold[1077]
Lung, **Heart**

Sang Shen Zi, Sang Shen, Sang Guo (Fructus Mori, Mulberry Fruit, White Mulberry Fruit)
Tonify Blood/Tonify Yin
Sweet
Cold
Heart,[1078] Liver, Kidney
Name (Shao Yin, Heart/Kidney) + Liver

Gui Ban (Plastrum Testudinis, Tortoise Plastron)
Tonify Yin
Salty, Sweet
Cold
Liver, Kidney, **Heart**, Ren[1079]
Name (Shao Yin, Kidney/Heart) + Liver, Ren

Astringe, Stabilize and Bind

Wu Wei Zi (Fructus Schisandrae Chinensis, Schizandra Fruit)
Astringe, Stabilize and Bind
Sour, Sweet,[1080] Acrid,[1081] Bitter,[1082] Salty,[1083] Astringent
Warm
Kidney, Lung, **Heart**, Dai[1084]
Name (Shao Yin, Kidney/Heart), Branch (You/Chicken, Lung/Kidney, 5PM-6:59PM) + Dai

Lian Zi, Ou Shi, Lian Shi, Pi Guo (Semen Nelumbinis, Lotus Seed)
Astringe, Stabilize and Bind
Sweet, Astringent
Neutral
Heart, Kidney, Spleen
Name (Shao Yin, Heart/Kidney), Clock Neighbor (Spleen/Heart)

He Ye (Folium Nelumbinis, Lotus Leaf)
Clear Heat Clean Toxin/Astringe, Stabilize and Bind
Bitter, slightly Sweet,[1085] Astringent, Aromatic[1086]
Neutral
Heart, Liver, Spleen
Clock Neighbor (Spleen/Heart), Branch (Chou/Ox, Spleen/Liver, 1AM-2:59AM)

Fu Xiao Mai (Semen Tritici Levis, Un-Ripened Wheat Grain)
Astringe, Stabilize and Bind
Sweet, slightly Salty,[1087] Astringent
Cool to Cold,[1088] new wheat is hot,[1089] old wheat is neutral[1090]
Heart
Branch (Wu/Horse, Heart/Heart, 11AM-12:59PM)

Lian Zi Xin (Plumula Nelumbinis, Lotus Plumule)
Clear Heat Purge Fire/Astringe, Stabilize and Bind
Bitter, Astringent
Slightly Cold to Cold[1091]
Heart, Pericardium

Lian Xu (Stamen Nelumbinis, Lotus Stamen)
Astringe, Stabilize and Bind
Sweet, Astringent
Neutral
Heart, Kidney, Liver[1092]
Name (Shao Yin, Heart/Kidney) + Liver

Emetic

Chang Shan (Radix Dichroae, Dichroa Root)
Expel Parasites/Emetic
Acrid, Bitter
Cold, Toxic*
Lung, **Heart**, Liver
Clock Neighbor (Liver/Lung) + Heart

Shu Qi (Folium Dichroae, Dichroa Leaves)
Emetic
Acrid, Bitter
Cold to Warm,[1093] Toxic*
Lung, **Heart**, Liver
Clock Neighbor (Liver/Lung) + Heart

External Application

Xiong Huang (Realgar)
External Application
Acrid, Bitter
Neutral to Warm, Toxic*
Heart, Liver, Kidney,[1094] Stomach,[1095] Lung,[1096] Large Intestine[1097]
Name (Shao Yin, Heart/Kidney, Yang Ming, Large Intestine/Stomach), Bie Jing (Jue Yin/Yang Ming, Liver/Large Intestine), Biao/Li (Large Intestine/Lung), Clock Opposite (Kidney/Large Intestine), Clock Neighbor (Large Intestine/Stomach, Liver/Lung), Branch (Mao/Rabbit, Liver/Large Intestine, 5AM-6:59AM, You/Chicken, Lung, Kidney, 5PM-6:59PM)

Chan Su (Venenum Bufonis, Poison Toad Venom)
External Application
Acrid, Sweet
Warm, Toxic*
Heart, Stomach[1098]

Zhang Nao (Camphora, Camphor)
External Application
Acrid, Aromatic
Hot, Toxic*
Heart, Spleen
Clock Neighbor (Spleen/Heart)

Qian Dan, Huang Dan (Minium, Lead Oxide)
External Application
Bitter, Acrid[1099]
Cool to slightly Cold,[1100] Toxic*
Heart, Liver, Spleen[1101]
Clock Neighbor (Spleen, Heart), Branch (Chou/Ox, Spleen/Liver, 1AM-2:59AM)

Xue Jie (Daemonoropis Resina, Sanguis Draconis, Dragon's Blood)
Vitalize Blood Transform Stasis/External Application
Sweet, Acrid,[1102] Salty,[1103] Aromatic
Neutral
Heart, Liver

Hand Tai Yang Small Intestine Herbs

Acrid Warm Exterior Releasing

Qiang Huo, Can Qiang, Zhu Jie Qiang (Rhizoma et Radix Notopterygii)
Acrid Warm Exterior Releasing
Acrid, Bitter, Aromatic
Warm to very Warm[1104]
Urinary Bladder, **Tai Yang**,[1105] Kidney, Liver,[1106] Du[1107]
Biao/Li (Urinary Bladder/Kidney), and possibly Name (Small Intestine/Urinary Bladder), Clock Opposite (Liver/Small Intestine) and Clock Neighbor (Small Intestine/Urinary Bladder) if Tai Yang[1108] really means Tai Yang. If Tai Yang only means the Foot Tai Yang Urinary Bladder Jing-channel, then + Liver, Du

Acrid Cool Exterior Releasing

Ge Gen (Radix Puerariae, Kudzu Root, Pueraria)
Acrid Cool Exterior Releasing
Sweet, Acrid, slightly Bitter[1109]
Cool
Spleen, Stomach, **Tai Yang**,[1110] Yang Ming[1111]
Biao/Li (Stomach/Spleen), possibly Name (Yang Ming Large Intestine/Stomach) and Clock Neighbor (Large Intestine/Stomach) if Yang Ming[1112] really means the entire Yang Ming Jing-channel, and possibly Name (Tai Yang, Small Intestine/Urinary Bladder), Bie Jing (Spleen, Small Intestine), Clock Neighbor (Small Intestine/Urinary Bladder) and Qian/Hou (Front/Back, Stomach/Urinary Bladder) if Tai Yang[1113] really means the entire Tai Yang Jing-channel.

Clear Heat Purge Fire

Wu Long Cha (Folium Camellia Sinensis Fermentata, 'Oolong' Tea)
Clear Heat Purge Fire
Bitter, Sweet
Cool
Heart, Lung, Stomach, **Small Intestine**
Biao/Li (Small Intestine/Heart) + Lung, Stomach

Ya Zhi Cao, Zhu Ye Shui Cao, Zhu Jie Cai (Herba Commelinae, Common Dayflower)
Clear Heat Purge Fire
Sweet, Bland
Cold
Lung, Stomach, **Small Intestine**

Dan Zhu Ye (Herba Lophatheri, Lophatherum)
Clear Heat Purge Fire
Sweet, Bland
Cold
Heart, Stomach, **Small Intestine**
Biao/Li (Small Intestine/Heart) + Stomach

Clear Heat Dry Dampness

Ku Shen, Ku Shen Gen, Ku Gu (Radix Sophorae Flavescentis, Flavescent Sophora Root)
Clear Heat Dry Dampness
Bitter to extremely Bitter[1114]
Cold
Heart, Liver, Stomach, Large Intestine, Urinary Bladder, **Small Intestine**[1115]
Name (Yang Ming, Large Intestine/Stomach, Tai Yang, Small Intestine/Urinary Bladder), Bie Jing (Jue Yin/Yang Ming, Liver/Large Intestine), Biao/Li (Small Intestine/Heart), Clock Opposite (Liver/Small Intestine), Clock Neighbor (Large Intestine/Stomach, Small Intestine/Urinary Bladder), Branch (Shen/Monkey, Large Intestine/Urinary Bladder, 3PM-4:59PM and Mao/Rabbit, Liver/Large Intestine, 5AM-6:59AM), Qian/Hou (Front/Back, Stomach/Urinary Bladder)

Ji Xue Cao, Beng Da Wan (Herba Centellae, Gotu Kola, Pennywort)
Clear Heat Dry Dampness/Clear Heat Clean Toxin
Acrid, Bitter
Cold
Liver, Spleen, Kidney, **Small Intestine**, Large Intestine
Bie Jing (Jue Yin/Yang Ming, Liver/Large Intestine, Tai Yin/Tai Yang, Spleen/Small Intestine), Clock Opposite (Liver/Small Intestine, Kidney/Large Intestine), Branch (Chou/Ox, Spleen/Liver, 1AM-2:59AM, Si/Snake, Small Intestine/Spleen, 9AM-10:59AM, Wei/Sheep, Spleen/Small Intestine, 1PM-2:59PM, Mao/Rabbit, Liver/Large Intestine, 5AM-6:59AM)

Clear Heat Clean Toxin

Chuan Xin Lian, Lan He Lian (Herba Andrographis, Green Chiretta, Kariyat)
Clear Heat Clean Toxin
Bitter
Cold
Lung, Stomach, Large Intestine, **Small Intestine**
Name (Yang Ming, Large Intestine/Stomach), Biao/Li (Large Intestine/Lung), Clock Neighbor (Large Intestine/Stomach) + Small Intestine

Hu Yao Huang (Herba Leucas Mollissimae, Leucas)
Clear Heat Clean Toxin
Bitter
Cool
Large Intestine, **Small Intestine**, Lung
Biao/Li (Large Intestine/Lung) + Small Intestine

Ban Bian Lian (Herba Lobeliae Chinensis)
Clear Heat Clean Toxin/Regulate Water Resolve Dampness
Acrid, Sweet,[1116] Bland[1117]
Slightly Cold[1118] to Cold, Toxic*[1119]
Heart, Lung, **Small Intestine**
Biao/Li (Small Intestine/Heart) + Lung

Bai Hua She She Cao (Herba Oldenlandia, Heydyotis)
Clear Heat Clean Toxin
Slightly Bitter, Sweet
Cold
Stomach, Large Intestine, **Small Intestine**, Liver[1120]
Name (Yang Ming, Large Intestine/Stomach), Bie Jing (Jue Yin/Yang Ming, Liver/Large Intestine), Clock Opposite (Liver/Small Intestine), Clock Neighbor (Large Intestine/Stomach), Branch (Mao/Rabbit, Liver/Large Intestine, 5AM-6:59AM)

Ji Xue Cao, Beng Da Wan (Herba Centellae, Gotu Kola, Pennywort)
Clear Heat Dry Dampness/Clear Heat Clean Toxin
Acrid, Bitter
Cold
Liver, Spleen, Kidney, **Small Intestine**, Large Intestine
Bie Jing (Jue Yin/Yang Ming, Liver/Large Intestine, Tai Yin/Tai Yang, Spleen/Small Intestine), Clock Opposite (Liver/Small Intestine, Kidney/Large Intestine), Branch (Chou/Ox, Spleen/Liver, 1AM-2:59AM, Si/Snake, Small Intestine/Spleen, 9AM-10:59AM, Wei/Sheep, Spleen/Small Intestine, 1PM-2:59PM, Mao/Rabbit, Liver/Large Intestine, 5AM-6:59AM)

Chui Pen Cao (Herba Sedi, Sedum, Hanging Stonecrop)
Clear Heat Clean Toxin
Sweet, Bland, slightly Sour
Cool
Liver, Gall Bladder, **Small Intestine**
Biao/Li (Gall Bladder/Liver), Clock Opposite (Liver/Small Intestine)

Moist Laxative

Yu Li Ren (Semen Pruni, Bush Cherry Kernel, Dwarf Flowering Cherry Kernel)
Moist Laxative
Acrid, Bitter, Sweet
Neutral
Spleen, Large Intestine, **Small Intestine**
Bie Jing (Tai Yin/Tai Yang, Spleen/Small Intestine), Branch (Si/Snake, Small Intestine/Spleen, 9AM-10:59AM and Wei/Sheep, Spleen/Small Intestine, 1PM-2:59PM) + Large Intestine

Cathartic

Qian Niu Zi (Semen Pharbitidis, Pharbitis, Morning Glory Seed)
Cathartic
Bitter, Acrid[1121]
Cold, Toxic*
Lung, Kidney, Large Intestine, **Small Intestine**[1122]
Biao/Li (Large Intestine/Lung), Clock Opposite (Kidney/Large Intestine), Branch (You/Chicken, Lung/Kidney, 5PM-6:59PM) + Small Intestine

Regulate Water Resolve Dampness

Dong Gua Zi (Semen Benincasae, White Gourd Seed, Winter Melon Seed)
Regulate Water Resolve Dampness
Sweet
Cool to Cold[1123]
Lung, Stomach, **Small Intestine**, Large Intestine
Name (Yang Ming, Large Intestine/Stomach), Biao/Li (Large Intestine/Lung), Clock Neighbor (Large Intestine/Stomach) + Small Intestine

Ze Qi (Herba Euphorbiae Helioscopiae, Euphorbia, Sun Spurge)
Regulate Water Resolve Dampness/Transform Phlegm
Sweet, Bitter, Acrid
Cool to slightly Cold,[1124] slightly Toxic[1125] to Toxic*
Large Intestine, **Small Intestine**, Lung
Biao/Li (Large Intestine/Lung) + Small Intestine

Deng Xin Cao (Medulla Junci, Juncus, Rush Pith)
Regulate Water Resolve Dampness
Sweet, Bland
Cool to slightly Cold[1126]
Heart, Lung, **Small Intestine**
Biao/Li (Small Intestine/Heart) + Lung

Ban Bian Lian (Herba Lobeliae Chinensis)
Clear Heat Clean Toxin/Regulate Water Resolve Dampness
Acrid, Sweet,[1127] Bland[1128]
Slightly Cold[1129] to Cold, Toxic*[1130]
Heart, Lung, **Small Intestine**
Biao/Li (Small Intestine/Heart) + Lung

Chuan Mu Tong (Caulis Clematidis Armandii, Armand's Clematis)
Regulate Water Resolve Dampness
Bitter, Bland[1131]
Cold
Urinary Bladder, Heart, Lung,[1132] **Small Intestine**
Name (Tai Yang, Small Intestine/Urinary Bladder), Bie Jing (Tai Yin/Tai Yang, Lung/Urinary Bladder), Biao/Li (Small Intestine/Heart), Clock Opposite (Lung/Urinary Bladder), Clock Neighbor (Small Intestine/Urinary Bladder)

Dong Gua Pi (Exocarpium Benincasae, White Gourd Rind, Winter Melon Rind)
Regulate Water Resolve Dampness
Sweet, Bland[1133]
Slightly Cold
Lung, **Small Intestine**

Che Qian Zi (Semen Plantaginis, Plantago Seed, Plantain Seed)
Regulate Water Resolve Dampness
Sweet, Bland[1134]
Cold
Kidney, Urinary Bladder, Liver, Lung, **Small Intestine**[1135]
Name (Tai Yang, Small Intestine/Urinary Bladder), Bie Jing (Tai Yin/Tai Yang, Lung/Urinary Bladder), Biao/Li (Urinary Bladder/Kidney), Clock Opposite (Lung/Urinary Bladder, Liver/Small Intestine), Clock Neighbor (Small Intestine/Urinary Bladder, Liver/Lung), Branch (You/Chicken, Lung/Kidney, 5PM-6:59PM)

Che Qian Cao (Herba Plantaginis)
Regulate Water Resolve Dampness
Sweet
Cold
Liver, Kidney, Lung, **Small Intestine**
Clock Opposite (Liver/Small Intestine), Clock Neighbor (Liver/Lung), Branch (You/Chicken, Lung/Kidney, 5PM-6:59PM)

Dong Kui Guo (Fructus Malvae, Mallow Fruit, Cluster Mallow Fruit)
Regulate Water Resolve Dampness
Sweet
Cold
Urinary Bladder, **Small Intestine**, Stomach,[1136] Large Intestine[1137]
Name (Tai Yang, Small Intestine/Urinary Bladder, Yang Ming, Large Intestine/Stomach), Clock Neighbor (Large Intestine/Stomach, Small Intestine/Urinary Bladder), Qian/Hou (Front/Back, Stomach/Urinary Bladder), Branch (Shen/Monkey, Large Intestine/Urinary Bladder, 3PM-4:59PM)

Dong Kui Zi (Semen Malvae, Malva, Mallow Seed, Whorled Mallow Seed)
Regulate Water Resolve Dampness
Sweet
Cold
Urinary Bladder, Large Intestine, **Small Intestine**
Name (Tai Yang, Small Intestine/Urinary Bladder), Clock Neighbor (Small Intestine/Urinary Bladder), Branch (Shen/Monkey, Large Intestine/Urinary Bladder, 3PM-4:59PM)

Chi Xiao Dou, Hong Dou (Semen Phaseoli, Phaseolus, Adzuki Bean, Rice Bean)
Regulate Water Resolve Dampness
Sweet, Sour
Neutral
Heart, **Small Intestine**
Biao/Li (Small Intestine/Heart)

Qu Mai (Herba Dianthi, Dianthus, Fringed Pink, Lilac Pink, Chinese Pink, Rainbow Pink)
Regulate Water Resolve Dampness
Bitter
Cold
Urinary Bladder, Heart, **Small Intestine**
Name (Tai Yang, Small Intestine/Urinary Bladder), Biao/Li (Small Intestine/Heart), Clock Neighbor (Small Intestine/Urinary Bladder)

Mu Tong (Caulis Akebiae, Akebia)
Regulate Water Resolve Dampness
Bitter
Slightly Cold
Urinary Bladder, Heart, **Small Intestine**
Name (Tai Yang, Small Intestine/Urinary Bladder), Biao/Li (Small Intestine/Heart), Clock Neighbor (Small Intestine/Urinary Bladder)

Hai Jin Sha (Spora Lygodi, Climbing Fern Spore)
Regulate Water Resolve Dampness
Sweet, Bland, Salty[1138]
Cold
Urinary Bladder, **Small Intestine**
Name (Tai Yang, Small Intestine/Urinary Bladder), Clock Neighbor (Small Intestine/Urinary Bladder)

Xian Feng Cao (Herba Bidentis, Bidens)
Regulate Water Resolve Dampness
Bland
Cold
Kidney, **Small Intestine**, Urinary Bladder
Name (Tai Yang, Small Intestine/Urinary Bladder), Biao/Li (Urinary Bladder/Kidney), Clock Neighbor (Small Intestine/Urinary Bladder)

Regulate and Rectify Qi

Da Fu Pi (Pericarpium Arecae, Areca Peel, Betel Husk)
Regulate and Rectify Qi
Acrid
Slightly Warm
Large Intestine, **Small Intestine**, Spleen, Stomach
Name (Yang Ming, Large Intestine/Stomach), Bie Jing (Tai Yin/Tai Yang, Spleen/Small Intestine), Biao/Li (Stomach/Spleen), Clock Neighbor (Large Intestine/Stomach), Branch (Si/Snake, Small Intestine/Spleen, 9AM-10:59AM, Wei/Sheep, Spleen/Small Intestine, 1PM-2:59PM)

Chuan Lian Zi, Jin Ling Zi (Fructus Toosendan, Sichuan Pagoda Tree Fruit, Sichuan Chinaberry)
Regulate and Rectify Qi
Bitter, slightly Sour[1139]
Cold, slightly Toxic*
Liver, **Small Intestine**, Stomach, Urinary Bladder
Name (Tai Yang, Small Intestine/Urinary Bladder), Clock Opposite (Liver/Small Intestine), Clock Neighbor (Small Intestine/Urinary Bladder), Qian/Hou (Front/Back, Stomach/Urinary Bladder)

Digestive

Ji Nei Jin (Endothelium Corneum Gigerae Galli, Chicken Gizzard Lining)
Digestive
Sweet
Neutral
Urinary Bladder, **Small Intestine**, Spleen, Stomach
Name (Tai Yang, Small Intestine/Urinary Bladder), Biao/Li (Stomach/Spleen), Bie Jing (Tai Yin/Tai Yang, Spleen/Small Intestine), Clock Neighbor (Small Intestine/Urinary Bladder), Qian/Hou (Front/Back, Stomach/Urinary Bladder), Branch (Si/Snake, Small Intestine/Spleen, 9AM-10:59AM and Wei/Sheep, Spleen/Small Intestine, 1PM-2:59PM)

Expel Parasites

He Cao Ya (Gemma Agrimoniae, Agrimonia, Hairy-Vein Agrimonia Bud)
Expel Parasites
Bitter, Astringent
Cool
Liver, **Small Intestine**, Large Intestine
Bie Jing (Jue Yin/Yang Ming, Liver/Large Intestine), Clock Opposite (Liver, Small Intestine)
Branch (Mao/Rabbit, Liver/Large Intestine, 5AM-6:59AM)

Stop Bleeding

Bai Mao Gen (Rhizoma Imperatae, Wolly Grass Rhizome, Cogon Rhizome)
Stop Bleeding
Sweet
Cold
Lung, Stomach, Urinary Bladder, **Small Intestine**[1140]
Name (Tai Yang, Small Intestine/Urinary Bladder), Bie Jing (Tai Yin/Tai Yang, Lung/Urinary Bladder), Clock Opposite (Lung/Urinary Bladder), Clock Neighbor (Small Intestine/Urinary Bladder), Qian/Hou (Front/Back, Stomach/Urinary Bladder)

Xiao Ji, Da Xiao Ji (Herba Cirisii, Cirsium, Field Thistle)
Stop Bleeding
Bitter,[1141] Sweet
Cool
Liver, Heart, **Small Intestine**,[1142] Urinary Bladder[1143]
Name (Tai Yang, Small Intestine/Urinary Bladder), Biao/Li (Small Intestine/Heart), Clock Opposite (Liver/Small Intestine), Clock Neighbor (Small Intestine/Urinary Bladder)

Transform Phlegm

Ze Qi (Herba Euphorbiae Helioscopiae, Euphorbia, Sun Spurge)
Regulate Water Resolve Dampness/Transform Phlegm
Sweet, Bitter, Acrid
Cool to slightly Cold,[1144] slightly Toxic[1145] to Toxic*
Large Intestine, **Small Intestine**, Lung
Biao/Li (Large Intestine/Lung) + Small Intestine

Tonify Qi

Sha Ji, Cu Liu Guo (Fructus Hippophae, Sea Buckthorn Fruit, Swallow Thorn Fruit)
Tonify Qi
Sour, slightly Sweet, Astringent
Warm
Lung, Spleen, Stomach, Large Intestine, Liver, **Small Intestine**[1146]
Name (Tai Yin, Lung/Spleen, Yang Ming, Large Intestine/Stomach), Bie Jing (Jue Yin/Yang Ming, Liver/Large Intestine, Tai Yin/Tai Yang, Spleen/Small Intestine), Biao/Li (Large Intestine/Lung, Stomach/Spleen), Clock Opposite (Liver/Small Intestine), Clock Neighbor (Liver/Lung, Large Intestine/Stomach), Branch (Chou/Ox, Spleen/Liver, 1AM-2:59AM, Mao/Rabbit, Liver/Large Intestine, 5AM-6:59AM, Si/Snake, Small Intestine/Spleen, 9AM-10:59AM, Wei/Sheep, Spleen/Small Intestine, 1PM-2:59PM)

External Application

Qing Fen (Calomelas, Calomel)
External Application
Acrid, Bland[1147]
Cold, very Toxic*
Liver, Kidney, Large Intestine,[1148] **Small Intestine**[1149]
Bie Jing (Jue Yin/Yang Ming, Liver/Large Intestine), Clock Opposite (Liver/Small Intestine, Kidney/Large Intestine), Branch (Mao/Rabbit, Liver/Large Intestine, 5AM-6:59AM)

Foot Tai Yang Urinary Bladder Herbs

Acrid Warm Exterior Releasing

Gui Zhi, Liu Gui (Ramulus Cinnamomi, Cassia Twig)
Acrid Warm Exterior Releasing
Acrid, Sweet
Warm
Heart, Lung, **Urinary Bladder**
Bie Jing (Tai Yin/Tai Yang, Lung/Urinary Bladder), Clock Opposite (Lung/Urinary Bladder) + Heart

Ma Huang, Ma Huang Cao (Herba Ephedrae, Ephedra Stem, Mormon Tea)
Acrid Warm Exterior Releasing
Acrid, slightly Bitter[1150] to Bitter, no big taste[1151]
Warm
Lung, **Urinary Bladder**, Yang Qiao[1152]
Bie Jing (Tai Yin/Tai Yang, Lung/Urinary Bladder), Clock Opposite (Lung/Urinary Bladder) + Yang Qiao

Fang Feng, Pang Feng (Radix Saposhnikoviae, and sometimes Ledebouriella Root as a substitute)
Acrid Warm Exterior Releasing
Acrid, Sweet, Aromatic
Slightly Warm
Urinary Bladder, Liver, Spleen, Du,[1153] Yang Qiao[1154]
Branch (Chou/Ox, Spleen/Liver,1AM-2:59AM) + Urinary Bladder, Du, Yang Qiao

Qiang Huo, Can Qiang, Zhu Jie Qiang (Rhizoma et Radix Notopterygii)
Acrid Warm Exterior Releasing
Acrid, Bitter, Aromatic
Warm to very Warm[1155]
Urinary Bladder, Tai Yang,[1156] Kidney, Liver,[1157] Du[1158]
Biao/Li (Urinary Bladder/Kidney), and possibly Name (Small Intestine/Urinary Bladder), Clock Opposite (Liver/Small Intestine) and Clock Neighbor (Small Intestine/Urinary Bladder) if Tai Yang[1159] really means Tai Yang. If Tai Yang only means the Foot Tai Yang Urinary Bladder Jing-channel, then + Liver, Du

Gao Ben (Rhizoma Ligustici, Chinese Lovage Root)
Acrid Warm Exterior Releasing
Acrid, Aromatic
Warm
Urinary Bladder, Du[1160]

Acrid Cool Exterior Releasing

Man Jing Zi, Jing Tiao Zi, Bai Bu Jing (Fructus Viticis, Vitex Fruit)
Acrid Cool Exterior Releasing
Acrid, Bitter
Both Cool and Warm[1161]
Lung,[1162] Liver, Stomach, **Urinary Bladder**,[1163] Gall Bladder,[1164] San Jiao[1165]
Name (Shao Yang, Gall Bladder/San Jiao), Bie Jing (Tai Yin/Tai Yang, Lung/Urinary Bladder), Biao/Li (Gall Bladder/Liver), Clock Opposite (Lung, Urinary Bladder), Clock Neighbor (San Jiao/Gall Bladder, Liver/Lung), Qian/Hou (Front/Back, Stomach/Urinary Bladder), Branch (Yin/Tiger, Gall Bladder/Lung, 3AM-4:59AM, Hai/Pig, Urinary Bladder/San Jiao, 9PM-10:59PM)

Fu Ping, Fu Piao, Qing Ping (Herba Spirodelae, Duckweed, Spirodela)
Acrid Cool Exterior Releasing
Acrid
Cold
Lung, **Urinary Bladder**
Bie Jing (Tai Yin/Tai Yang, Lung/Urinary Bladder), Clock Opposite (Lung/Urinary Bladder)

Ge Gen (Radix Puerariae, Kudzu Root, Pueraria)
Acrid Cool Exterior Releasing
Sweet, Acrid, slightly Bitter[1166]
Cool
Spleen, Stomach, **Tai Yang**,[1167] Yang Ming[1168]
Biao/Li (Stomach/Spleen), possibly Name (Yang Ming Large Intestine/Stomach) and Clock Neighbor (Large Intestine/Stomach) if Yang Ming[1169] really means the entire Yang Ming Jing-channel, and possibly Name (Tai Yang, Small Intestine/Urinary Bladder), Bie Jing (Spleen, Small Intestine), Clock Neighbor (Small Intestine/Urinary Bladder) and Qian/Hou (Front/Back, Stomach/Urinary Bladder) if Tai Yang[1170] really means the entire Tai Yang Jing-channel.

Clear Heat Purge Fire

Xi Gua (Fructus Citrulli, Watermelon Fruit)
Clear Heat Purge Fire
Sweet
Cold
Heart, Stomach, **Urinary Bladder**, Lung[1171]
Bie Jing (Tai Yin/Tai Yang, Lung/Urinary Bladder), Clock Opposite (Lung/Urinary Bladder), Qian/Hou (Front/Back, Stomach/Urinary Bladder) + Heart

Shi Lian Zi (Herba Sinocrassulae Indicae, Indian Sinocrassula)
Clear Heat Purge Fire
Bitter
Cold
Large Intestine, **Urinary Bladder**, Stomach
Name (Yang Ming, Large Intestine/Stomach), Clock Neighbor (Large Intestine/Stomach), Qian/Hou (Front/Back, Stomach/Urinary Bladder), Branch (Shen/Monkey, Large Intestine/Urinary Bladder, 3PM-4:59PM)

Xi Gua Pi (Exocarpium Citrulli, Watermelon Rind)
Clear Heat Purge Fire
Sweet
Cold
Heart, Stomach, **Urinary Bladder**
Qian/Hou (Front/Back, Stomach/Urinary Bladder) + Heart

Clear Heat Dry Dampness

Ku Shen, Ku Shen Gen, Ku Gu (Radix Sophorae Flavescentis, Flavescent Sophora Root)
Clear Heat Dry Dampness
Bitter to extremely Bitter[1172]
Cold
Heart, Liver, Stomach, Large Intestine, **Urinary Bladder**, Small Intestine[1173]
Name (Yang Ming, Large Intestine/Stomach, Tai Yang, Small Intestine/Urinary Bladder), Bie Jing (Jue Yin/Yang Ming, Liver/Large Intestine), Biao/Li (Small Intestine/Heart), Clock Opposite (Liver/Small Intestine), Clock Neighbor (Large Intestine/Stomach, Small Intestine/Urinary Bladder), Qian/Hou (Front/Back, Stomach/Urinary Bladder), Branch (Shen/Monkey, Large Intestine/Urinary Bladder, 3PM-4:59PM and Mao/Rabbit, Liver/Large Intestine, 5AM-6:59AM)

Huang Bai, Huang Bo (Cortex Phellodendri, Amur Cork Tree Bark, Phellodendron Bark)
Clear Heat Dry Dampness
Bitter
Cold
Kidney, **Urinary Bladder**, Large Intestine
Biao/Li (Urinary Bladder/Kidney), Clock Opposite (Kidney/Large Intestine), Branch (Shen/Monkey, Large Intestine/Urinary Bladder, 3PM-4:59PM)

Long Dan Cao, Long Dan, Dan Cao (Radix Gentianae, Chinese Gentian Root, Gentiana)
Clear Heat Dry Dampness
Bitter, Astringing[1174]
Cold
Liver, Gall Bladder, Stomach, **Urinary Bladder**[1175]
Biao/Li (Gall Bladder/Liver), Qian/Hou (Front/Back, Stomach/Urinary Bladder)

Clear Heat Clean Toxin

Long Kui, Ku Kui (Herba Solanum Nigrum, Black Nightshade)
Clear Heat Clean Toxin
Slightly Bitter, slightly Sweet[1176]
Cold, non-Toxic[1177] to slightly Toxic*
Lung, **Urinary Bladder**, Stomach[1178]
Bie Jing (Tai Yin/Tai Yang, Lung/Urinary Bladder), Clock Opposite (Lung/Urinary Bladder), Qian/Hou (Front/Back, Stomach/Urinary Bladder)

Pao Zai Cao, Deng Long Cao (Herba Physalis Angulatae)
Clear Heat Clean Toxin
Bitter
Cool
Lung, **Urinary Bladder**, Liver, Kidney
Bie Jing (Tai Yin/Tai Yang, Lung/Urinary Bladder), Biao/Li (Urinary Bladder/Kidney), Clock Neighbor (Liver/Lung), Clock Opposite (Lung/Urinary Bladder), Branch (You/Chicken, Lung/Kidney, 5PM-6:59PM)

Dao Diao Jin Zhong, Feng Fang Ran (Melothria Maderospatana, Melothria)
Clear Heat Clean Toxin
Sweet, Bitter
Cool
Lung, Liver, **Urinary Bladder**
Bie Jing (Tai Yin/Tai Yang, Lung/Urinary Bladder), Clock Opposite (Lung/Urinary Bladder), Clock Neighbor (Liver/Lung)

Feng Wei Cao, Feng Huang Cao (Herba Pteris, Chinese Brake, Huguenot Fern, Spider Brake)
Clear Heat Clean Toxin
Bitter
Cold
Large Intestine, **Urinary Bladder**
Branch (Shen/Monkey, Large Intestine/Urinary Bladder, 3PM-4:59PM)

Tian Kui Zi, Tian Kui, Zi Bei Tian Kui (Radix Semiaquilegiae, Muskroot-like Semiaquilegia Root)
Clear Heat Clean Toxin
Sweet, Bitter
Cold
Liver, Spleen, **Urinary Bladder**
Branch (Chou/Ox, Spleen/Liver, 1AM-2:59AM) + Urinary Bladder

Cathartic

Shang Lu (Radix Phytolaccae, Poke Root)
Cathartic
Bitter
Cold, highly Toxic*
Lung, Spleen,[1179] Kidney, Large Intestine, **Urinary Bladder**[1180]
Name (Tai Yin, Lung/Spleen), Bie Jing (Tai Yin/Tai Yang, Lung/Urinary Bladder), Biao/Li (Large Intestine/Lung, Urinary Bladder/Kidney), Clock Opposite (Kidney/Large Intestine, Lung/Urinary Bladder), Branch (You/Chicken, Lung/Kidney, 5PM-6:59PM, Shen/Monkey, Large Intestine/Urinary Bladder, 3PM-4:59PM)

Dispel Wind Dampness, Open Channels and Luo-Network Vessels and Relieve Pain

Han Fang Ji/Fen Fang Ji (Radix Stephaniae Tetandrae, Stephania Root)
Dispel Wind Dampness, Open Channels and Luo-Network Vessels and Relieve Pain
Acrid, Bitter to very Bitter[1181]
Cold to very Cold[1182]
Urinary Bladder, Lung,[1183] Spleen,[1184] Kidney, Yang Qiao,[1185] and possibly San Jiao[1186]
Name (Tai Yin, Spleen/Lung), Bie Jing (Tai Yin/Tai Yang, Lung/Urinary Bladder), Biao/Li (Urinary Bladder/Kidney), Clock Opposite (Lung/Urinary Bladder), Branch (You/Chicken, Lung/Kidney, 5PM-6:59PM) and possibly Bie Jing (Shao Yin/Shao Yang, Kidney/San Jiao), Clock Opposite (San Jiao/Spleen), Branch (Hai/Pig, Urinary Bladder/San Jiao, 9PM-10:59PM) + Yang Qiao

Guang Fang Ji (Radix Aristolochiae Fangchi)
Dispel Wind Dampness, Open Channels and Luo-Network Vessels and Relieve Pain
Acrid, Bitter
Cold, Toxic*
Urinary Bladder, Lung, Yang Qiao[1187]
Bie Jing (Tai Yin/Tai Yang, Lung/Urinary Bladder), Clock Opposite (Lung/Urinary Bladder) + Yang Qiao

Mu Fang Ji (Radix Cocculi, Cocculus Root)
Dispel Wind Dampness, Open Channels and Luo-Network Vessels and Relieve Pain
Bitter, Acrid
Cold
Urinary Bladder, Kidney, Spleen
Biao/Li (Urinary Bladder/Kidney) + Spleen

Wei Ling Xian, Lao Hu Xu, Ling Xian Gen (Radix Clematidis, Clematis Root, Chinese Clematis)
Dispel Wind Dampness, Open Channels and Luo-Network Vessels and Relieve Pain
Acrid, Salty
Warm, slightly Toxic*[1188]
Urinary Bladder

Du Huo, Da Huo, Rou Du Huo (Radix Angelicae Pubescentis, Angelica Root)
Dispel Wind Dampness, Open Channels and Luo-Network Vessels and Relieve Pain
Acrid, Bitter, Aromatic
Slightly Warm to very Warm[1189]
Liver, Kidney,[1190] **Urinary Bladder**, Du[1191]
Biao/Li (Urinary Bladder/Kidney) + Liver, Du

Regulate Water Resolve Dampness

Chuan Mu Tong (Caulis Clematidis Armandii, Armand's Clematis)
Regulate Water Resolve Dampness
Bitter, Bland[1192]
Cold
Urinary Bladder, Heart, Lung,[1193] Small Intestine
Name (Tai Yang, Small Intestine/Urinary Bladder), Bie Jing (Tai Yin/Tai Yang, Lung/Urinary Bladder), Biao/Li (Small Intestine/Heart), Clock Opposite (Lung/Urinary Bladder), Clock Neighbor (Small Intestine/Urinary Bladder)

Che Qian Zi (Semen Plantaginis, Plantago Seed, Plantain Seed)
Regulate Water Resolve Dampness
Sweet, Bland[1194]
Cold
Kidney, **Urinary Bladder**, Liver, Lung, Small Intestine[1195]
Name (Tai Yang, Small Intestine/Urinary Bladder), Bie Jing (Tai Yin/Tai Yang, Lung/Urinary Bladder), Biao/Li (Urinary Bladder/Kidney), Clock Opposite (Lung/Urinary Bladder, Liver/Small Intestine), Clock Neighbor (Small Intestine/Urinary Bladder, Liver/Lung), Branch (You/Chicken, Lung/Kidney, 5PM-6:59PM)

Shi Wei, Shi Lan, Fei Xin Cao (Folium Pyrrosiae, Pyrrosia, Japanese Felt Fern)
Regulate Water Resolve Dampness
Bitter, Sweet
Cool to slightly Cold[1196]
Urinary Bladder, Lung
Bie Jing (Tai Yin/Tai Yang, Lung/Urinary Bladder), Clock Opposite (Urinary Bladder/Lung)

Dong Kui Guo (Fructus Malvae, Mallow Fruit, Cluster Mallow Fruit)
Regulate Water Resolve Dampness
Sweet
Cold
Urinary Bladder, Small Intestine, Stomach,[1197] Large Intestine[1198]
Name (Tai Yang, Small Intestine/Urinary Bladder, Yang Ming, Large Intestine/Stomach), Clock Neighbor (Large Intestine/Stomach, Small Intestine/Urinary Bladder), Qian/Hou (Front/Back, Stomach/Urinary Bladder), Branch (Shen/Monkey, Large Intestine/Urinary Bladder, 3PM-4:59PM)

Dong Kui Zi (Semen Malvae, Malva, Mallow Seed, Whorled Mallow Seed)
Regulate Water Resolve Dampness
Sweet
Cold
Urinary Bladder, Large Intestine, Small Intestine
Name (Tai Yang, Small Intestine/Urinary Bladder), Clock Neighbor (Small Intestine/Urinary Bladder), Branch (Shen/Monkey, Large Intestine/Urinary Bladder, 3PM-4:59PM)

Qing Ma Zi, Bai Ma Zi, Kui Zi (Semen Abutili, Abutilon Seed, Indian Mallow Seed)
Regulate Water Resolve Dampness
Bitter
Neutral
Urinary Bladder, Large Intestine, Liver
Bie Jing (Yang Ming/Jue Yin, Large Intestine/Liver), Branch (Shen/Monkey, Large Intestine/Urinary Bladder, 3PM-4:59PM and Mao/Rabbit, Liver/Large Intestine, 5AM-6:59AM)

Hua Shi, Fei Hua Shi (Talcum)
Regulate Water Resolve Dampness
Sweet, Bland
Cold
Stomach, **Urinary Bladder**
Qian/Hou (Front/Back, Stomach/Urinary Bladder)

Bi Xie (Rhizoma Dioscoriae Hypoglaucae, Fish Poison Yam, Tokoro)
Regulate Water Resolve Dampness
Bitter
Neutral
Urinary Bladder, Liver, Stomach
Qian/Hou (Front/Back, Stomach/Urinary Bladder) + Liver

Qu Mai (Herba Dianthi, Dianthus, Fringed Pink, Lilac Pink, Chinese Pink, Rainbow Pink)
Regulate Water Resolve Dampness
Bitter
Cold
Urinary Bladder, Heart, Small Intestine
Name (Tai Yang, Small Intestine/Urinary Bladder), Biao/Li (Small Intestine/Heart), Clock Neighbor (Small Intestine/Urinary Bladder)

Mu Tong (Caulis Akebiae, Akebia)
Regulate Water Resolve Dampness
Bitter
Slightly Cold
Urinary Bladder, Heart, Small Intestine
Name (Tai Yang, Small Intestine/Urinary Bladder), Biao/Li (Small Intestine/Heart), Clock Neighbor (Small Intestine/Urinary Bladder)

Hai Jin Sha (Spora Lygodi, Climbing Fern Spore)
Regulate Water Resolve Dampness
Sweet, Bland, Salty[1199]
Cold
Urinary Bladder, Small Intestine
Name (Tai Yang, Small Intestine/Urinary Bladder), Clock Neighbor (Small Intestine/Urinary Bladder)

Xian Feng Cao (Herba Bidentis, Bidens)
Regulate Water Resolve Dampness
Bland
Cold
Kidney, Small Intestine, **Urinary Bladder**
Name (Tai Yang, Small Intestine/Urinary Bladder), Biao/Li (Urinary Bladder/Kidney), Clock Neighbor (Small Intestine/Urinary Bladder)

Bian Xu (Herba Polygoni Avicularis, Common Knotgrass)
Regulate Water Resolve Dampness
Bitter
Cool to slightly Cold[1200]
Urinary Bladder

Di Fu Zi (Fructus Kochiae, Summer Cypress Fruit, Burning Bush Fruit)
Regulate Water Resolve Dampness
Sweet,[1201] Bitter, Acrid[1202]
Cold
Urinary Bladder, Kidney
Biao/Li (Urinary Bladder/Kidney)

Bi Zi Cao (Herba Pogonantheri Criniti, Crinite Pogonatherum)
Regulate Water Resolve Dampness
Sweet
Cool
Kidney, **Urinary Bladder**
Biao/Li (Urinary Bladder/Kidney)

Shui Ding Xiang (Herba Ludwigiae Prostratae, Ludwigia)
Regulate Water Resolve Dampness
Sweet, Bland
Very Cold
Kidney, **Urinary Bladder**
Biao/Li (Urinary Bladder/Kidney)

Zhu Ling (Polyporus, Pore Fungus)
Regulate Water Resolve Dampness
Sweet, Bland
Neutral
Kidney, **Urinary Bladder**
Biao/Li (Urinary Bladder, Kidney)

Ze Xie (Rhizoma Alismatis, Water Plantain Rhizome)
Regulate Water Resolve Dampness
Sweet, Salty,[1203] Bland
Cold
Kidney, **Urinary Bladder**
Biao/Li (Urinary Bladder/Kidney)

Yu Mi Xu, Yu Mai Xu (Stigma Maydis, Corn Stigma, Corn Silk)
Regulate Water Resolve Dampness
Sweet, Bland
Neutral
Urinary Bladder, Kidney, Liver, Gall Bladder[1204]
Biao/Li (Urinary Bladder/Kidney, Gall Bladder/Liver), Branch (Zi/Rat, Kidney/Gall Bladder, 11PM-12:59AM)

Jin Qian Cao (Herba Lysimachiae, Lysimachia, Loose Strife Herb)
Regulate Water Resolve Dampness
Sweet, Salty, Bland[1205]
Cool to slightly Cold[1206]
Urinary Bladder, Gall Bladder, Kidney, Liver
Biao/Li (Urinary Bladder/Kidney, Gall Bladder/Liver), Branch (Zi/Rat, Kidney/Gall Bladder, 11PM-12:59AM)

Hua Shi Cao (Herba Orthosiphon Aristatus, Orthosiphon, Cat's Whiskers)
Regulate Water Resolve Dampness
Bitter
Cold
Liver, Kidney, **Urinary Bladder**
Biao/Li (Urinary Bladder/Kidney) + Liver

Guang Jin Qian Cao (Herba Desmodii Styracifolii, Desmodium, Snowbell Leaf Tick Clover)
Regulate Water Resolve Dampness
Sweet, Bland
Cool
Liver, Kidney, **Urinary Bladder**
Biao/Li (Urinary Bladder/Kidney) + Liver

Warm Interior

Jiao Mu (Semen Zanthoxyli, Zanthoxylum Seed, Sichuan Peppercorn Seed)
Warm Interior
Bitter
Cold, Toxic*
Spleen, **Urinary Bladder**, Lung, Kidney
Name (Tai Yin, Spleen/Lung), Bie Jing (Tai Yin/Tai Yang, Lung/Urinary Bladder), Biao/Li (Urinary Bladder/Kidney), Clock Opposite (Lung/Urinary Bladder), Branch (You/Chicken, Lung/Kidney, 5PM-6:59PM)

Bi Cheng Qie, Cheng Qie Zi (Fructus Litseae, Cubeb Fruit)
Warm Interior
Acrid, Aromatic[1207]
Warm
Spleen, Stomach, Kidney, **Urinary Bladder**
Biao/Li (Stomach/Spleen, Urinary Bladder/Kidney), Qian/Hou (Front/Back, Stomach/Urinary Bladder)

Regulate and Rectify Qi

Wu Yao, Tai Wu Yao, Tai Wu (Radix Linderae, Lindera Root)
Regulate and Rectify Qi
Acrid, Aromatic[1208]
Warm
Urinary Bladder, Kidney, Lung, Spleen
Name (Tai Yin, Lung/Spleen), Bie Jing (Tai Yin/Tai Yang, Lung/Urinary Bladder), Biao/Li (Urinary Bladder/Kidney), Clock Opposite (Lung/Urinary Bladder), Branch (You/Chicken, Lung/Kidney, 5PM-6:59PM)

Chuan Lian Zi, Jin Ling Zi (Fructus Toosendan, Sichuan Pagoda Tree Fruit, Sichuan Chinaberry)
Regulate and Rectify Qi
Bitter, slightly Sour[1209]
Cold, slightly Toxic*
Liver, Small Intestine, Stomach, **Urinary Bladder**
Name (Tai Yang, Small Intestine/Urinary Bladder), Clock Opposite (Liver/Small Intestine), Clock Neighbor (Small Intestine/Urinary Bladder), Qian/Hou (Front/Back, Stomach/Urinary Bladder)

Ju He, Ju Zi He, Ju Zi Ren, Ju Ren (Citri Reticulatae Semen, Tangerine/Orange Seed)
Regulate and Rectify Qi
Bitter
Neutral
Liver, Kidney,[1210] **Urinary Bladder**[1211]
Biao/Li (Urinary Bladder/Kidney) + Liver

Digestive

Ji Nei Jin (Endothelium Corneum Gigerae Galli, Chicken Gizzard Lining)
Digestive
Sweet
Neutral
Urinary Bladder, Small Intestine, Spleen, Stomach
Name (Tai Yang, Small Intestine/Urinary Bladder), Biao/Li (Stomach/Spleen), Bie Jing (Tai Yin/Tai Yang, Spleen/Small Intestine), Clock Neighbor (Small Intestine/Urinary Bladder), Qian/Hou (Front/Back, Stomach/Urinary Bladder), Branch (Si/Snake, Small Intestine/Spleen, 9AM-10:59AM and Wei/Sheep, Spleen/Small Intestine, 1PM-2:59PM)

Stop Bleeding

Bai Mao Gen (Rhizoma Imperatae, Wolly Grass Rhizome, Cogon Rhizome)
Stop Bleeding
Sweet
Cold
Lung, Stomach, **Urinary Bladder**, Small Intestine[1212]
Name (Tai Yang, Small Intestine/Urinary Bladder), Bie Jing (Tai Yin/Tai Yang, Lung/Urinary Bladder), Clock Opposite (Lung/Urinary Bladder), Clock Neighbor (Small Intestine/Urinary Bladder), Qian/Hou (Front/Back, Stomach/Urinary Bladder)

Zhu Fan Hua Tou, Su Xiang (Rhizoma Mirabilidis, Mirabilis)
Stop Bleeding
Sweet, Bitter, Astringent
Neutral
Lung, Stomach, **Urinary Bladder**
Bie Jing (Tai Yin/Tai Yang, Lung/Urinary Bladder), Clock Opposite (Lung/Urinary Bladder), Qian/Hou (Front/Back, Stomach/Urinary Bladder)

Xiao Ji, Da Xiao Ji (Herba Cirisii, Cirsium, Field Thistle)
Stop Bleeding
Bitter,[1213] Sweet
Cool
Liver, Heart, Small Intestine,[1214] **Urinary Bladder**[1215]
Name (Tai Yang, Small Intestine/Urinary Bladder), Biao/Li (Small Intestine/Heart), Clock Opposite (Liver/Small Intestine), Clock Neighbor (Small Intestine/Urinary Bladder)

Vitalize Blood Transform Stasis

Wang Bu Liu Xing (Semen Vaccariae, Vaccaria Seeds, Cow Soapwort Seed)
Vitalize Blood Transform Stasis
Acrid,[1216] Bitter
Neutral
Liver, Stomach, **Urinary Bladder**[1217]
Qian/Hou (Front/Back, Stomach/Urinary Bladder) + Liver

Yi Mu Cao (Herba Leonuri, Chinese Motherwort)
Vitalize Blood Transform Stasis
Acrid, Bitter
Cool to slightly Cold[1218]
Heart, Liver, **Urinary Bladder**

Shui Zhi (Hirudo, Leech)
Vitalize Blood Transform Stasis
Salty, Bitter
Neutral, slightly Toxic*
Liver, **Urinary Bladder**[1219]

Relieve Cough and Wheezing/Panting

Ting Li Zi (Semen Descurainiae seu Lepidii, Descurainia seed, Lepidium Seed)
Relieve Cough and Wheezing/Panting
Acrid, Bitter
Very Cold
Lung, **Urinary Bladder**
Bie Jing (Tai Yin/Tai Yang, Lung/Urinary Bladder), Clock Opposite (Lung/Urinary Bladder)

Sang Bai Pi, Sang Pi (Cortex Mori, Mulberry Bark)
Relieve Cough and Wheezing/Panting
Sweet
Cold
Lung, **Urinary Bladder**[1220]
Bie Jing (Tai Yin/Tai Yang, Lung/Urinary Bladder), Clock Opposite (Lung/Urinary Bladder)

Calm Shen Sedative

Hu Po (Succinum, Amber)
Calm Shen Sedative
Sweet, Bland[1221]
Neutral
Heart, Liver, **Urinary Bladder**[1222]

Calm Liver Extinguish Wind

Di Long, Qiu Yin (Pheretima, Earthworm)
Calm Liver Extinguish Wind
Salty
Cold
Liver, Spleen, Kidney,[1223] **Urinary Bladder**, Lung[1224]
Name (Tai Yin, Spleen/Lung), Bie Jing (Tai Yin/Tai Yang, Lung/Urinary Bladder), Biao/Li (Urinary Bladder/Kidney), Clock Opposite (Lung/Urinary Bladder), Clock Neighbor (Liver/Lung), Branch (Chou/Ox, Spleen/Liver, 1AM-2:59AM)

Astringe, Stabilize and Bind

Jin Ying Zi (Fructus Rosae Laevigatae, Cherokee Rosehip)
Astringe, Stabilize and Bind
Sour, Astringent
Neutral to Warm[1225]
Kidney, **Urinary Bladder**, Large Intestine
Biao/Li (Urinary Bladder/Kidney), Clock Opposite (Kidney/Large Intestine), Branch (Shen/Monkey, Large Intestine/Urinary Bladder, 3PM-4:59PM)

Foot Shao Yin Kidney Herbs

Acrid Warm Exterior Releasing

Xi Xin (Radix et Rhizoma Asari, Asarum, Chinese Wild Ginger)
Acrid Warm Exterior Releasing
Acrid to extremely Acrid,[1226] Aromatic
Warm, slightly Toxic*
Lung, Heart, **Kidney**, Du,[1227] all channels[1228]
Name (Shao Yin, Heart/Kidney), Branch (You/Chicken, Lung/Kidney, 5PM-6:59PM) + Du

Qiang Huo, Can Qiang, Zhu Jie Qiang (Rhizoma et Radix Notopterygii)
Acrid Warm Exterior Releasing
Acrid, Bitter, Aromatic
Warm to very Warm[1229]
Urinary Bladder, Tai Yang,[1230] **Kidney**, Liver,[1231] Du[1232]
Biao/Li (Urinary Bladder/Kidney), and possibly Name (Small Intestine/Urinary Bladder), Clock Opposite (Liver/Small Intestine) and Clock Neighbor (Small Intestine/Urinary Bladder) if Tai Yang[1233] really means Tai Yang. If Tai Yang only means the Foot Tai Yang Urinary Bladder Jing-channel, then + Liver, Du

Clear Heat Purge Fire

Zhi Mu (Radix Anemarrhenae, Anemarrhena)
Clear Heat Purge Fire
Bitter, Sweet
Cold
Lung, Stomach, **Kidney**
Branch (You/Chicken, Lung/Kidney, 5PM-6:59PM) + Stomach

Jue Ming Zi, Cao Jue Ming (Semen Cassiae, Cassia Seeds, Foetid Cassia Seeds)
Clear Heat Purge Fire/Calm Liver Extinguish Wind
Sweet, Bitter, Salty[1234]
Cool to slightly Cold
Liver, Large Intestine, **Kidney**[1235]
Bie Jing (Jue Yin/Yang Ming, Liver/Large Intestine), Clock Opposite (Kidney/Large Intestine), Branch (Mao/Rabbit, Liver/Large Intestine, 5AM-6:59AM)

Han Shui Shi, Yan Jing Shi (Glauberitum, Calcitum, Calcite)
Clear Heat Purge Fire
Acrid,[1236] Salty
Very Cold
Stomach, **Kidney**

Clear Heat Dry Dampness

Ji Xue Cao, Beng Da Wan (Herba Centellae, Gotu Kola, Pennywort)
Clear Heat Dry Dampness/Clear Heat Clean Toxin
Acrid, Bitter
Cold
Liver, Spleen, **Kidney**, Small Intestine, Large Intestine
Bie Jing (Jue Yin/Yang Ming, Liver/Large Intestine, Tai Yin/Tai Yang, Spleen/Small Intestine), Clock Opposite (Liver/Small Intestine, Kidney/Large Intestine), Branch (Chou/Ox, Spleen/Liver, 1AM-2:59AM, Si/Snake, Small Intestine/Spleen, 9AM-10:59AM, Wei/Sheep, Spleen/Small Intestine, 1PM-2:59PM, Mao/Rabbit, Liver/Large Intestine, 5AM-6:59AM)

Huang Bai, Huang Bo (Cortex Phellodendri, Amur Cork Tree Bark, Phellodendron Bark)
Clear Heat Dry Dampness
Bitter
Cold
Kidney, Urinary Bladder, Large Intestine
Biao/Li (Urinary Bladder/Kidney), Clock Opposite (Kidney/Large Intestine), Branch (Shen/Monkey, Large Intestine/Urinary Bladder, 3PM-4:59PM)

Clear Heat Cool Blood

Xuan Shen, Yuan Shen, Hei Shen (Radix Scrophulariae, Ningpo Figwort Root)
Clear Heat Cool Blood
Bitter, Sweet, Salty
Cold
Lung, Stomach, **Kidney**
Branch (You/Chicken, Lung/Kidney, 5PM-6:59PM) + Stomach

Ji Guan Hua (Flos Celosiae Cristatae, Cock's Comb Flower)
Clear Heat Cool Blood/Astringe, Stabilize and Bind
Sweet, Astringent[1237]
Cool
Large Intestine, Liver, **Kidney**[1238]
Bie Jing (Jue Yin/Yang Ming, Liver/Large Intestine), Clock Opposite (Kidney/Large Intestine), Branch (Mao/Rabbit, Liver/Large Intestine, 5AM-6:59AM)

Mu Dan Pi, Mu Shao Yao (Cortex Moutan, Peony Tree Root Cortex)
Clear Heat Cool Blood/Vitalize Blood Transform Stasis
Bitter, Acrid, Aromatic
Cool to slightly Cold
Heart, Liver, **Kidney**, Pericardium[1239]
Name (Shao Yin, Heart/Kidney, Jue Yin, Liver/Pericardium), Clock Neighbor (Kidney/Pericardium)

Sheng Di Huang (Radix Rehmanniae, Chinese Foxglove Root)
Clear Heat Cool Blood
Sweet, Bitter
Cold
Heart, Liver, **Kidney**
Name (Shao Yin, Heart/Kidney) + Liver

Clear Heat Clean Toxin

Ban Zhi Lian (Herba Scutellariae Barbatae, Barbat Skullcap, Barbed Skullcap)
Clear Heat Clean Toxin
Acrid, slightly Bitter
Cool
Liver, Lung, Stomach, **Kidney**,[1240] Large Intestine[1241]
Name (Yang Ming, Large Intestine/Stomach), Bie Jing (Jue Yin/Yang Ming, Liver/Large Intestine), Biao/Li (Large Intestine/Lung), Clock Opposite (Kidney/Large Intestine), Clock Neighbor (Large Intestine/Stomach, Liver/Lung), Branch (You/Chicken, Lung/Kidney, 5PM-6:59PM, Mao/Rabbit, Liver/Large Intestine, 5AM-6:59AM)

Pao Zai Cao, Deng Long Cao (Herba Physalis Angulatae)
Clear Heat Clean Toxin
Bitter
Cool
Lung, Urinary Bladder, Liver, **Kidney**
Bie Jing (Tai Yin/Tai Yang, Lung/Urinary Bladder), Biao/Li (Urinary Bladder/Kidney), Clock Neighbor (Liver/Lung), Clock Opposite (Lung/Urinary Bladder), Branch (You/Chicken, Lung/Kidney, 5PM-6:59PM)

Tu Niu Xi (Radix Achyranthes Longiflora, Native Achyranthis Root)
Clear Heat Clean Toxin/Vitalize Blood Transform Stasis
Bitter, Sour, Acrid[1242]
Neutral to Cold,[1243] slightly Toxic[1244]
Lung, Liver, **Kidney**
Clock Neighbor (Liver/Lung), Branch (You/Chicken, Lung/Kidney, 5PM-6:59PM)

Ji Xue Cao, Beng Da Wan (Herba Centellae, Gotu Kola, Pennywort)
Clear Heat Dry Dampness/Clear Heat Clean Toxin
Acrid, Bitter
Cold
Liver, Spleen, **Kidney**, Small Intestine, Large Intestine
Bie Jing (Jue Yin/Yang Ming, Liver/Large Intestine, Tai Yin/Tai Yang, Spleen/Small Intestine), Clock Opposite (Liver/Small Intestine, Kidney/Large Intestine), Branch (Chou/Ox, Spleen/Liver, 1AM-2:59AM, Si/Snake, Small Intestine/Spleen, 9AM-10:59AM, Wei/Sheep, Spleen/Small Intestine, 1PM-2:59PM, Mao/Rabbit, Liver/Large Intestine, 5AM-6:59AM)

Clear Deficient Heat

Bai Wei (Radix Cynanchi Atrati, Black Swallow-Wort Root)
Clear Deficient Heat
Bitter, Salty
Cold
Stomach, Liver, **Kidney**,[1245] Lung,[1246] Ren and Chong[1247]
Clock Neighbor (Liver/Lung), Branch (You/Chicken, Lung/Kidney, 5PM-6:59PM) + Stomach, Ren, Chong

Di Gu Pi (Cortex Lycii, Wolfberry Root Cortex)
Clear Deficient Heat
Sweet, Bland, Bitter[1248]
Cold
Lung, **Kidney**, Liver[1249]
Clock Neighbor (Liver/Lung), Branch (You/Chicken, Lung/Kidney, 5PM-6:59PM)

Qing Hao (Herba Artemesiae Annuae, Sweet Wormwood)
Clear Deficient Heat
Bitter, Acrid, Aromatic
Cold
Liver, Gall Bladder, Stomach,[1250] **Kidney**[1251]
Biao/Li (Gall Bladder/Liver), Branch (Zi/Rat, Kidney/Gall Bladder, 11PM-12:59AM) + Stomach

Cathartic

Shang Lu (Radix Phytolaccae, Poke Root)
Cathartic
Bitter
Cold, highly Toxic*
Lung, Spleen,[1252] **Kidney**, Large Intestine, Urinary Bladder[1253]
Name (Tai Yin, Lung/Spleen), Bie Jing (Tai Yin/Tai Yang, Lung/Urinary Bladder), Biao/Li (Large Intestine/Lung, Urinary Bladder/Kidney), Clock Opposite (Kidney/Large Intestine, Lung/Urinary Bladder), Branch (You/Chicken, Lung/Kidney, 5PM-6:59PM, Shen/Monkey, Large Intestine/Urinary Bladder, 3PM-4:59PM)

Da Ji (Radix Euphorbiae seu Knoxiae)
Cathartic
Bitter, Acrid
Cold, extremely Toxic*
Spleen,[1254] Lung,[1255] **Kidney**, Large Intestine, Liver,[1256] Gall Bladder[1257]
Name (Tai Yin, Lung/Spleen), Bie Jing (Jue Yin/Yang Ming, Liver/Large Intestine), Biao/Li (Large Intestine/Lung, Gall Bladder/Liver), Clock Opposite (Kidney/Large Intestine), Clock Neighbor (Liver/Lung), Branch (Zi/Rat, Kidney/Gall Bladder, 11PM-12:59AM, Chou/Ox, Spleen/Liver, 1AM-2:59AM, Mao/Rabbit, Liver/Large Intestine, 5AM-6:59AM, and You/Chicken, Lung/Kidney, 5PM-6:59PM)

Qian Niu Zi (Semen Pharbitidis, Pharbitis, Morning Glory Seed)
Cathartic
Bitter, Acrid[1258]
Cold, Toxic*
Lung, **Kidney**, Large Intestine, Small Intestine[1259]
Biao/Li (Large Intestine/Lung), Clock Opposite (Kidney/Large Intestine), Branch (You/Chicken, Lung/Kidney, 5PM-6:59PM) + Small Intestine

Gan Sui (Radix Euphorbiae Kansui, Kan Sui Root)
Cathartic
Bitter, Sweet
Cold, Toxic*
Lung, **Kidney**, Large Intestine
Biao/Li (Large Intestine/Lung), Clock Opposite (Kidney/Large Intestine), Branch (You/Chicken, Lung/Kidney, 5PM-6:59PM)

Yuan Hua, Lao Shu Hua (Flos Genkwa, Genkwa Flower, Lilac Daphne Flower Bud)
Cathartic
Acrid, Bitter
Warm, Toxic*
Lung, **Kidney**, Large Intestine
Biao/Li (Large Intestine/Lung), Clock Opposite (Kidney/Large Intestine), Branch (You/Chicken, Lung/Kidney, 5PM-6:59PM)

Dispel Wind Dampness, Open Channels and Luo-Network Vessels and Relieve Pain

Han Fang Ji/Fen Fang Ji (Radix Stephaniae Tetandrae, Stephania Root)
Dispel Wind Dampness, Open Channels and Luo-Network Vessels and Relieve Pain
Acrid, Bitter to very Bitter[1260]
Cold to very Cold[1261]
Urinary Bladder, Lung,[1262] Spleen,[1263] **Kidney**, Yang Qiao,[1264] and possibly San Jiao[1265]
Name (Tai Yin, Spleen/Lung), Bie Jing (Tai Yin/Tai Yang, Lung/Urinary Bladder), Biao/Li (Urinary Bladder/Kidney), Clock Opposite (Lung/Urinary Bladder), Branch (You/Chicken, Lung/Kidney, 5PM-6:59PM) and possibly Bie Jing (Shao Yin/Shao Yang, Kidney/San Jiao), Clock Opposite (San Jiao/Spleen), Branch (Hai/Pig, Urinary Bladder/San Jiao, 9PM-10:59PM) + Yang Qiao

Lao Guan Cao (Herba Erodi seu Geranii, Geranium, Common Heron's Bill Herb)
Dispel Wind Dampness, Open Channels and Luo-Network Vessels and Relieve Pain
Acrid, Bitter
Neutral
Liver, Large Intestine, **Kidney**,[1266] Spleen[1267]
Bie Jing (Jue Yin/Yang Ming, Liver/Large Intestine), Clock Opposite (Kidney/Large Intestine), Branch (Mao/Rabbit, Liver/Large Intestine, 5AM-6:59AM, Chou/Ox, Spleen/Liver, 1AM-2:59AM)

Ma An Teng (Herba Ipomoea Pes-caprae, Beach Morning Glory)
Dispel Wind Dampness, Open Channels and Luo-Network Vessels and Relieve Pain
Acrid, Bitter
Neutral
Liver, **Kidney**, Large Intestine
Bie Jing (Jue Yin/Yang Ming, Liver/Large Intestine), Clock Opposite (Kidney/Large Intestine), Branch (Mao/Rabbit, Liver/Large Intestine, 5AM-6:59AM)

Mu Fang Ji (Radix Cocculi, Cocculus Root)
Dispel Wind Dampness, Open Channels and Luo-Network Vessels and Relieve Pain
Bitter, Acrid
Cold
Urinary Bladder, **Kidney**, Spleen
Biao/Li (Urinary Bladder/Kidney) + Spleen

Tou Gu Cao (Caulis Impatientis, Garden Balsam)
Dispel Wind Dampness, Open Channels and Luo-Network Vessels and Relieve Pain
Bitter, slightly Sweet, Acrid
Cool
Liver, Spleen, **Kidney**
Branch (Chou/Ox, Spleen/Liver, 1AM-2:59AM) + Kidney

Hai Tong Pi (Cortex Erythrinae, Coral Bean Bark)
Dispel Wind Dampness, Open Channels and Luo-Network Vessels and Relieve Pain
Bitter, Acrid
Neutral
Liver, Spleen,[1268] **Kidney**[1269]
Branch (Chou/Ox, Spleen/Liver, 1AM-2:59AM) + Kidney

Shen Jin Cao, Shi Song, Shi Wu Gong (Herba Lycopodii, Ground Pine, Staghorn Moss, Wolf's Claw Club Moss)
Dispel Wind Dampness, Open Channels and Luo-Network Vessels and Relieve Pain
Bitter, Acrid
Warm
Liver, Spleen,[1270] **Kidney**[1271]
Branch (Chou/Ox, Spleen/Liver, 1AM-2:59AM) + Kidney

Hai Feng Teng (Caulis Piperis Kadsurae, Kadsura Pepper Stem, Futokadsura Stem)
Dispel Wind Dampness, Open Channels and Luo-Network Vessels and Relieve Pain
Acrid, Bitter, Aromatic
Slightly Warm
Liver, Heart,[1272] **Kidney**[1273]
Name (Shao Yin, Heart/Kidney) + Liver

Du Huo, Da Huo, Rou Du Huo (Radix Angelicae Pubescentis, Angelica Root)
Dispel Wind Dampness, Open Channels and Luo-Network Vessels and Relieve Pain
Acrid, Bitter, Aromatic
Slightly Warm to very Warm[1274]
Liver, **Kidney**,[1275] Urinary Bladder, Du[1276]
Biao/Li (Urinary Bladder/Kidney) + Liver, Du

Hai Fu Rong (Herba Limonium Wrightii, Limonium)
Dispel Wind Dampness, Open Channels and Luo-Network Vessels and Relieve Pain
Acrid, Bitter
Cold
Liver, **Kidney**

Xi Xian Cao (Herba Siegesbeckiae, Siegesbeckia, Common St. Paul's Wort)
Dispel Wind Dampness, Open Channels and Luo-Network Vessels and Relieve Pain
Bitter, Acrid[1277]
Cold, slightly Toxic*[1278]
Kidney, Liver

Song Jie (Lignum Pini Nodi, Knotty Pine Wood)
Dispel Wind Dampness, Open Channels and Luo-Network Vessels and Relieve Pain
Bitter, Acrid[1279]
Warm
Liver, **Kidney**[1280]

Qian Nian Jian (Rhizoma Homalomenae, Homalomena)
Dispel Wind Dampness, Open Channels and Luo-Network Vessels and Relieve Pain/Dispel Wind-Dampness Strengthen Sinew/Tendon and Bone
Bitter, Acrid, Aromatic[1281]
Warm, Toxic*[1282]
Kidney, Liver

Yi Tiao Gen (Radix Moghaniae, Moghania)
Dispel Wind Dampness, Open Channels and Luo-Network Vessels and Relieve Pain
Acrid
Warm
Liver, **Kidney**

Dispel Wind-Dampness Strengthen Sinew/Tendon and Bone

Shi Nan Teng (Ramulus Piper, Piper Vine)
Dispel Wind-Dampness Strengthen Sinew/Tendon and Bone
Acrid
Warm
Liver, Lung, **Kidney**
Clock Neighbor (Liver/Lung), Branch (You/Chicken, Lung/Kidney, 5PM-6:59PM)

Xiang Jia Pi (Cortex Periplocae, Chinese Silkvine Root Bark)
Dispel Wind-Dampness Strengthen Sinew/Tendon and Bone
Acrid, Bitter
Warm, Toxic*
Liver, **Kidney**, Heart
Name (Shao Yin, Kidney/Heart) + Liver

Sang Ji Sheng (Herba Taxilli, Taxillus, Mulberry Mistletoe Stem, Mistletoe)
Dispel Wind-Dampness Strengthen Sinew/Tendon and Bone
Bitter, Sweet,[1283] Sour[1284]
Neutral
Liver, **Kidney**

Hu Ji Sheng, Bei Ji Sheng (Herba Visci, Colored Mistletoe)
Dispel Wind-Dampness Strengthen Sinew/Tendon and Bone
Bitter
Neutral, slightly Toxic*[1285]
Liver, **Kidney**

Lu Han Cao, Lu Xian Cao, Lu Ti Cao (Herba Pyrolae, Pyrola)
Dispel Wind-Dampness Strengthen Sinew/Tendon and Bone
Sweet, Bitter
Warm
Liver, **Kidney**

Wu Jia Pi (Cortex Acanthopanacis/Eleutherococcus, Eleutherococcus Root Bark, Acanthopanax Root Bark)
Dispel Wind-Dampness Strengthen Sinew/Tendon and Bone
Acrid, Bitter
Warm
Kidney, Liver

Qian Nian Jian (Rhizoma Homalomenae, Homalomena)
Dispel Wind Dampness, Open Channels and Luo-Network Vessels and Relieve Pain/Dispel Wind-Dampness Strengthen Sinew/Tendon and Bone
Bitter, Acrid, Aromatic[1286]
Warm, Toxic*[1287]
Kidney, Liver

Regulate Water Resolve Dampness

Yi Yi Ren (Semen Coicis, Job's Tears)
Regulate Water Resolve Dampness
Sweet, Bland
Cool to slightly Cold
Spleen, Stomach, Lung, **Kidney**[1288]
Name (Tai Yin, Spleen/Lung), Biao/Li (Stomach/Spleen), Branch (You/Chicken, Lung/Kidney, 5PM-6:59PM)

Fu Ling, Yun Ling (Poria, Hoelen, China Root)
Regulate Water Resolve Dampness
Sweet, Bland
Neutral
Heart, Spleen, **Kidney**, Lung[1289]
Name (Shao Yin, Heart/Kidney, Tai Yin, Spleen/Lung), Clock Neighbor (Spleen/Heart)

Che Qian Zi (Semen Plantaginis, Plantago Seed, Plantain Seed)
Regulate Water Resolve Dampness
Sweet, Bland[1290]
Cold
Kidney, Urinary Bladder, Liver, Lung, Small Intestine[1291]
Name (Tai Yang, Small Intestine/Urinary Bladder), Bie Jing (Tai Yin/Tai Yang, Lung/Urinary Bladder), Biao/Li (Urinary Bladder/Kidney), Clock Opposite (Lung/Urinary Bladder, Liver/Small Intestine), Clock Neighbor (Small Intestine/Urinary Bladder, Liver/Lung), Branch (You/Chicken, Lung/Kidney, 5PM-6:59PM)

Che Qian Cao (Herba Plantaginis)
Regulate Water Resolve Dampness
Sweet
Cold
Liver, **Kidney**, Lung, Small Intestine
Clock Opposite (Liver/Small Intestine), Clock Neighbor (Liver/Lung), Branch (You/Chicken, Lung/Kidney, 5PM-6:59PM)

Bai Long Chuan Hua Tou (Radix Clerodendron Paniculatum, Clerodendron, Scarlet Glory Bower)
Regulate Water Resolve Dampness
Slightly Bitter
Warm
Lung, Liver, **Kidney**
Clock Neighbor (Liver/Lung), Branch (You/Chicken, Lung/Kidney, 5PM-6:59PM)

Liu Zhi Huang (Herba Solidaginis, Solidago)
Regulate Water Resolve Dampness
Bitter, Sweet
Cold
Lung, Liver, **Kidney**
Clock Neighbor (Liver/Lung), Branch (You/Chicken, Lung/Kidney, 5PM-6:59PM)

Shan Pu Tao (Radix Vitis Amurensis, Viticis)
Regulate Water Resolve Dampness
Sweet
Cold
Lung, Liver, **Kidney**
Clock Neighbor (Liver/Lung), Branch (You/Chicken, Lung/Kidney, 5PM-6:59PM)

Ding Shu Xiu (Herba Elephantopus Scaber, Elephantopi)
Regulate Water Resolve Dampness
Sweet, Bitter
Cold
Liver, **Kidney**, Large Intestine
Bie Jing (Jue Yin/Yang Ming, Liver/Large Intestine), Clock Opposite (Kidney/Large Intestine), Branch (Mao/Rabbit, Liver/Large Intestine, 5AM-6:59AM)

Xian Feng Cao (Herba Bidentis, Bidens)
Regulate Water Resolve Dampness
Bland
Cold
Kidney, Small Intestine, Urinary Bladder
Name (Tai Yang, Small Intestine/Urinary Bladder), Biao/Li (Urinary Bladder/Kidney), Clock Neighbor (Small Intestine/Urinary Bladder)

Di Fu Zi (Fructus Kochiae, Summer Cypress Fruit, Burning Bush Fruit)
Regulate Water Resolve Dampness
Sweet,[1292] Bitter, Acrid[1293]
Cold
Urinary Bladder, **Kidney**
Biao/Li (Urinary Bladder/Kidney)

Bi Zi Cao (Herba Pogonantheri Criniti, Crinite Pogonatherum)
Regulate Water Resolve Dampness
Sweet
Cool
Kidney, Urinary Bladder
Biao/Li (Urinary Bladder/Kidney)

Shui Ding Xiang (Herba Ludwigiae Prostratae, Ludwigia)
Regulate Water Resolve Dampness
Sweet, Bland
Very Cold
Kidney, Urinary Bladder
Biao/Li (Urinary Bladder/Kidney)

Zhu Ling (Polyporus, Pore Fungus)
Regulate Water Resolve Dampness
Sweet, Bland
Neutral
Kidney, Urinary Bladder
Biao/Li (Urinary Bladder, Kidney)

Ze Xie (Rhizoma Alismatis, Water Plantain Rhizome)
Regulate Water Resolve Dampness
Sweet, Salty,[1294] Bland
Cold
Kidney, Urinary Bladder
Biao/Li (Urinary Bladder/Kidney)

Yu Mi Xu, Yu Mai Xu (Stigma Maydis, Corn Stigma, Corn Silk)
Regulate Water Resolve Dampness
Sweet, Bland
Neutral
Urinary Bladder, **Kidney**, Liver, Gall Bladder[1295]
Biao/Li (Urinary Bladder/Kidney, Gall Bladder/Liver), Branch (Zi/Rat, Kidney/Gall Bladder, 11PM-12:59AM)

Jin Qian Cao (Herba Lysimachiae, Lysimachia, Loose Strife Herb)
Regulate Water Resolve Dampness
Sweet, Salty, Bland[1296]
Cool to slightly Cold[1297]
Urinary Bladder, Gall Bladder, **Kidney**, Liver
Biao/Li (Urinary Bladder/Kidney, Gall Bladder/Liver), Branch (Zi/Rat, Kidney/Gall Bladder, 11PM-12:59AM)

Hua Shi Cao (Herba Orthosiphon Aristatus, Orthosiphon, Cat's Whiskers)
Regulate Water Resolve Dampness
Bitter
Cold
Liver, **Kidney**, Urinary Bladder
Biao/Li (Urinary Bladder/Kidney) + Liver

Guang Jin Qian Cao (Herba Desmodii Styracifolii, Desmodium, Snowbell Leaf Tick Clover)
Regulate Water Resolve Dampness
Sweet, Bland
Cool
Liver, **Kidney**, Urinary Bladder
Biao/Li (Urinary Bladder/Kidney) + Liver

Mo Gu Xiao (Caulis Hyptis Capitatae, Hyptis)
Regulate Water Resolve Dampness
Bland
Cold
Liver, **Kidney**

Huang Jin Gui (Caulis Vanieriae, Vanieria)
Regulate Water Resolve Dampness
Bland
Cool
Liver, **Kidney**

Warm Interior

Jiao Mu (Semen Zanthoxyli, Zanthoxylum Seed, Sichuan Peppercorn Seed)
Warm Interior
Bitter
Cold, Toxic*
Spleen, Urinary Bladder, Lung, **Kidney**
Name (Tai Yin, Spleen/Lung), Bie Jing (Tai Yin/Tai Yang, Lung/Urinary Bladder), Biao/Li (Urinary Bladder/Kidney), Clock Opposite (Lung/Urinary Bladder), Branch (You/Chicken, Lung/Kidney, 5PM-6:59PM)

Xi Xin (Radix et Rhizoma Asari, Asarum, Chinese Wild Ginger)
Acrid Warm Exterior Releasing/Warm Interior
Acrid to extremely Acrid,[1298] Aromatic
Warm, slightly Toxic*
Lung, Heart, **Kidney**, Du,[1299] all channels[1300]
Name (Shao Yin, Heart/Kidney), Branch (You/Chicken, Lung/Kidney, 5PM-6:59PM) + Du

Bi Cheng Qie, Cheng Qie Zi (Fructus Litseae, Cubeb Fruit)
Warm Interior
Acrid, Aromatic[1301]
Warm
Spleen, Stomach, **Kidney**, Urinary Bladder
Biao/Li (Stomach/Spleen, Urinary Bladder/Kidney), Qian/Hou (Front/Back, Stomach/Urinary Bladder)

Ding Xiang (Flos Caryophylli, Clove Flower Bud)
Warm Interior
Acrid, Aromatic
Warm
Kidney, Spleen, Stomach
Biao/Li (Stomach/Spleen) + Kidney

Hua Jiao, Chuan Jiao (Pericarpium Zanthoxyli, Sichuan Peppercorn)
Warm Interior
Acrid
Warm[1302] to Hot, slightly Toxic*
Kidney, Spleen, Stomach
Biao/Li (Stomach/Spleen) + Kidney

Wu Zhu Yu, Wu Yu (Fructus Evodiae, Evodia Fruit)
Warm Interior
Acrid, Bitter, Aromatic
Hot, slightly Toxic*
Liver, Spleen, Stomach, **Kidney**[1303]
Biao/Li (Stomach/Spleen), Branch (Chou/Ox, Spleen/Liver, 1AM-2:59AM) + Kidney

Xiao Hui Xiang, Gui Hui Xiang (Fructus Foeniculi, Fennel Seed)
Warm Interior
Acrid, Aromatic
Warm
Liver, **Kidney**, Spleen, Stomach
Biao/Li (Stomach/Spleen), Branch (Chou/Ox, Spleen/Liver, 1AM-2:59AM) + Kidney

Zhi Cao Wu (Radix Aconiti Kusnezoffii, Wild Aconite Root)
Warm Interior
Acrid, Bitter
Hot, extremely Toxic**
Heart, Liver, Spleen, **Kidney**[1304]
Name (Shao Yin, Kidney/Heart), Clock Neighbor (Spleen/Heart), Branch (Chou/Ox, Spleen/Liver, 1AM-2:59AM)

Rou Gui (Cortex Cinnamomi, Cinnamon Bark, Cassia Bark)
Warm Interior
Acrid to highly Acrid,[1305] Sweet, Aromatic
Greatly Warming[1306] to Hot
Heart, **Kidney**, Liver, Spleen
Name (Shao Yin, Heart/Kidney), Clock Neighbor (Spleen/Heart), Branch (Chou/Ox, Spleen/Liver, 1AM-2:59AM)

Zhi Fu Zi, Tian Xiong (Radix Aconiti Lateralis Praeparata, Aconite, Prepared/Processed Aconite Accessory Root)
Warm Interior
Acrid to extremely Acrid,[1307] Sweet[1308]
Hot to very Hot,[1309] Toxic*
Heart, **Kidney**, Spleen, Du[1310]
Name (Shao Yin, Heart/Kidney), Clock Neighbor (Spleen/Heart) + Du

Da Hui Xiang, Ba Jiao Hui, Ba Jiao Hui Xiang (Fructus Anisi Stellati, Star Anis)
Warm Interior
Acrid, Sweet, Aromatic
Warm
Liver, **Kidney**, Spleen
Branch (Chou/Ox, Spleen/Liver, 1AM-2:59AM) + Kidney

Regulate and Rectify Qi

Tian Xian Teng, Ma Dou Ling Teng (Herba Aristolochiae, Aristolochia, Dutchman's Pipe)
Regulate and Rectify Qi
Bitter
Warm, Toxic*
Heart, Lung, Spleen, **Kidney**
Name (Shao Yin, Heart/Kidney, Tai Yin, Spleen/Lung)
Clock Neighbor (Spleen/Heart), Branch (You/Chicken, Lung/Kidney, 5PM-6:59PM)

Wu Yao, Tai Wu Yao, Tai Wu (Radix Linderae, Lindera Root)
Regulate and Rectify Qi
Acrid, Aromatic[1311]
Warm
Urinary Bladder, **Kidney**, Lung, Spleen
Name (Tai Yin, Lung/Spleen), Bie Jing (Tai Yin/Tai Yang, Lung/Urinary Bladder), Biao/Li (Urinary Bladder/Kidney), Clock Opposite (Lung/Urinary Bladder), Branch (You/Chicken, Lung/Kidney, 5PM-6:59PM)

Dao Dou (Semen Canavaliae, Sword Bean)
Regulate and Rectify Qi
Sweet
Warm
Stomach, Spleen,[1312] **Kidney**, Large Intestine[1313]
Name (Yang Ming, Large Intestine/Stomach), Biao/Li (Stomach/Spleen), Clock Opposite (Kidney/Large Intestine), Clock Neighbor (Large Intestine/Stomach)

Chen Xiang (Lignum Aquilariae Resinatum, Aloeswood)
Regulate and Rectify Qi
Acrid, Bitter, Aromatic
Warm
Kidney, Spleen, Stomach
Biao/Li (Stomach/Spleen) + Kidney

Po Bu Zi Ye (Folium Cordia Dichotoma, Sebastan Plum Cordia Leaf)
Regulate and Rectify Qi
Bitter, slightly Astringent
Cool
Liver, **Kidney**, Stomach

Jiu Ceng Ta (Herba Ocimi Basilici, Basil)
Regulate and Rectify Qi
Acrid
Warm
Stomach, Liver, **Kidney**

Jiu Xiang Chong, Da Pi Chong (Aspongopus, Stinkbug)
Regulate and Rectify Qi
Salty
Warm
Spleen, Liver, **Kidney**
Branch (Chou/Ox, Spleen/Liver, 1AM-2:59AM) + Kidney

Ju He, Ju Zi He, Ju Zi Ren, Ju Ren (Citri Reticulatae Semen, Tangerine/Orange Seed)
Regulate and Rectify Qi
Bitter
Neutral
Liver, **Kidney**,[1314] Urinary Bladder[1315]
Biao/Li (Urinary Bladder/Kidney) + Liver

Stop Bleeding

Xue Yu Tan (Crinis Carbonitsatus, Charred Human Hair)
Stop Bleeding
Bitter, Astringent[1316]
Neutral
Liver, Stomach, Heart,[1317] **Kidney**[1318]
Name (Shao Yin, Heart/Kidney) + Liver, Stomach

Lian Fang (Receptaculum Nelumbinis, Lotus Peduncle)
Stop Bleeding
Bitter, Astringent
Warm
Liver, Spleen, **Kidney**
Branch (Chou/Ox, Spleen/Liver, 1AM-2:59AM) + Kidney

Ai Ye (Folium Artemisiae Argyi, Mugwort Leaf, Moxa)
Stop Bleeding
Bitter, Acrid, Aromatic
Warm
Spleen, Liver, **Kidney**, Dai[1319]
Branch (Chou/Ox, Spleen/Liver, 1AM-2:59AM) + Kidney, Dai

Vitalize Blood Transform Stasis

Tu Niu Xi (Radix Achyranthes Longiflora, Native Achyranthis Root)
Clear Heat Clean Toxin/Vitalize Blood Transform Stasis
Bitter, Sour, Acrid[1320]
Neutral to Cold,[1321] slightly Toxic[1322]
Lung, Liver, **Kidney**
Clock Neighbor (Liver/Lung), Branch (You/Chicken, Lung/Kidney, 5PM-6:59PM)

Mu Dan Pi, Mu Shao Yao (Cortex Moutan, Peony Tree Root Cortex)
Clear Heat Cool Blood/Vitalize Blood Transform Stasis
Bitter, Acrid, Aromatic
Cool to slightly Cold
Heart, Liver, **Kidney**, Pericardium[1323]
Name (Shao Yin, Heart/Kidney, Jue Yin, Liver/Pericardium), Clock Neighbor (Kidney/Pericardium)

Huai Niu Xi (Radix Achyranthis Bidentatae, Achyranthes Root)
Vitalize Blood Transform Stasis
Bitter, Sour
Neutral
Liver, **Kidney**

Chuan Niu Xi (Radix Cyathulae, Cyathula)
Vitalize Blood Transform Stasis
Bitter, Sour, Sweet[1324]
Neutral
Liver, **Kidney**

Ding Jing Cao (Herba Linderniae)
Vitalize Blood Transform Stasis
Sweet, slightly Bitter
Neutral
Liver, **Kidney**

Niao Bu Su (Ramus Kalopanax Pictus, Kalopanacis)
Vitalize Blood Transform Stasis
Acrid, Bitter
Warm, slightly Toxic*
Liver, **Kidney**

Transform Phlegm

Hai Zao (Sargassum, Seaweed, Gulfweed)
Transform Phlegm
Bitter,[1325] Salty
Cold
Liver, **Kidney**, Stomach,[1326] Lung[1327]
Clock Neighbor (Liver/Lung), Branch (You/Chicken, Lung/Kidney, 5PM-6:59PM) + Stomach

Fu Shi, Shi Hua (Pumex, Pumice) and Fu Hai Shi, Hai Fu Shi, Fu Shui Shi (Os Costaziae, Costaziae Skeletons)
Transform Phlegm
Salty
Cold
Lung, **Kidney**[1328]
Branch (You/Chicken, Lung/Kidney, 5PM-6:59PM)

Kun Bu (Thallus Laminariae seu Eckloniae, Kelp)
Transform Phlegm
Salty
Cold
Liver, Stomach, **Kidney**

Relieve Cough and Wheezing/Panting

Zhong Ru Shi (Stalactitum, Stalactite Tip)
Relieve Cough and Wheezing/Panting/Tonify Yang
Sweet, Acrid[1329]
Warm
Lung, **Kidney**, Stomach
Branch (You/Chicken, Lung/Kidney, 5PM-6:59PM) + Stomach

Bai Guo, Yin Xing (Semen Ginkgo, Ginkgo Nut)
Relieve Cough and Wheezing/Panting/Astringe, Stabilize and Bind
Sweet, Bitter, Astringent
Neutral, slightly Toxic*
Lung, **Kidney**[1330]
Branch (You/Chicken, Lung/Kidney, 5PM-6:59PM)

Nourish and Calm Shen

Yuan Zhi (Radix Polygalae, Senega Root)
Nourish and Calm Shen
Acrid, Bitter
Slightly Warm
Lung, Heart, **Kidney**[1331]
Name (Shao Yin, Heart/Kidney), Branch (You/Chicken, Lung/Kidney, 5PM-6:59PM)

Bai Zi Ren (Semen Platycadi, Arbor-Vitae Seed, Biota)
Nourish and Calm Shen
Sweet, Acrid,[1332] Aromatic[1333]
Neutral to Cool[1334]
Heart, **Kidney**, Large Intestine
Name (Shao Yin, Kidney/Heart), Clock Opposite (Kidney/Large Intestine)

Calm Shen Sedative

Ci Shi (Magnetitum, Magnetite, Loadstone)
Calm Shen Sedative
Acrid,[1335] Salty
Cold
Liver, **Kidney**, Heart
Name (Shao Yin, Kidney/Heart) + Liver

Long Gu (Os Draconis, Fossilia Mastodi Ossis, Fossilized Bones)
Calm Shen Sedative
Sweet, slightly Acrid,[1336] Astringent[1337]
Neutral[1338] to Cool to slightly Cold[1339]
Heart, Liver, **Kidney**,[1340] Dai[1341]
Name (Shao Yin, Heart/Kidney) + Liver, Dai

Mu Li, Mu Li Ke (Concha Ostreae, Oyster Shell)
Calm Shen Sedative/Calm Liver Extinguish Wind
Salty, Astringent
Cool to slightly Cold[1342]
Liver, **Kidney**

Calm Liver Extinguish Wind

Di Long, Qiu Yin (Pheretima, Earthworm)
Calm Liver Extinguish Wind
Salty
Cold
Liver, Spleen, **Kidney**,[1343] Urinary Bladder, Lung[1344]
Name (Tai Yin, Spleen/Lung), Bie Jing (Tai Yin/Tai Yang, Lung/Urinary Bladder), Biao/Li (Urinary Bladder/Kidney), Clock Opposite (Lung/Urinary Bladder), Clock Neighbor (Liver/Lung), Branch (Chou/Ox, Spleen/Liver, 1AM-2:59AM)

Jue Ming Zi, Cao Jue Ming (Semen Cassiae, Cassia Seeds, Foetid Cassia Seeds)
Clear Heat Purge Fire/Calm Liver Extinguish Wind
Sweet, Bitter, Salty[1345]
Cool to slightly Cold
Liver, Large Intestine, **Kidney**[1346]
Bie Jing (Jue Yin/Yang Ming, Liver/Large Intestine), Clock Opposite (Kidney/Large Intestine), Branch (Mao/Rabbit, Liver/Large Intestine, 5AM-6:59AM)

Hei Dou (Semen Glycinis, Black Soybean)
Calm Liver Extinguish Wind
Sweet
Neutral
Spleen, **Kidney**

Mu Li, Mu Li Ke (Concha Ostreae, Oyster Shell)
Calm Shen Sedative/Calm Liver Extinguish Wind
Salty, Astringent
Cool to slightly Cold[1347]
Liver, **Kidney**

Shi Jue Ming, Qian Li Guang (Concha Haliotidis, Abalone Shell)
Calm Liver Extinguish Wind
Salty
Cold
Liver, **Kidney**[1348]

Tonify Qi

Xi Yang Shen, Hua Qi Shen (Radix Panacis Quinquefoli, American Ginseng Root)
Tonify Qi/Tonify Yin
Sweet, slightly Bitter[1349] to Bitter to very Bitter[1350]
Cold
Kidney, Heart, Lung, Spleen[1351]
Name (Shao Yin, Kidney/Heart, Tai Yin, Spleen/Lung), Clock Neighbor (Spleen/Heart), Branch (You/Chicken, Lung/Kidney, 5PM-6:59PM)

Ren Shen (Radix Ginseng, Ginseng Root)
Tonify Qi
Sweet, slightly Bitter
Slightly Warm
Lung, Spleen, Heart,[1352] **Kidney**[1353]
Name (Tai Yin, Lung/Spleen, Shao Yin, Kidney/Heart), Clock Neighbor (Spleen/Heart), Branch (You/Chicken, Lung/Kidney, 5PM-6:59PM)

Ci Wu Jia, Wu Jia Shen (Radix et Caulis Acanthopanacis Senticosi, Siberian Ginseng, Eleutherococcus Ginseng)
Tonify Qi
Acrid, slightly Bitter
Warm
Spleen, **Kidney**, Heart, Lung[1354]
Name (Tai Yin, Spleen/Lung, Shao Yin, Kidney/Heart), Clock Neighbor (Spleen/Heart), Branch (You/Chicken, Lung/Kidney, 5PM-6:59PM)

Shan Yao, Huai Shan Yao, Huai Shan, Shan Shu (Rhizoma Dioscoriae, Chinese Yam)
Tonify Qi
Sweet, Sour,[1355] slightly Astringent
Neutral
Kidney, Lung, Spleen, Dai[1356]
Name (Tai Yin, Lung/Spleen), Branch (You/Chicken, Lung/Kidney, 5PM-6:59PM) + Dai

Tonify Yang

Hu Tao Ren, He Tao Ren, Hu Tao Rou (Semen Juglandis, Walnut Nut)
Tonify Yang
Sweet, Astringent[1357]
Warm
Kidney, Lung, Large Intestine
Biao/Li (Large Intestine/Lung), Clock Opposite (Kidney/Large Intestine), Branch (You/Chicken, Lung/Kidney, 5PM-6:59PM)

Zhong Ru Shi (Stalactitum, Stalactite Tip)
Relieve Cough and Wheezing/Panting/Tonify Yang
Sweet, Acrid[1358]
Warm
Lung, **Kidney**, Stomach
Branch (You/Chicken, Lung/Kidney, 5PM-6:59PM) + Stomach

Dong Chong Xia Cao, Dong Chong Cao (Cordyceps, Caterpillar Fungus, Aweto)
Tonify Yang
Sweet
Neutral to Warm
Lung, **Kidney**
Branch (You/Chicken, Lung/Kidney, 5PM-6:59PM)

Ge Jie, Xian Dan (Gecko, Tokay)
Tonify Yang
Salty
Neutral
Lung, **Kidney**
Branch (You/Chicken, Lung/Kidney, 5PM-6:59PM)

Zi He Che (Placenta Hominis, Human Placenta)
Tonify Yang
Sweet, Salty
Warm
Kidney, Lung, Liver
Clock Neighbor (Liver/Lung), Branch (You/Chicken, Lung/Kidney, 5PM-6:59PM)

Rou Cong Rong, Cong Rong, Da Yun (Herba Cistanches, Fleshy Stem of Broomrape)
Tonify Yang
Sweet, Salty
Warm
Kidney, Large Intestine
Clock Opposite (Kidney/Large Intestine)

Yin Yang Huo, Xian Ling Pi (Herba Epimedii, Arial Parts of Epimedium, Horny Goat Weed)
Tonify Yang
Acrid, Sweet, Aromatic[1359]
Warm
Kidney, Liver, and possibly Large Intestine, Stomach and San Jiao[1360]
Possibly Name (Yang Ming, Large Intestine/Stomach), Bie Jing (Jue Yin/Yang Ming, Liver/Large Intestine, Shao Yin/Shao Yang, Kidney/San Jiao), Clock Opposite (Kidney/Large Intestine), Clock Neighbor (Large Intestine/Stomach), Branch (Mao/Rabbit, Liver/Large Intestine, 5AM-6:59AM)

Suo Yang, Di Mao Qiu (Herba Cynomorii, Fleshy Stem of Cynomorium)
Tonify Yang
Sweet
Warm
Liver, **Kidney**, Large Intestine
Bie Jing (Jue Yin/Yang Ming, Liver/Large Intestine), Clock Opposite (Kidney/Large Intestine), Branch (Mao/Rabbit, Liver/Large Intestine, 5AM-6:59AM)

Bu Gu Zhi, Gu Zi, Po Gu Zhi (Fructus Psoraleae, Psoralea Fruit)
Tonify Yang
Bitter, Acrid, Astringent[1361]
Very Warm to Hot
Kidney, Spleen

Yi Zhi Ren, Yi Zhi, Yi Zhi Zi (Fructus Alpiniae Oxyphyllae, Black Cardamon)
Tonify Yang
Acrid, Astringent,[1362] Aromatic
Warm
Kidney, Spleen

Xian Mao (Rhizoma Curculiginis, Golden Eye Grass Rhizome)
Tonify Yang
Acrid
Warm[1363] to Hot, Toxic*
Kidney, Liver,[1364] Spleen[1365] and possibly San Jiao[1366]
Branch (Chou/Ox, Spleen/Liver, 1AM-2:59AM) + Kidney
and possibly Bie Jing (Shao Yin/Shao Yang, Kidney/San Jiao), Clock Opposite (Spleen/San Jiao)

Tu Si Zi (Semen Cuscutae, Chinese Dodder Seeds)
Tonify Yang
Acrid, Sweet, Astringent[1367]
Neutral to Warm[1368]
Liver, **Kidney**, Spleen[1369]
Branch (Chou/Ox, Spleen/Liver, 1AM-2:59AM) + Kidney

Hai Shen, Hai Shu, Ci Shen (Strichopus Japonicus, Sea Cucumber, Sea Slug, Trepang)
Tonify Yang
Sweet, Salty
Warm
Heart, **Kidney**
Name (Shao Yin, Heart/Kidney)

Lu Jiao Shuang (Cornu Cervi Degelatinatium)
Tonify Yang
Sweet, Salty, Astringent[1370]
Slightly Warm
Kidney, Liver, Heart, Pericardium
Name (Shao Yin, Kidney/Heart, Jue Yin, Liver/Pericardium), Clock Neighbor (Kidney/Pericardium)

Hai Long (Syngnathus, Pipe Fish)
Tonify Yang
Sweet, Salty
Slightly Warm
Kidney

Yang Qi Shi, Bai Shi, Shi Sheng (Actinolitum, Actinolite)
Tonify Yang
Salty
Slightly Warm
Kidney

Jiu Cai Zi, Jiu Zi, Jiu Cai Ren (Semen Alli Tuberosi, Chinese Leek Seed, Allium Seed)
Tonify Yang
Acrid, Sweet, Sour,[1371] Astringent[1372]
Warm
Liver, **Kidney**

Gu Sui Bu, Hou Jiang, Mao Jiang, Shen Jiang (Rhizoma Drynariae, Drynaria Rhizome)
Tonify Yang
Bitter
Warm
Liver, **Kidney**

Hu Lu Ba (Semen Trigonellae, Fenugreek seed)
Tonify Yang
Bitter, Aromatic
Warm to very Warm[1373]
Kidney, Liver[1374]

Gou Ji, Jin Gou Ji (Rhizoma Cibotii, Lamb of Tartary Rhizome, Scythian Lamb Rhizome, Chain Fern Rhizome)
Tonify Yang
Sweet, Bitter, Astringent[1375]
Neutral[1376] to Warm
Liver, **Kidney**

Du Zhong, Si Mian Pi, Yu Zi Pi, Mu Mian (Cortex Eucommiae, Eucommia Bark)
Tonify Yang
Sweet, slightly Acrid[1377]
Warm
Kidney, Liver

Sha Yuan Zi, Sha Yuan Ji Li (Semen Astragali Complanati, Milkvetch Seed, Astragalus Seed)
Tonify Yang
Sweet, Astringent[1378]
Warm
Kidney, Liver

Hai Ma (Hippocampus, Sea Horse)
Tonify Yang
Sweet, Salty
Warm
Kidney, Liver

Lu Jiao Jiao, Bai Jiao (Gelatinum Cornu Cervi, Deer Antler Glue)
Tonify Yang
Sweet, Salty
Warm
Liver, **Kidney**

Lu Jiao (Cornu Cervi, Deer Antler)
Tonify Yang
Salty
Warm
Kidney, Liver

Hai Gou Shen, Wa Na Qi (Testes et Penis Otariae, Seal Testicles and Penis)
Tonify Yang
Salty
Hot
Kidney, Liver

Ba Ji Tian, Ba Ji, Ji Yan Teng (Radix Morindae Officinalis, Morinda Root)
Tonify Yang
Acrid, Sweet, Bitter[1379]
Slightly Warm
Kidney, Liver,[1380] Chong[1381]

Lu Rong (Cornu Cervi Pantotrichum, Elk/Deer Horn Velvet)
Tonify Yang
Sweet, Salty
Warm
Kidney, Liver, Du[1382]

Xu Duan, Chuan Duan (Radix Dipsaci, Japanese Teasel Root)
Tonify Yang
Bitter, Sweet, Acrid, Astringent
Slightly Warm
Liver, **Kidney**, Dai[1383]

Tonify Blood

Gou Qi Zi, Di Gu Zi (Fructus Lycii, Chinese Wolfberry Fruit, Matrimony Vine Fruit, Boxthorn Fruit)
Tonify Blood/Tonify Yin
Sweet
Neutral
Liver, **Kidney**, Lung
Clock Neighbor (Liver/Lung), Branch (You/Chicken, Lung/Kidney, 5PM-6:59PM)

E Jiao, Lu Pi Jiao (Colla Corii Asini, Donkey-Hide Glue, Gelatin)
Tonify Blood
Sweet
Neutral
Lung, Liver, **Kidney**
Clock Neighbor (Liver/Lung), Branch (You/Chicken, Lung/Kidney, 5PM-6:59PM)

Sang Shen Zi, Sang Shen, Sang Guo (Fructus Mori, Mulberry Fruit, White Mulberry Fruit)
Tonify Blood/Tonify Yin
Sweet
Cold
Heart,[1384] Liver, **Kidney**
Name (Shao Yin, Heart/Kidney) + Liver

Shu Di Huang (Radix Rehmanniae Preparata, Cooked and Cured Rehmannia, Cooked and Cured Chinese Foxglove Root)
Tonify Blood
Sweet
Slightly Warm
Liver, **Kidney**, Heart[1385]
Name (Shao Yin, Heart/Kidney) + Liver

He Shou Wu, Zhi He Shou Wu (Radix Polygoni Multiflori Preparata, Prepared Polygonum, Prepared Fleeceflower Root)
Tonify Blood
Sweet, Bitter, Astringent
Neutral to slightly Warm
Kidney, Liver

Tonify Yin

Tian Men Dong, Tian Dong (Radix Asparagi, Asparagus Tuber)
Tonify Yin
Sweet, Bitter
Cold to very Cold
Lung, **Kidney**, Stomach[1386]
Branch (You/Chicken, Lung/Kidney, 5PM-6:59PM) + Stomach

Xi Yang Shen, Hua Qi Shen (Radix Panacis Quinquefoli, American Ginseng Root)
Tonify Qi/Tonify Yin
Sweet, slightly Bitter[1387] to Bitter to very Bitter[1388]
Cold
Kidney, Heart, Lung, Spleen[1389]
Name (Shao Yin, Kidney/Heart, Tai Yin, Spleen/Lung), Clock Neighbor (Spleen/Heart), Branch (You/Chicken, Lung/Kidney, 5PM-6:59PM)

Huang Jing, Mi Pu (Rhizoma Polygonati, Siberian Solomon Seal Rhizome)
Tonify Yin
Sweet
Neutral
Spleen, Lung, **Kidney**
Name (Tai Yin, Spleen/Lung), Branch (You/Chicken, Lung/Kidney, 5PM-6:59PM)

Gou Qi Zi, Di Gu Zi (Fructus Lycii, Chinese Wolfberry Fruit, Matrimony Vine Fruit, Boxthorn Fruit)
Tonify Blood/Tonify Yin
Sweet
Neutral
Liver, **Kidney**, Lung
Clock Neighbor (Liver/Lung), Branch (You/Chicken, Lung/Kidney, 5PM-6:59PM)

Hei Zhi Ma, Hu Ma Zi, Hu Ma Ren, Zhi Ma (Semen Sesame Nigrum, Black Sesame Seed)
Tonify Yin
Sweet, Aromatic[1390]
Neutral
Liver, **Kidney**, Large Intestine[1391]
Bie Jing (Jue Yin/Yang Ming, Liver/Large Intestine), Clock Opposite (Kidney/Large Intestine), Branch (Mao/Rabbit, Liver/Large Intestine, 5AM-6:59AM)

Shi Hu (Herba Dendrobii, Dendrobium Stem)
Tonify Yin
Sweet, slightly Salty,[1392] Bland[1393]
Slightly Cold
Kidney, Stomach

Chu Shi Zi, Chu Shi, Chu Shi Mi (Fructus Broussonetiae, Paper Mulberry Fruit)
Tonify Yin
Sweet
Cold
Kidney, Liver, Spleen[1394]
Branch (Chou/Ox, Spleen/Liver, 1AM-2:59AM) + Kidney

Bie Jia (Carapax Trionycis, Chinese Soft Shell Turtle Shell)
Tonify Yin
Salty
Slightly Cold[1395] to Cold
Liver, **Kidney**,[1396] Spleen,[1397] Chong[1398]
Branch (Chou/Ox, Spleen/Liver, 1AM-2:59AM) + Kidney, Chong

Sang Shen Zi, Sang Shen, Sang Guo (Fructus Mori, Mulberry Fruit, White Mulberry Fruit)
Tonify Blood/Tonify Yin
Sweet
Cold
Heart,[1399] Liver, **Kidney**
Name (Shao Yin, Heart/Kidney) + Liver

Gui Ban (Plastrum Testudinis, Tortoise Plastron)
Tonify Yin
Salty, Sweet
Cold
Liver, **Kidney**, Heart, Ren[1400]
Name (Shao Yin, Kidney/Heart) + Liver, Ren

Han Lian Cao, Mo Han Lian (Herba Ecliptae)
Tonify Yin
Sweet, Sour, Aromatic[1401]
Cool[1402] to Cold
Liver, **Kidney**

Nu Zhen Zi (Fructus Ligustri Lucidi, Japanese Privet Fruit, Wax Tree Fruit)
Tonify Yin
Sweet, Bitter
Cool
Liver, **Kidney**

Astringe, Stabilize and Bind

Ying Su Ke (Pericarpium Papaveris, Opium Poppy Husk)
Astringe, Stabilize and Bind
Sour, Astringent
Neutral, Toxic*
Kidney, Large Intestine, Lung
Biao/Li (Large Intestine/Lung), Clock Opposite (Kidney/Large Intestine), Branch (You/Chicken, Lung/Kidney, 5PM-6:59PM)

Wu Bei Zi, Wen Ge, Bai Chong Chong (Galla Chinensis, Gallnut of Chinese Sumac)
Astringe, Stabilize and Bind
Salty, Sour, Astringent
Cold, slightly Toxic*[1403]
Lung, Large Intestine, **Kidney**
Biao/Li (Large Intestine/Lung), Clock Opposite (Kidney/Large Intestine), Branch (You/Chicken, Lung/Kidney, 5PM-6:59PM)

Wu Wei Zi (Fructus Schisandrae Chinensis, Schizandra Fruit)
Astringe, Stabilize and Bind
Sour, Sweet,[1404] Acrid,[1405] Bitter,[1406] Salty,[1407] Astringent
Warm
Kidney, Lung, Heart, Dai[1408]
Name (Shao Yin, Kidney/Heart), Branch (You/Chicken, Lung/Kidney, 5PM-6:59PM) + Dai

Bai Guo, Yin Xing (Semen Ginkgo, Ginkgo Nut)
Relieve Cough and Wheezing/Panting/Astringe, Stabilize and Bind
Sweet, Bitter, Astringent
Neutral, slightly Toxic*
Lung, **Kidney**[1409]
Branch (You/Chicken, Lung/Kidney, 5PM-6:59PM)

Nuo Dao Gen, Nuo Dao Gen Xu (Radix Oryzae Glutinosae, Glutinous Rice Root)
Astringe, Stabilize and Bind
Sweet, Acrid[1410]
Neutral
Lung, Liver, **Kidney**[1411]
Clock Neighbor (Liver/Lung), Branch (You/Chicken, Lung/Kidney, 5PM-6:59PM)

Jin Ying Zi (Fructus Rosae Laevigatae, Cherokee Rosehip)
Astringe, Stabilize and Bind
Sour, Astringent
Neutral to Warm[1412]
Kidney, Urinary Bladder, Large Intestine
Biao/Li (Urinary Bladder/Kidney), Clock Opposite (Kidney/Large Intestine), Branch (Shen/Monkey, Large Intestine/Urinary Bladder, 3PM-4:59PM)

Ji Guan Hua (Flos Celosiae Cristatae, Cock's Comb Flower)
Clear Heat Cool Blood/Astringe, Stabilize and Bind
Sweet, Astringent[1413]
Cool
Large Intestine, Liver, **Kidney**[1414]
Bie Jing (Jue Yin/Yang Ming, Liver/Large Intestine), Clock Opposite (Kidney/Large Intestine), Branch (Mao/Rabbit, Liver/Large Intestine, 5AM-6:59AM)

Hai Piao Xiao, Wu Zei Gu (Endoconcha Sepiae, Cuttlefish Bone)
Astringe, Stabilize and Bind
Salty, Astringent
Slightly Warm
Liver, **Kidney**, Stomach[1415]

Lian Zi, Ou Shi, Lian Shi, Pi Guo (Semen Nelumbinis, Lotus Seed)
Astringe, Stabilize and Bind
Sweet, Astringent
Neutral
Heart, **Kidney**, Spleen
Name (Shao Yin, Heart/Kidney), Clock Neighbor (Spleen/Heart)

Qian Shi (Semen Euryales, Euryale Seed)
Astringe, Stabilize and Bind
Sweet, Astringent
Neutral
Kidney, Spleen, Dai[1416]

Lian Xu (Stamen Nelumbinis, Lotus Stamen)
Astringe, Stabilize and Bind
Sweet, Astringent
Neutral
Heart, **Kidney**, Liver[1417]
Name (Shao Yin, Heart/Kidney) + Liver

Shan Zhu Yu, Shan Yu Rou (Fructus Corni, Asiatic Cornelian Cherry Fruit)
Astringe, Stabilize and Bind
Sour, Acrid,[1418] Astringent
Slightly Warm
Kidney, Liver

Fu Pen Zi (Fructus Rubi, Chinese Raspberry)
Astringe, Stabilize and Bind
Sweet, Sour, Astringent
Neutral[1419] to slightly Warm
Kidney, Liver, Dai[1420]

Sang Piao Xiao, Sang Xiao (Ootheca Mantidis, Praying Mantis Egg Case)
Astringe, Stabilize and Bind
Sweet, Salty, Astringent[1421]
Neutral
Liver, **Kidney**, Dai[1422]

External Application

Xiong Huang (Realgar)
External Application
Acrid, Bitter
Neutral to Warm, Toxic*
Heart, Liver, **Kidney**,[1423] Stomach,[1424] Lung,[1425] Large Intestine[1426]
Name (Shao Yin, Heart/Kidney, Yang Ming, Large Intestine/Stomach), Bie Jing (Jue Yin/Yang Ming, Liver/Large Intestine), Biao/Li (Large Intestine/Lung), Clock Opposite (Kidney/Large Intestine), Clock Neighbor (Large Intestine/Stomach, Liver/Lung), Branch (Mao/Rabbit, Liver/Large Intestine, 5AM-6:59AM, You/Chicken, Lung, Kidney, 5PM-6:59PM)

Qing Fen (Calomelas, Calomel)
External Application
Acrid, Bland[1427]
Cold, very Toxic*
Liver, **Kidney**, Large Intestine,[1428] Small Intestine[1429]
Bie Jing (Jue Yin/Yang Ming, Liver/Large Intestine), Clock Opposite (Liver/Small Intestine, Kidney/Large Intestine), Branch (Mao/Rabbit, Liver/Large Intestine, 5AM-6:59AM)

Liu Huang (Sulfur)
External Application
Sour, Sweet[1430]
Warm to Hot,[1431] Toxic*
Kidney, Large Intestine, Pericardium[1432]
Clock Opposite (Kidney/Large Intestine), Clock Neighbor (Kidney, Pericardium)

Da Feng Zi (Semen Hydnocarpi, Hydnocarpus Seed, Chaulmoogra Seed)
External Application
Acrid, Bitter[1433]
Hot, extremely Toxic*
Liver, Spleen, **Kidney**
Branch (Chou/Ox, Spleen/Liver,1AM-2:59AM) + Kidney

She Chuang Zi (Fructus Cnidii, Cnidium Seed)
External Application
Acrid, Bitter, Aromatic
Warm, slightly Toxic*
Kidney

Wu Ming Yi (Pyrolusitum, Pyrolusite)
External Application
Sweet
Neutral
Liver, **Kidney**

Hand Jue Yin Pericardium Herbs

Acrid Cool Exterior Releasing

Chai Hu (Radix Bupeuri, Thorowax Root, Bupleurum, Hare's Ear Root)
Acrid Cool Exterior Releasing
Bitter, Acrid, Aromatic[1434]
Neutral[1435] to Cool to slightly Cold[1436]
Liver, Gall Bladder, **Pericardium**,[1437] San Jiao[1438]
Name (Jue Yin, Liver/Pericardium, Shao Yang, San Jiao/Gall Bladder), Biao/Li (Gall Bladder/Liver, San Jiao/Pericardium), Clock Neighbor (San Jiao/Gall Bladder)

Clear Heat Purge Fire

Lian Zi Xin (Plumula Nelumbinis, Lotus Plumule)
Clear Heat Purge Fire/Astringe, Stabilize and Bind
Bitter, Astringent
Slightly Cold to Cold[1439]
Heart, **Pericardium**

Clear Heat Cool Blood

Mu Dan Pi, Mu Shao Yao (Cortex Moutan, Peony Tree Root Cortex)
Clear Heat Cool Blood/Vitalize Blood Transform Stasis
Bitter, Acrid, Aromatic
Cool to slightly Cold
Heart, Liver, Kidney, **Pericardium**[1440]
Name (Shao Yin, Heart/Kidney, Jue Yin, Liver/Pericardium), Clock Neighbor (Kidney/Pericardium)

Clear Heat Clean Toxin

Zi Hua Di Ding, Jian Tou Cao, Di Ding Cao (Herba Violae, Yedeon's Violet)
Clear Heat Clean Toxin
Bitter, Acrid
Cold
Heart, Liver, Stomach,[1441] **Pericardium**[1442]
Name (Jue Yin, Pericardium/Liver), Bie Jing (Jue Yin/Yang Ming, Pericardium/Stomach), Clock Opposite (Pericardium/Stomach), Branch (Shu/Dog, Stomach/Pericardium, 7PM-8:59PM) + Heart

Stop Bleeding

San Qi, Tian Qi (Radix Notoginseng, Pseudoginseng Root)
Stop Bleeding
Sweet, slightly Bitter
Warm
Liver, Stomach,[1443] Spleen,[1444] Large Intestine,[1445] **Pericardium**[1446]
Name (Yang Ming, Large Intestine/Stomach and Jue Yin, Liver/Pericardium), Bie Jing (Jue Yin/Yang Ming, Pericardium/Stomach and Liver/Large Intestine), Biao/Li (Stomach/Spleen), Clock Opposite (Pericardium/Stomach), Clock Neighbor (Large Intestine/Stomach), Branch (Chou/Ox, Spleen/Liver, 1AM-2:59AM, Mao/Rabbit, Liver/Large Intestine, 5AM-6:59AM and Shu/Dog, Stomach/Pericardium, 7PM-8:59PM)

Pu Huang (Pollen Typhae, Cattail Pollen, Bulrush Pollen)
Stop Bleeding
Sweet, Acrid,[1447] Astringent,[1448] Aromatic[1449]
Neutral
Liver, **Pericardium**,[1450] Heart,[1451] Spleen[1452]
Name (Jue Yin, Liver/Pericardium), Clock Neighbor (Spleen/Heart), Branch (Chou/Ox, Spleen/Liver, 1AM-2:59AM)

Vitalize Blood Transform Stasis

Mu Dan Pi, Mu Shao Yao (Cortex Moutan, Peony Tree Root Cortex)
Clear Heat Cool Blood/Vitalize Blood Transform Stasis
Bitter, Acrid, Aromatic
Cool to slightly Cold
Heart, Liver, Kidney, **Pericardium**[1453]
Name (Shao Yin, Heart/Kidney, Jue Yin, Liver/Pericardium), Clock Neighbor (Kidney/Pericardium)

Dan Shen (Radix Salviae Miltiorrhizae, Salvia Root)
Vitalize Blood Transform Stasis
Bitter
Cool to slightly Cold[1454] to Warm[1455]
Heart, **Pericardium**,[1456] Liver
Name (Jue Yin, Pericardium/Liver) + Heart

Chuan Xiong, Xiong Qiong, Fu Xiong (Rhizoma Ligustici Chuanxiong, Szechuan Lovage Root)
Vitalize Blood Transform Stasis
Acrid, Bitter,[1457] Aromatic
Warm
Liver, Gall Bladder, **Pericardium**, San Jiao,[1458] Chong[1459]
Name (Jue Yin, Liver/Pericardium, Shao Yang, San Jiao/Gall Bladder), Biao/Li (Gall Bladder/Liver, San Jiao/Pericardium), Clock Neighbor (San Jiao/Gall Bladder) + Chong

Ling Xiao Hua, Ling Xiao, Zi Wei (Flos Campsis, Campsis Flower, Trumpet Creeper)
Vitalize Blood Transform Stasis
Sweet, Sour, Salty[1460]
Slightly Cold
Liver, **Pericardium**
Name (Jue Yin, Liver/Pericardium)

Calm Liver Extinguish Wind

Dai Zhe Shi, Zhe Shi (Haematitum, Hematite)
Calm Liver Extinguish Wind
Bitter
Cold
Heart, Liver, **Pericardium**[1461]
Name (Jue Yin, Liver/Pericardium) + Heart

Gou Teng (Ramulus Uncariae cum Uncis, Gambir Vine Stems and Thorns)
Calm Liver Extinguish Wind
Sweet
Cool to slightly Cold[1462]
Liver, **Pericardium**, Heart[1463]
Name (Jue Yin, Liver/Pericardium) + Heart

Tonify Yang

Lu Jiao Shuang (Cornu Cervi Degelatinatium)
Tonify Yang
Sweet, Salty, Astringent[1464]
Slightly Warm
Kidney, Liver, Heart, **Pericardium**
Name (Shao Yin, Kidney/Heart, Jue Yin, Liver/Pericardium), Clock Neighbor (Kidney/Pericardium)

Astringe, Stabilize and Bind

Lian Zi Xin (Plumula Nelumbinis, Lotus Plumule)
Clear Heat Purge Fire/Astringe, Stabilize and Bind
Bitter, Astringent
Slightly Cold to Cold[1465]
Heart, **Pericardium**

External Application

Liu Huang (Sulfur)
External Application
Sour, Sweet[1466]
Warm to Hot,[1467] Toxic*
Kidney, Large Intestine, **Pericardium**[1468]
Clock Opposite (Kidney/Large Intestine), Clock Neighbor (Kidney, Pericardium)

Hand Shao Yang San Jiao Herbs

Acrid Warm Exterior Releasing

Jing Jie (Herba Schizonepitae, Schizonepeta)
Acrid Warm Exterior Releasing
Acrid, Aromatic
Slightly Warm
Lung, Liver, Gall Bladder,[1469] **San Jiao**,[1470] Du[1471]
Name (Shao Yang, Gall Bladder/San Jiao), Biao/Li (Gall Bladder/Liver), Clock Neighbor (San Jiao/Gall Bladder, Liver/Lung), Branch (Yin/Tiger, Gall Bladder/Lung, 3AM-4:59AM) + Du

Acrid Cool Exterior Releasing

Man Jing Zi, Jing Tiao Zi, Bai Bu Jing (Fructus Viticis, Vitex Fruit)
Acrid Cool Exterior Releasing
Acrid, Bitter
Both Cool and Warm[1472]
Lung,[1473] Liver, Stomach, Urinary Bladder,[1474] Gall Bladder,[1475] **San Jiao**[1476]
Name (Shao Yang, Gall Bladder/San Jiao), Bie Jing (Tai Yin/Tai Yang, Lung/Urinary Bladder), Biao/Li (Gall Bladder/Liver), Clock Opposite (Lung, Urinary Bladder), Clock Neighbor (San Jiao/Gall Bladder, Liver/Lung), Qian/Hou (Front/Back, Stomach/Urinary Bladder), Branch (Yin/Tiger, Gall Bladder/Lung, 3AM-4:59AM, Hai/Pig, Urinary Bladder/San Jiao, 9PM-10:59PM)

Chai Hu (Radix Bupleuri, Thorowax Root, Bupleurum, Hare's Ear Root)
Acrid Cool Exterior Releasing
Bitter, Acrid, Aromatic[1477]
Neutral[1478] to Cool to slightly Cold[1479]
Liver, Gall Bladder, Pericardium,[1480] **San Jiao**[1481]
Name (Jue Yin, Liver/Pericardium, Shao Yang, San Jiao/Gall Bladder), Biao/Li (Gall Bladder/Liver, San Jiao/Pericardium), Clock Neighbor (San Jiao/Gall Bladder)

Clear Heat Purge Fire

Shan Zhi Zi, Zhi Zi (Fructus Gardeniae, Cape Jasmine Fruit, Gardenia Fruit)
Clear Heat Purge Fire
Bitter
Cold
Heart, Lung, Stomach, **San Jiao**, Liver[1482]
Clock Neighbor (Liver/Lung) + Heart, Stomach, San Jiao

Clear Heat Clean Toxin

Ma Chi Xian, Chang Shou Cai, Wu Xing Cai (Herba Portulacae, Purslane, Portulaca)
Clear Heat Clean Toxin
Sour
Cold
Large Intestine, Liver, and possibly **San Jiao**[1483]
Bie Jing (Jue Yin/Yang Ming, Liver/Large Intestine), Branch (Mao/Rabbit, Liver/Large Intestine, 5AM-6:59AM) + possibly San Jiao

Cha Chi Huang (Herba Stellariae Aquaticae)
Clear Heat Clean Toxin
Acrid, slightly Bitter
Neutral
Liver, Large Intestine, **San Jiao**
Bie Jing (Jue Yin/Yang Ming, Liver/Large Intestine), Branch (Mao/Rabbit, Liver/Large Intestine, 5AM-6:59AM) + San Jiao

Dispel Wind Dampness, Open Channels and Luo-Network Vessels and Relieve Pain

Han Fang Ji/Fen Fang Ji (Radix Stephaniae Tetandrae, Stephania Root)
Dispel Wind Dampness, Open Channels and Luo-Network Vessels and Relieve Pain
Acrid, Bitter to very Bitter[1484]
Cold to very Cold[1485]
Urinary Bladder, Lung,[1486] Spleen,[1487] Kidney, Yang Qiao,[1488] and possibly **San Jiao**[1489]
Name (Tai Yin, Spleen/Lung), Bie Jing (Tai Yin/Tai Yang, Lung/Urinary Bladder), Biao/Li (Urinary Bladder/Kidney), Clock Opposite (Lung/Urinary Bladder), Branch (You/Chicken, Lung/Kidney, 5PM-6:59PM) and possibly Bie Jing (Shao Yin/Shao Yang, Kidney/San Jiao), Clock Opposite (San Jiao/Spleen), Branch (Hai/Pig, Urinary Bladder/San Jiao, 9PM-10:59PM) + Yang Qiao

Aromatic Dissolve Dampness

Bai Dou Kou (Fructus Amomi Rotundus, Round Cardamom Fruit)
Aromatic Dissolve Dampness
Intensely[1490] Acrid, not Astringent,[1491] Aromatic
Warm
Lung, Spleen, Stomach and possibly **San Jiao**[1492]
Name (Tai Yin, Lung/Spleen), Biao/Li (Stomach/Spleen) and possibly Clock Opposite (Spleen/San Jiao)

Regulate and Rectify Qi

Mu Xiang (Radix Aucklandiae, Costus Root)
Regulate and Rectify Qi
Acrid, Bitter, slightly Astringent[1493] Aromatic
Warm
Gall Bladder, Large Intestine, Spleen, Stomach, **San Jiao**[1494]
Name (Yang Ming, Large Intestine/Stomach, Shao Yang, Gall Bladder/San Jiao), Biao/Li (Stomach/Spleen), Clock Opposite (Spleen/San Jiao), Clock Neighbor (Large Intestine/Stomach, San Jiao/Gall Bladder)

Qing Pi, Qing Ju Pi (Pericarpium Citri Reticulatae Viride, Green or Unripened Tangerine Peel)
Regulate and Rectify Qi
Acrid, Bitter, slightly Sour,[1495] Aromatic
Warm
Liver, Gall Bladder, Stomach, **San Jiao**[1496]
Name (Shao Yang, San Jiao/Gall Bladder), Biao/Li (Gall Bladder/Liver), Clock Neighbor (San Jiao/Gall Bladder) + Stomach

Xiang Fu (Rhizoma Cyperi, Cyperus Rhizome, Nut Grass Rhizome)
Regulate and Rectify Qi
Acrid to intensely Acrid,[1497] slightly Bitter, slightly Sweet, Aromatic
Neutral
Liver, Spleen,[1498] **San Jiao**, Gall Bladder,[1499] some sources indicate that it enters all channels.
Name (Shao Yang, San Jiao/Gall Bladder), Biao/Li (Gall Bladder/Liver), Clock Opposite (Spleen/San Jiao), Clock Neighbor (San Jiao/Gall Bladder), Branch (Chou/Ox, Spleen/Liver, 1AM-2:59AM)

Vitalize Blood Transform Stasis

Chuan Xiong, Xiong Qiong, Fu Xiong (Rhizoma Ligustici Chuanxiong, Szechuan Lovage Root)
Vitalize Blood Transform Stasis
Acrid, Bitter,[1500] Aromatic
Warm
Liver, Gall Bladder, Pericardium, **San Jiao**,[1501] Chong[1502]
Name (Jue Yin, Liver/Pericardium, Shao Yang, San Jiao/Gall Bladder), Biao/Li (Gall Bladder/Liver, San Jiao/Pericardium), Clock Neighbor (San Jiao/Gall Bladder) + Chong

Tonify Qi

Huang Qi (Radix Astragali, Astragalus Root, Milk Vetch Root)
Tonify Qi
Sweet
Slightly Warm
Spleen, Lung, **San Jiao**[1503]
Name (Tai Yin, Spleen/Lung), Clock Opposite (Spleen/San Jiao)

Tonify Yang

Yin Yang Huo, Xian Ling Pi (Herba Epimedii, Arial Parts of Epimedium, Horny Goat Weed)
Tonify Yang
Acrid, Sweet, Aromatic[1504]
Warm
Kidney, Liver, and possibly Large Intestine, Stomach and **San Jiao**[1505]
Possibly Name (Yang Ming, Large Intestine/Stomach), Bie Jing (Jue Yin/Yang Ming, Liver/Large Intestine, Shao Yin/Shao Yang, Kidney/San Jiao), Clock Opposite (Kidney/Large Intestine), Clock Neighbor (Large Intestine/Stomach), Branch (Mao/Rabbit, Liver/Large Intestine, 5AM-6:59AM)

Xian Mao (Rhizoma Curculiginis, Golden Eye Grass Rhizome)
Tonify Yang
Acrid
Warm[1506] to Hot, Toxic*
Kidney, Liver,[1507] Spleen[1508] and possibly **San Jiao**[1509]
Branch (Chou/Ox, Spleen/Liver, 1AM-2:59AM) + Kidney
and possibly Bie Jing (Shao Yin/Shao Yang, Kidney/San Jiao), Clock Opposite (Spleen/San Jiao)

Foot Shao Yang Gall Bladder Herbs

Acrid Warm Exterior Releasing

Jing Jie (Herba Schizonepitae, Schizonepeta)
Acrid Warm Exterior Releasing
Acrid, Aromatic
Slightly Warm
Lung, Liver, **Gall Bladder**,[1510] San Jiao,[1511] Du[1512]
Name (Shao Yang, Gall Bladder/San Jiao), Biao/Li (Gall Bladder/Liver), Clock Neighbor (San Jiao/Gall Bladder, Liver/Lung), Branch (Yin/Tiger, Gall Bladder/Lung, 3AM-4:59AM) + Du

Acrid Cool Exterior Releasing

Man Jing Zi, Jing Tiao Zi, Bai Bu Jing (Fructus Viticis, Vitex Fruit)
Acrid Cool Exterior Releasing
Acrid, Bitter
Both Cool and Warm[1513]
Lung,[1514] Liver, Stomach, Urinary Bladder,[1515] **Gall Bladder**,[1516] San Jiao[1517]
Name (Shao Yang, Gall Bladder/San Jiao), Bie Jing (Tai Yin/Tai Yang, Lung/Urinary Bladder), Biao/Li (Gall Bladder/Liver), Clock Opposite (Lung, Urinary Bladder), Clock Neighbor (San Jiao/Gall Bladder, Liver/Lung), Qian/Hou (Front/Back, Stomach/Urinary Bladder), Branch (Yin/Tiger, Gall Bladder/Lung, 3AM-4:59AM, Hai/Pig, Urinary Bladder/San Jiao, 9PM-10:59PM)

Mao Zi Dun Tou (Herba Abutilon Indicum, Indian Abutilon)
Acrid Cool Exterior Releasing
Sweet
Neutral, slightly Toxic*
Lung, Liver, **Gall Bladder**, Spleen
Name (Tai Yin, Lung/Spleen), Biao/Li (Gall Bladder, Liver), Clock Neighbor (Liver/Lung), Branch (Yin/Tiger, Gall Bladder/Lung, 3AM-4:59AM, and Chou/Ox, Spleen/Liver, 1AM-2:59AM)

Mu Zei, Jie Gu Cao, Jie Jie Cao (Herba Equesti Hiemalis, Scouring Rush, Shave Grass, Horsetail)
Acrid Cool Exterior Releasing
Sweet, Bitter
Neutral to slightly Cold
Lung, Liver, **Gall Bladder**[1518]
Biao/Li (Gall Bladder/Liver), Clock Neighbor (Liver/Lung), Branch (Yin/Tiger, Gall Bladder/Lung, 3AM-4:59AM)

Chai Hu (Radix Bupleuri, Thorowax Root, Bupleurum, Hare's Ear Root)
Acrid Cool Exterior Releasing
Bitter, Acrid, Aromatic[1519]
Neutral[1520] to Cool to slightly Cold[1521]
Liver, **Gall Bladder**, Pericardium,[1522] San Jiao[1523]
Name (Jue Yin, Liver/Pericardium, Shao Yang, San Jiao/Gall Bladder), Biao/Li (Gall Bladder/Liver, San Jiao/Pericardium), Clock Neighbor (San Jiao/Gall Bladder)

Clear Heat Purge Fire

Xia Ku Cao (Spica Prunellae, Selfheal Spike, Prunella)
Clear Heat Purge Fire
Bitter, Acrid
Cold
Liver, **Gall Bladder**
Biao/Li (Gall Bladder/Liver)

Clear Heat Dry Dampness

Huang Qin (Radix Scutellariae, Baical Skullcap Root, Scutellaria, Scute)
Clear Heat Dry Dampness
Bitter
Cold
Lung, **Gall Bladder**, Stomach, Large Intestine and possibly San Jiao[1524]
Name (Yang Ming, Large Intestine/Stomach) Biao/Li (Large Intestine/Lung), Clock Neighbor (Large Intestine/Stomach), Branch (Yin/Tiger, Gall Bladder/Lung, 3AM-4:59AM), and possibly Name (Shao Yang, San Jiao/Gall Bladder), Clock Neighbor (San Jiao/Gall Bladder)

Qin Pi (Cortex Fraxini, Bark of Korean Ash Branch)
Clear Heat Dry Dampness/Clear Heat Clean Toxin
Bitter, Acrid,[1525] Astringent[1526]
Cold
Gall Bladder, Liver, Large Intestine, Stomach[1527]
Name (Yang Ming, Large Intestine/Stomach), Bie Jing (Jue Yin/Yang Ming, Liver/Large Intestine), Biao/Li (Gall Bladder/Liver), Clock Neighbor (Large Intestine/Stomach), Branch (Mao/Rabbit, Liver/Large Intestine, 5AM-6:59AM)

Long Dan Cao, Long Dan, Dan Cao (Radix Gentianae, Chinese Gentian Root, Gentiana)
Clear Heat Dry Dampness
Bitter, Astringing[1528]
Cold
Liver, **Gall Bladder**, Stomach, Urinary Bladder[1529]
Biao/Li (Gall Bladder/Liver), Qian/Hou (Front/Back, Stomach/Urinary Bladder)

Clear Heat Clean Toxin

Lian Qiao (Fructus Forsythiae, Forsythia Fruit)
Clear Heat Clean Toxin
Bitter, slightly Acrid[1530]
Cool to slightly Cold[1531]
Lung, Heart, **Gall Bladder**
Bie Jing (Shao Yin/Shao Yang, Heart/Gall Bladder), Clock Opposite (Heart/Gall Bladder), Branch (Yin/Tiger, Gall Bladder/Lung, 3AM-4:59AM)

Qin Pi (Cortex Fraxini, Bark of Korean Ash Branch)
Clear Heat Dry Dampness/Clear Heat Clean Toxin
Bitter, Acrid,[1532] Astringent[1533]
Cold
Gall Bladder, Liver, Large Intestine, Stomach[1534]
Name (Yang Ming, Large Intestine/Stomach), Bie Jing (Jue Yin/Yang Ming, Liver/Large Intestine), Biao/Li (Gall Bladder/Liver), Clock Neighbor (Large Intestine/Stomach), Branch (Mao/Rabbit, Liver/Large Intestine, 5AM-6:59AM)

Niu Huang (Calculus Bovis, Cattle Bezoar, Cattle Gallstone)
Clear Heat Clean Toxin/Open Orifices
Bitter, Aromatic
Cool to Cold[1535]
Liver, Heart, **Gall Bladder**[1536]
Bie Jing (Shao Yin/Shao Yang, Heart/Gall Bladder), Biao/Li (Gall Bladder/Liver), Clock Opposite (Heart/Gall Bladder)

Chui Pen Cao (Herba Sedi, Sedum, Hanging Stonecrop)
Clear Heat Clean Toxin
Sweet, Bland, slightly Sour
Cool
Liver, **Gall Bladder**, Small Intestine
Biao/Li (Gall Bladder/Liver), Clock Opposite (Liver/Small Intestine)

Ji Gu Cao, Huang Tou Cao, Hong Mu Ji Cao (Herba Abri, Abrus)
Clear Heat Clean Toxin
Sweet
Neutral[1537] to Cool
Liver, **Gall Bladder**
Biao/Li (Gall Bladder/Liver)

Clear Deficient Heat

Qing Hao (Herba Artemesiae Annuae, Sweet Wormwood)
Clear Deficient Heat
Bitter, Acrid, Aromatic
Cold
Liver, **Gall Bladder**, Stomach,[1538] Kidney[1539]
Biao/Li (Gall Bladder/Liver), Branch (Zi/Rat, Kidney/Gall Bladder, 11PM-12:59AM) + Stomach

Cathartic

Da Ji (Radix Euphorbiae seu Knoxiae)
Cathartic
Bitter, Acrid
Cold, extremely Toxic*
Spleen,[1540] Lung,[1541] Kidney, Large Intestine, Liver,[1542] **Gall Bladder**[1543]
Name (Tai Yin, Lung/Spleen), Bie Jing (Jue Yin/Yang Ming, Liver/Large Intestine), Biao/Li (Large Intestine/Lung, Gall Bladder/Liver), Clock Opposite (Kidney/Large Intestine), Clock Neighbor (Liver/Lung), Branch (Zi/Rat, Kidney/Gall Bladder, 11PM-12:59AM, Chou/Ox, Spleen/Liver, 1AM-2:59AM, Mao/Rabbit, Liver/Large Intestine, 5AM-6:59AM, and You/Chicken, Lung/Kidney, 5PM-6:59PM)

Dispel Wind Dampness, Open Channels and Luo-Network Vessels and Relieve Pain

Qin Jiao (Radix Gentianae Macrophyllae, Gentiana)
Dispel Wind Dampness, Open Channels and Luo-Network Vessels and Relieve Pain
Bitter, Acrid, Aromatic[1544]
Neutral[1545] to Cool to slightly Cold
Stomach, Liver, **Gall Bladder,** Spleen[1546]
Biao/Li (Gall Bladder/Liver, Stomach/Spleen), Branch (Chou/Ox, Spleen/Liver, 1AM-2:59AM)

Regulate Water Resolve Dampness

Yin Chen Hao, Yin Chen (Herba Artemesia Scopariae, Virgate Wormwood, Capillary Wormwood)
Regulate Water Resolve Dampness
Bitter, Aromatic
Cool to Cold[1547]
Liver, Spleen, **Gall Bladder**, Stomach
Biao/Li (Gall Bladder/Liver, Stomach/Spleen), Branch (Chou/Ox, Spleen/Liver, 1AM-2:59AM)

Yu Mi Xu, Yu Mai Xu (Stigma Maydis, Corn Stigma, Corn Silk)
Regulate Water Resolve Dampness
Sweet, Bland
Neutral
Urinary Bladder, Kidney, Liver, **Gall Bladder**[1548]
Biao/Li (Urinary Bladder/Kidney, Gall Bladder/Liver), Branch (Zi/Rat, Kidney/Gall Bladder, 11PM-12:59AM)

Jin Qian Cao (Herba Lysimachiae, Lysimachia, Loose Strife Herb)
Regulate Water Resolve Dampness
Sweet, Salty, Bland[1549]
Cool to slightly Cold[1550]
Urinary Bladder, **Gall Bladder**, Kidney, Liver
Biao/Li (Urinary Bladder/Kidney, Gall Bladder/Liver), Branch (Zi/Rat, Kidney/Gall Bladder, 11PM-12:59AM)

Regulate and Rectify Qi

Mu Xiang (Radix Aucklandiae, Costus Root)
Regulate and Rectify Qi
Acrid, Bitter, slightly Astringent,[1551] Aromatic
Warm
Gall Bladder, Large Intestine, Spleen, Stomach, San Jiao[1552]
Name (Yang Ming, Large Intestine/Stomach, Shao Yang, Gall Bladder/San Jiao), Biao/Li (Stomach/Spleen), Clock Opposite (Spleen/San Jiao), Clock Neighbor (Large Intestine/Stomach, San Jiao/Gall Bladder)

Qing Pi, Qing Ju Pi (Pericarpium Citri Reticulatae Viride, Green or Unripened Tangerine Peel)
Regulate and Rectify Qi
Acrid, Bitter, slightly Sour,[1553] Aromatic
Warm
Liver, **Gall Bladder**, Stomach, San Jiao[1554]
Name (Shao Yang, San Jiao/Gall Bladder), Biao/Li (Gall Bladder/Liver), Clock Neighbor (San Jiao/Gall Bladder) + Stomach

Xiang Fu (Rhizoma Cyperi, Cyperus Rhizome, Nut Grass Rhizome)
Regulate and Rectify Qi
Acrid to intensely Acrid,[1555] slightly Bitter, slightly Sweet, Aromatic
Neutral
Liver, Spleen,[1556] San Jiao, **Gall Bladder**,[1557] some sources indicate that it enters all channels.
Name (Shao Yang, San Jiao/Gall Bladder), Biao/Li (Gall Bladder/Liver), Clock Opposite (Spleen/San Jiao), Clock Neighbor (San Jiao/Gall Bladder), Branch (Chou/Ox, Spleen/Liver, 1AM-2:59AM)

Stop Bleeding

Huai Jiao (Fructus Sophorae, Sophora Fruit)
Stop Bleeding
Bitter, Aromatic[1558]
Cold
Liver, **Gall Bladder**, Large Intestine
Bie Jing (Jue Yin/Yang Ming, Liver/Large Intestine), Biao/Li (Gall Bladder/Liver), Branch (Mao/Rabbit, Liver/Large Intestine, 5AM-6:59AM)

Vitalize Blood Transform Stasis

Yu Jin (Radix Curcumae, Aromatic Tumeric Tuber)
Vitalize Blood Transform Stasis
Acrid, Bitter, Aromatic
Cold
Heart, Liver, **Gall Bladder**, Lung[1559]
Bie Jing (Shao Yin/Shao Yang, Heart/Gall Bladder), Biao/Li (Gall Bladder/Liver), Clock Opposite (Heart/Gall Bladder), Clock Neighbor (Liver/Lung), Branch (Yin/Tiger, Gall Bladder/Lung, 3AM-4:59AM)

Hu Zhang (Rhizoma Polygoni Cuspidati, Bushy Knotweed Rhizome, Japanese Knotweed Rhizome, Giant Knotweed Rhizome)
Vitalize Blood Transform Stasis
Bitter
Cold
Liver, **Gall Bladder**, Lung
Biao/Li (Gall Bladder/Liver), Clock Neighbor (Liver/Lung), Branch (Yin/Tiger, Gall Bladder/Lung, 3AM-4:59AM)

Chuan Xiong, Xiong Qiong, Fu Xiong (Rhizoma Ligustici Chuanxiong, Szechuan Lovage Root)
Vitalize Blood Transform Stasis
Acrid, Bitter,[1560] Aromatic
Warm
Liver, **Gall Bladder**, Pericardium, San Jiao,[1561] Chong[1562]
Name (Jue Yin, Liver/Pericardium, Shao Yang, San Jiao/Gall Bladder), Biao/Li (Gall Bladder/Liver, San Jiao/Pericardium), Clock Neighbor (San Jiao/Gall Bladder) + Chong

Transform Phlegm

Zhu Ru (Caulis Bambusae in Taenia, Bamboo Shavings)
Transform Phlegm
Sweet, Bitter[1563]
Cool to slightly Cold[1564]
Lung, Stomach, **Gall Bladder**
Branch (Yin/Tiger, Gall Bladder/Lung, 3AM-4:59AM) + Stomach

Dan Nan Xing, Dan Xing (Arisaema cum Bile)
Transform Phlegm
Bitter, slightly Acrid[1565]
Cool, slightly Toxic*
Liver, Lung,[1566] Spleen,[1567] **Gall Bladder**[1568]
Name (Tai Yin, Spleen/Lung), Biao/Li (Gall Bladder/Liver), Clock Neighbor (Liver/Lung), Branch (Chou/Ox, Spleen/Liver, 1AM-2:59AM and Yin/Tiger, Gall Bladder/Lung, 3AM-4:59AM)

Qian Hu (Radix Peucedani, Hogfennel Root)
Transform Phlegm
Bitter, Acrid
Cool to slightly Cold[1569]
Lung, Liver,[1570] **Gall Bladder**[1571]
Biao/Li (Gall Bladder/Liver), Clock Neighbor (Liver/Lung), Branch (Yin/Tiger, Gall Bladder/Lung, 3AM-4:59AM)

Tian Zhu Huang (Concretio Silicea Bambusae, Siliceous Secretions of Bamboo, Bamboo Sugar, Tabasheer)
Transform Phlegm
Sweet, Bitter[1572]
Cold
Gall Bladder, Heart, Liver
Bie Jing (Shao Yin/Shao Yang, Heart/Gall Bladder), Biao/Li (Gall Bladder/Liver), Clock Opposite (Heart/Gall Bladder)

Nourish and Calm Shen

Suan Zao Ren, Dong Zao (Semen Zizyphi Spinosae, Sour Jujube Seed)
Nourish and Calm Shen
Sweet, Sour[1573]
Neutral
Heart, Liver, **Gall Bladder**,[1574] Spleen[1575]
Bie Jing (Shao Yin/Shao Yang, Heart/Gall Bladder), Biao/Li (Gall Bladder/Liver), Clock Opposite (Heart/Gall Bladder), Clock Neighbor (Spleen/Heart), Branch (Chou/Ox, Spleen/Liver, 1AM-2:59AM)

Open Orifices

Niu Huang (Calculus Bovis, Cattle Bezoar, Cattle Gallstone)
Clear Heat Clean Toxin/Open Orifices
Bitter, Aromatic
Cool to Cold[1576]
Liver, Heart, **Gall Bladder**[1577]
Bie Jing (Shao Yin/Shao Yang, Heart/Gall Bladder), Biao/Li (Gall Bladder/Liver), Clock Opposite (Heart/Gall Bladder)

Foot Jue Yin Liver Herbs

Acrid Warm Exterior Releasing

Jing Jie (Herba Schizonepitae, Schizonepeta)
Acrid Warm Exterior Releasing
Acrid, Aromatic
Slightly Warm
Lung, **Liver**, Gall Bladder,[1578] San Jiao,[1579] Du[1580]
Name (Shao Yang, Gall Bladder/San Jiao), Biao/Li (Gall Bladder/Liver), Clock Neighbor (San Jiao/Gall Bladder, Liver/Lung), Branch (Yin/Tiger, Gall Bladder/Lung, 3AM-4:59AM) + Du

Ji Xiang Teng (Caulis Paederiae, Paederia)
Acrid Warm Exterior Releasing
Sweet
Neutral to slightly Warm[1581] to Warm
Lung, **Liver**
Clock Neighbor (Liver/Lung)

E Bu Shi Cao, Nue Ji Cao, Di Hu Jiao (Herba Centipedae)
Acrid Warm Exterior Releasing
Acrid
Slightly Warm[1582] to Warm
Lung, **Liver**
Clock Neighbor (Liver/Lung)

Cang Er Zi (Fructus Xanthii, Cocklebur Fruit, Xanthium Fruit)
Acrid Warm Exterior Releasing
Sweet,[1583] Bitter, Acrid
Warm, slightly Toxic*
Lung, **Liver**,[1584] Du[1585]
Clock Neighbor (Liver/Lung) + Du

Fang Feng, Pang Feng (Radix Saposhnikoviae, and sometimes Ledebouriella Root as a substitute)
Acrid Warm Exterior Releasing
Acrid, Sweet, Aromatic
Slightly Warm
Urinary Bladder, **Liver**, Spleen, Du,[1586] Yang Qiao[1587]
Branch (Chou/Ox, Spleen/Liver,1AM-2:59AM) + Urinary Bladder, Du, Yang Qiao

Qiang Huo, Can Qiang, Zhu Jie Qiang (Rhizoma et Radix Notopterygii)
Acrid Warm Exterior Releasing
Acrid, Bitter, Aromatic
Warm to very Warm[1588]
Urinary Bladder, Tai Yang,[1589] Kidney, **Liver**,[1590] Du[1591]
Biao/Li (Urinary Bladder/Kidney), and possibly Name (Small Intestine/Urinary Bladder), Clock Opposite (Liver/Small Intestine) and Clock Neighbor (Small Intestine/Urinary Bladder) if Tai Yang[1592] really means Tai Yang. If Tai Yang only means the Foot Tai Yang Urinary Bladder Jing-channel, then + Liver, Du

Acrid Cool Exterior Releasing

Sang Ye (Folium Mori, White Mulberry Leaf)
Acrid Cool Exterior Releasing
Bitter, Sweet, Acrid,[1593] Aromatic
Cold
Lung, **Liver**, Large Intestine,[1594] Stomach[1595]
Name (Yang Ming, Large Intestine/Stomach), Biao/Li (Large Intestine/Lung), Bie Jing (Jue Yin/Yang Ming, Liver/Large Intestine), Clock Neighbor (Liver/Lung, Large Intestine/Stomach), Branch (Mao/Rabbit, Liver/Large Intestine, 5AM-6:59AM)

Man Jing Zi, Jing Tiao Zi, Bai Bu Jing (Fructus Viticis, Vitex Fruit)
Acrid Cool Exterior Releasing
Acrid, Bitter
Both Cool and Warm[1596]
Lung,[1597] **Liver**, Stomach, Urinary Bladder,[1598] Gall Bladder,[1599] San Jiao[1600]
Name (Shao Yang, Gall Bladder/San Jiao), Bie Jing (Tai Yin/Tai Yang, Lung/Urinary Bladder), Biao/Li (Gall Bladder/Liver), Clock Opposite (Lung, Urinary Bladder), Clock Neighbor (San Jiao/Gall Bladder, Liver/Lung), Qian/Hou (Front/Back, Stomach/Urinary Bladder), Branch (Yin/Tiger, Gall Bladder/Lung, 3AM-4:59AM, Hai/Pig, Urinary Bladder/San Jiao, 9PM-10:59PM)

Mao Zi Dun Tou (Herba Abutilon Indicum, Indian Abutilon)
Acrid Cool Exterior Releasing
Sweet
Neutral, slightly Toxic*
Lung, **Liver**, Gall Bladder, Spleen
Name (Tai Yin, Lung/Spleen), Biao/Li (Gall Bladder, Liver), Clock Neighbor (Liver/Lung), Branch (Yin/Tiger, Gall Bladder/Lung, 3AM-4:59AM, and Chou/Ox, Spleen/Liver, 1AM-2:59AM)

Mu Zei, Jie Gu Cao, Jie Jie Cao (Herba Equesti Hiemalis, Scouring Rush, Shave Grass, Horsetail)
Acrid Cool Exterior Releasing
Sweet, Bitter
Neutral to slightly Cold
Lung, **Liver**, Gall Bladder[1601]
Biao/Li (Gall Bladder/Liver), Clock Neighbor (Liver/Lung), Branch (Yin/Tiger, Gall Bladder/Lung, 3AM-4:59AM)

Ju Hua (Flos Chrysanthemi, Chrysanthemum Flower)
Acrid Cool Exterior Releasing
Acrid,[1602] Sweet, Bitter, Aromatic[1603]
Cool to slightly Cold[1604]
Lung, **Liver**
Clock Neighbor (Liver/Lung)

Ye Ju Hua, Ku Yi (Flos Chrysanthemi Indici, Wild Chrysanthemum Flower)
Acrid Cool Exterior Releasing/Clear Heat Clean Toxin
Bitter, Acrid
Cool to slightly Cold[1605]
Lung, **Liver**
Clock Neighbor (Liver/Lung)

Yi Zhi Xiang (Herba Vernoniae Cinereae, Vernonia)
Acrid Cool Exterior Releasing
Acrid, Bitter
Cool
Lung, **Liver**
Clock Neighbor (Liver/Lung)

Chan Tui, Chan Yi (Periostracum Cicadae, Cicada Moulting)
Acrid Cool Exterior Releasing
Sweet, Salty, Bland[1606]
Slightly Cold[1607] to Cold
Liver, Lung
Clock Neighbor (Liver/Lung)

Bo He (Herba Menthae, Field Mint)
Acrid Cool Exterior Releasing
Acrid, Aromatic
Cool
Lung, **Liver**
Clock Neighbor (Liver/Lung)

Chai Hu (Radix Bupleuri, Thorowax Root, Bupleurum, Hare's Ear Root)
Acrid Cool Exterior Releasing
Bitter, Acrid, Aromatic[1608]
Neutral[1609] to Cool to slightly Cold[1610]
Liver, Gall Bladder, Pericardium,[1611] San Jiao[1612]
Name (Jue Yin, Liver/Pericardium, Shao Yang, San Jiao/Gall Bladder), Biao/Li (Gall Bladder/Liver, San Jiao/Pericardium), Clock Neighbor (San Jiao/Gall Bladder)

Clear Heat Purge Fire

Shan Zhi Zi, Zhi Zi (Fructus Gardeniae, Cape Jasmine Fruit, Gardenia Fruit)
Clear Heat Purge Fire
Bitter
Cold
Heart, Lung, Stomach, San Jiao, **Liver**[1613]
Clock Neighbor (Liver/Lung) + Heart, Stomach, San Jiao

Da Ding Huang (Caulis Euonymi, Euonymus)
Clear Heat Purge Fire
Bitter
Cold
Liver, Lung
Clock Neighbor (Liver/Lung)

Jue Ming Zi, Cao Jue Ming (Semen Cassiae, Cassia Seeds, Foetid Cassia Seeds)
Clear Heat Purge Fire/Calm Liver Extinguish Wind
Sweet, Bitter, Salty[1614]
Cool to slightly Cold
Liver, Large Intestine, Kidney[1615]
Bie Jing (Jue Yin/Yang Ming, Liver/Large Intestine), Clock Opposite (Kidney/Large Intestine), Branch (Mao/Rabbit, Liver/Large Intestine, 5AM-6:59AM)

Gu Jing Cao (Flos Eriocauli, Pipewort Scapus and Inflorescence)
Clear Heat Purge Fire
Sweet, Acrid[1616]
Cool[1617] to Neutral to Warm[1618]
Liver, Stomach

Xia Ku Cao (Spica Prunellae, Selfheal Spike, Prunella)
Clear Heat Purge Fire
Bitter, Acrid
Cold
Liver, Gall Bladder
Biao/Li (Gall Bladder/Liver)

Qing Xiang Zi (Semen Celosiae, Celosia Seeds)
Clear Heat Purge Fire
Bitter
Cool to slightly Cold[1619]
Liver

Rui Ren, Rui Ren Rou, Rui Zi (Semen Prinsepiae)
Clear Heat Purge Fire
Sweet
Cool
Liver

Mi Meng Hua, Chong Jian Si (Flos Buddlejae, Buddleia Flower Bud)
Clear Heat Purge Fire
Sweet
Slightly Cool[1620] to Cool, slightly Toxic*[1621]
Liver

Clear Heat Dry Dampness

Ku Shen, Ku Shen Gen, Ku Gu (Radix Sophorae Flavescentis, Flavescent Sophora Root)
Clear Heat Dry Dampness
Bitter to extremely Bitter[1622]
Cold
Heart, **Liver**, Stomach, Large Intestine, Urinary Bladder, Small Intestine[1623]
Name (Yang Ming, Large Intestine/Stomach, Tai Yang, Small Intestine/Urinary Bladder), Bie Jing (Jue Yin/Yang Ming, Liver/Large Intestine), Biao/Li (Small Intestine/Heart), Clock Opposite (Liver/Small Intestine), Clock Neighbor (Large Intestine/Stomach, Small Intestine/Urinary Bladder), Qian/Hou (Front/Back, Stomach/Urinary Bladder), Branch (Shen/Monkey, Large Intestine/Urinary Bladder, 3PM-4:59PM and Mao/Rabbit, Liver/Large Intestine, 5AM-6:59AM)

Huang Lian (Rhizoma Coptidis, Goldthread Rhizome, Coptis Root)
Clear Heat Dry Dampness
Very Bitter, purely Bitter[1624]
Very Cold
Heart, **Liver**, Stomach, Large Intestine, Du[1625]
Name (Yang Ming, Large Intestine/Stomach), Bie Jing (Jue Yin/Yang Ming, Liver/Large Intestine), Clock Neighbor (Large Intestine/Stomach), Branch (Mao/Rabbit, Liver/Large Intestine, 5AM-6:59AM) + Heart, Du

Qin Pi (Cortex Fraxini, Bark of Korean Ash Branch)
Clear Heat Dry Dampness/Clear Heat Clean Toxin
Bitter, Acrid,[1626] Astringent[1627]
Cold
Gall Bladder, **Liver**, Large Intestine, Stomach[1628]
Name (Yang Ming, Large Intestine/Stomach), Bie Jing (Jue Yin/Yang Ming, Liver/Large Intestine), Biao/Li (Gall Bladder/Liver), Clock Neighbor (Large Intestine/Stomach), Branch (Mao/Rabbit, Liver/Large Intestine, 5AM-6:59AM)

Ji Xue Cao, Beng Da Wan (Herba Centellae, Gotu Kola, Pennywort)
Clear Heat Dry Dampness/Clear Heat Clean Toxin
Acrid, Bitter
Cold
Liver, Spleen, Kidney, Small Intestine, Large Intestine
Bie Jing (Jue Yin/Yang Ming, Liver/Large Intestine, Tai Yin/Tai Yang, Spleen/Small Intestine), Clock Opposite (Liver/Small Intestine, Kidney/Large Intestine), Branch (Chou/Ox, Spleen/Liver, 1AM-2:59AM, Si/Snake, Small Intestine/Spleen, 9AM-10:59AM, Wei/Sheep, Spleen/Small Intestine, 1PM-2:59PM, Mao/Rabbit, Liver/Large Intestine, 5AM-6:59AM)

Long Dan Cao, Long Dan, Dan Cao (Radix Gentianae, Chinese Gentian Root, Gentiana)
Clear Heat Dry Dampness
Bitter, Astringing[1629]
Cold
Liver, Gall Bladder, Stomach, Urinary Bladder[1630]
Biao/Li (Gall Bladder/Liver), Qian/Hou (Front/Back, Stomach/Urinary Bladder)

Clear Heat Cool Blood

Ji Guan Hua (Flos Celosiae Cristatae, Cock's Comb Flower)
Clear Heat Cool Blood/Astringe, Stabilize and Bind
Sweet, Astringent[1631]
Cool
Large Intestine, **Liver**, Kidney[1632]
Bie Jing (Jue Yin/Yang Ming, Liver/Large Intestine), Clock Opposite (Kidney/Large Intestine), Branch (Mao/Rabbit, Liver/Large Intestine, 5AM-6:59AM)

Shui Niu Jiao (Bubali Cornu, Water Buffalo Horn)
Clear Heat Cool Blood
Salty, Bitter[1633]
Cold
Heart, **Liver**, Stomach

Chi Shao (Radix Paeoniae Rubrae, Red Peony Root)
Clear Heat Cool Blood/Vitalize Blood Transform Stasis
Bitter, Sour[1634]
Cool to slightly Cold
Liver, Spleen[1635]
Branch (Chou/Ox, Spleen/Liver, 1AM-2:59AM)

Mu Dan Pi, Mu Shao Yao (Cortex Moutan, Peony Tree Root Cortex)
Clear Heat Cool Blood/Vitalize Blood Transform Stasis
Bitter, Acrid, Aromatic
Cool to slightly Cold
Heart, **Liver**, Kidney, Pericardium[1636]
Name (Shao Yin, Heart/Kidney, Jue Yin, Liver/Pericardium), Clock Neighbor (Kidney/Pericardium)

Sheng Di Huang (Radix Rehmanniae, Chinese Foxglove Root)
Clear Heat Cool Blood
Sweet, Bitter
Cold
Heart, **Liver**, Kidney
Name (Shao Yin, Heart/Kidney) + Liver

Zi Cao, Zi Cao Gen (Radix Lithospermi, Arnebia, Groomwell Root)
Clear Heat Cool Blood
Sweet, Salty,[1637] Bitter[1638]
Cold
Heart, **Liver**

Huang Teng (Caulis Fibraurea, Fibraurea)
Clear Heat Cool Blood
Bitter
Cold
Liver

Clear Heat Clean Toxin

Ban Zhi Lian (Herba Scutellariae Barbatae, Barbat Skullcap, Barbed Skullcap)
Clear Heat Clean Toxin
Acrid, slightly Bitter
Cool
Liver, Lung, Stomach, Kidney,[1639] Large Intestine[1640]
Name (Yang Ming, Large Intestine/Stomach), Bie Jing (Jue Yin/Yang Ming, Liver/Large Intestine), Biao/Li (Large Intestine/Lung), Clock Opposite (Kidney/Large Intestine), Clock Neighbor (Large Intestine/Stomach, Liver/Lung), Branch (You/Chicken, Lung/Kidney, 5PM-6:59PM, Mao/Rabbit, Liver/Large Intestine, 5AM-6:59AM)

Qian Li Guang (Herba Senecionis Scandens, Climbing Groundsel, Ragwort)
Clear Heat Clean Toxin
Bitter
Cold
Lung, **Liver**, Large Intestine
Biao/Li (Large Intestine/Lung), Bie Jing (Jue Yin/Yang Ming, Liver/Large Intestine), Clock Neighbor (Liver/Lung), Branch (Mao/Rabbit, Liver/Large Intestine, 5AM-6:59AM)

Da Qing Ye (Folium Isatidis, Woad Leaf, Indigo Leaf)
Clear Heat Clean Toxin
Bitter, Salty[1641]
Very Cold
Heart, Lung, Stomach, **Liver**[1642]
Clock Neighbor (Liver/Lung) + Heart, Stomach

Nan Ban Lan Ye, Ma Lian Ye (Folium Baphicacanthis)
Clear Heat Clean Toxin
Bitter, Salty
Cold
Lung, Stomach, Heart, **Liver**
Clock Neighbor (Liver/Lung) + Stomach, Heart

Qing Dai (Indigo Naturalis)
Clear Heat Clean Toxin
Salty
Cold to very Cold[1643]
Liver, Lung, Stomach
Clock Neighbor (Liver/Lung) + Stomach

Shan Ma Ti (Radix Rauvolfiae, Devil Pepper Root)
Clear Heat Clean Toxin
Bitter
Cold, slightly Toxic*
Lung, **Liver**, Heart
Clock Neighbor (Liver/Lung) + Heart

Pao Zai Cao, Deng Long Cao (Herba Physalis Angulatae)
Clear Heat Clean Toxin
Bitter
Cool
Lung, Urinary Bladder, **Liver**, Kidney
Bie Jing (Tai Yin/Tai Yang, Lung/Urinary Bladder), Biao/Li (Urinary Bladder/Kidney), Clock Neighbor (Liver/Lung), Clock Opposite (Lung/Urinary Bladder), Branch (You/Chicken, Lung/Kidney, 5PM-6:59PM)

Dao Diao Jin Zhong, Feng Fang Ran (Melothria Maderospatana, Melothria)
Clear Heat Clean Toxin
Sweet, Bitter
Cool
Lung, **Liver**, Urinary Bladder
Bie Jing (Tai Yin/Tai Yang, Lung/Urinary Bladder), Clock Opposite (Lung/Urinary Bladder), Clock Neighbor (Liver/Lung)

Tu Niu Xi (Radix Achyranthes Longiflora, Native Achyranthis Root)
Clear Heat Clean Toxin/Vitalize Blood Transform Stasis
Bitter, Sour, Acrid[1644]
Neutral to Cold,[1645] slightly Toxic[1646]
Lung, **Liver**, Kidney
Clock Neighbor (Liver/Lung), Branch (You/Chicken, Lung/Kidney, 5PM-6:59PM)

Ye Ju Hua, Ku Yi (Flos Chrysanthemi Indici, Wild Chrysanthemum Flower)
Acrid Cool Exterior Releasing/Clear Heat Clean Toxin
Bitter, Acrid
Cool to slightly Cold[1647]
Lung, **Liver**
Clock Neighbor (Liver/Lung)

Zhu Zi Cao (Herba Euphorbiae Thymifoliae)
Clear Heat Clean Toxin
Sweet
Cool
Liver, Lung
Clock Neighbor (Liver/Lung)

Bai Hua She She Cao (Herba Oldenlandia, Heydyotis)
Clear Heat Clean Toxin
Slightly Bitter, Sweet
Cold
Stomach, Large Intestine, Small Intestine, **Liver**[1648]
Name (Yang Ming, Large Intestine/Stomach), Bie Jing (Jue Yin/Yang Ming, Liver/Large Intestine), Clock Opposite (Liver/Small Intestine), Clock Neighbor (Large Intestine/Stomach), Branch (Mao/Rabbit, Liver/Large Intestine, 5AM-6:59AM)

Qin Pi (Cortex Fraxini, Bark of Korean Ash Branch)
Clear Heat Dry Dampness/Clear Heat Clean Toxin
Bitter, Acrid,[1649] Astringent[1650]
Cold
Gall Bladder, **Liver**, Large Intestine, Stomach[1651]
Name (Yang Ming, Large Intestine/Stomach), Bie Jing (Jue Yin/Yang Ming, Liver/Large Intestine), Biao/Li (Gall Bladder/Liver), Clock Neighbor (Large Intestine/Stomach), Branch (Mao/Rabbit, Liver/Large Intestine, 5AM-6:59AM)

Bai Jiang Cao (Herba cum Radice Patriniae, Patrinia, Thlaspi)
Clear Heat Clean Toxin
Acrid, Bitter, Salty[1652]
Cool to slightly Cold
Stomach, Large Intestine, **Liver**
Name (Yang Ming, Large Intestine/Stomach), Bie Jing (Yang Ming/Jue Yin, Large Intestine/Liver), Clock Neighbor (Large Intestine/Stomach), Branch (Mao/Rabbit, Liver/Large Intestine, 5AM-6:59AM)

Quan Shen (Rhizoma Bistortae)
Clear Heat Clean Toxin
Bitter, Astringent
Cool, slightly Toxic*
Liver, Stomach, Large Intestine
Name (Yang Ming, Large Intestine/Stomach), Bie Jing (Jue Yin/Yang Ming, Liver/Large Intestine), Clock Neighbor (Large Intestine/Stomach), Branch (Mao/Rabbit, Liver/Large Intestine, 5AM-6:59AM)

Ji Xue Cao, Beng Da Wan (Herba Centellae, Gotu Kola, Pennywort)
Clear Heat Dry Dampness/Clear Heat Clean Toxin
Acrid, Bitter
Cold
Liver, Spleen, Kidney, Small Intestine, Large Intestine
Bie Jing (Jue Yin/Yang Ming, Liver/Large Intestine, Tai Yin/Tai Yang, Spleen/Small Intestine), Clock Opposite (Liver/Small Intestine, Kidney/Large Intestine), Branch (Chou/Ox, Spleen/Liver, 1AM-2:59AM, Si/Snake, Small Intestine/Spleen, 9AM-10:59AM, Wei/Sheep, Spleen/Small Intestine, 1PM-2:59PM, Mao/Rabbit, Liver/Large Intestine, 5AM-6:59AM)

Ma Chi Xian, Chang Shou Cai, Wu Xing Cai (Herba Portulacae, Purslane, Portulaca)
Clear Heat Clean Toxin
Sour
Cold
Large Intestine, **Liver**, and possibly San Jiao[1653]
Bie Jing (Jue Yin/Yang Ming, Liver/Large Intestine), Branch (Mao/Rabbit, Liver/Large Intestine, 5AM-6:59AM) + possibly San Jiao

Cha Chi Huang (Herba Stellariae Aquaticae)
Clear Heat Clean Toxin
Acrid, slightly Bitter
Neutral
Liver, Large Intestine, San Jiao
Bie Jing (Jue Yin/Yang Ming, Liver/Large Intestine), Branch (Mao/Rabbit, Liver/Large Intestine, 5AM-6:59AM) + San Jiao

Ya Dan Zi, Ku Dan Zi, Ku Zi, Ku Shen Zi (Fructus Bruceae, Java Brucea Fruit, Brucea)
Clear Heat Clean Toxin
Bitter
Cold, slightly to very Toxic*
Large Intestine, **Liver**
Bie Jing (Jue Yin/Yang Ming, Liver/Large Intestine), Branch (Mao/Rabbit, Liver/Large Intestine, 5AM-6:59AM)

Wei Ling Cai, Tian Qing Di Bai, Fan Bai Cao (Herba Potentillae Chinensis, Chinese Sliverweed, Chinese Cinquefoil)
Clear Heat Clean Toxin
Bitter
Neutral[1654] to Cold
Liver, Large Intestine
Bie Jing (Jue Yin/Yang Ming, Liver/Large Intestine), Branch (Mao/Rabbit, Liver/Large Intestine, 5AM-6:59AM)

Hong Teng, Da Xue Teng (Caulis Sargentodoxae, Sargentodoxa Vine)
Clear Heat Clean Toxin
Bitter
Neutral
Large Intestine, **Liver**[1655]
Bie Jing (Jue Yin/Yang Ming, Liver/Large Intestine), Branch (Mao/Rabbit, Liver/Large Intestine, 5AM-6:59AM)

Bai Lian, Bai Cao, Tu He, Kun Lun, Mao Er Luan (Radix Ampelopsis)
Clear Heat Clean Toxin
Bitter, Acrid, Sweet[1656]
Neutral to Cool to Cold[1657]
Heart, Stomach, **Liver**, Spleen[1658]
Biao/Li (Stomach/Spleen), Clock Neighbor (Spleen/Heart), Branch (Chou/Ox, Spleen/Liver, 1AM-2:59AM)

Guan Zhong, Mian Ma Guan Zhong (Rhizoma Dryopteridis, Dryopteris Root, Shield-Fern Root)
Clear Heat Clean Toxin/Expel Parasites
Bitter
Cool to Cold,[1659] slightly Toxic*
Liver, Spleen, Stomach[1660]
Biao/Li (Stomach/Spleen), Branch (Chou/Ox, Spleen/Liver, 1AM-2:59AM)

Dong Ling Cao (Herba Rabdosiae, Rabdosia)
Clear Heat Clean Toxin
Bitter, Sweet
Cool
Liver, Spleen, Stomach
Biao/Li (Stomach/Spleen), Branch (Chou/Ox, Spleen/Liver, 1AM-2:59AM)

Zi Hua Di Ding, Jian Tou Cao, Di Ding Cao (Herba Violae, Yedeon's Violet)
Clear Heat Clean Toxin
Bitter, Acrid
Cold
Heart, **Liver**, Stomach,[1661] Pericardium[1662]
Name (Jue Yin, Pericardium/Liver), Bie Jing (Jue Yin/Yang Ming, Pericardium/Stomach), Clock Opposite (Pericardium/Stomach), Branch (Shu/Dog, Stomach/Pericardium, 7PM-8:59PM) + Heart

Nan Ban Lan Gen (Rhizoma et Radix Baphicacathis)
Clear Heat Clean Toxin
Bitter
Cold
Heart, **Liver**, Stomach

Pu Gong Ying, Huang Hua Di Ding (Herba Taraxaci, Dandelion)
Clear Heat Clean Toxin
Bitter, Sweet
Cold
Liver, Stomach

Tu Fu Ling (Rhizoma Smilacis Glabrae, Glabrous Greenbrier Rhizome, Smilax)
Clear Heat Clean Toxin
Sweet, Bland
Neutral
Liver, Stomach

Shan Ci Gu, Mao Ci Gu, Guang Ci Gu (Psuedobulbus Cremastrae/Pleiones, Cremastra)
Clear Heat Clean Toxin
Sweet, Bland,[1663] slightly Acrid
Cold, slightly Toxic*
Liver, Stomach

He Ye (Folium Nelumbinis, Lotus Leaf)
Clear Heat Clean Toxin/Astringe, Stabilize and Bind
Bitter, slightly Sweet,[1664] Astringent, Aromatic[1665]
Neutral
Heart, **Liver**, Spleen
Clock Neighbor (Spleen/Heart), Branch (Chou/Ox, Spleen/Liver, 1AM-2:59AM)

Tian Kui Zi, Tian Kui, Zi Bei Tian Kui (Radix Semiaquilegiae, Muskroot-like Semiaquilegia Root)
Clear Heat Clean Toxin
Sweet, Bitter
Cold
Liver, Spleen, Urinary Bladder
Branch (Chou/Ox, Spleen/Liver, 1AM-2:59AM) + Urinary Bladder

Su Bai Jiang, Xi Ming (Herba Thlaspi, Thlaspi)
Clear Heat Clean Toxin
Bitter, Sweet
Slightly Cold
Liver, Spleen
Branch (Chou/Ox, Spleen/Liver, 1AM-2:59AM)

Niu Huang (Calculus Bovis, Cattle Bezoar, Cattle Gallstone)
Clear Heat Clean Toxin/Open Orifices
Bitter, Aromatic
Cool to Cold[1666]
Liver, Heart, Gall Bladder[1667]
Bie Jing (Shao Yin/Shao Yang, Heart/Gall Bladder), Biao/Li (Gall Bladder/Liver), Clock Opposite (Heart/Gall Bladder)

Chui Pen Cao (Herba Sedi, Sedum, Hanging Stonecrop)
Clear Heat Clean Toxin
Sweet, Bland, slightly Sour
Cool
Liver, Gall Bladder, Small Intestine
Biao/Li (Gall Bladder/Liver), Clock Opposite (Liver/Small Intestine)

Ji Gu Cao, Huang Tou Cao, Hong Mu Ji Cao (Herba Abri, Abrus)
Clear Heat Clean Toxin
Sweet
Neutral[1668] to Cool
Liver, Gall Bladder
Biao/Li (Gall Bladder/Liver)

Liu Ye (Folium Salicis Babylonicae, Weeping Willow Leaves)
Clear Heat Clean Toxin
Bitter
Cold
Liver

Chong Lou, Qi Ye Yi Zhi Hua, Zao Xiu (Rhizoma Paridis, Paris Rhizome)
Clear Heat Clean Toxin
Bitter
Cool to slightly Cold, slightly Toxic*
Liver

Shi Shang Bai (Herba Selaginellae Doederleini, Selaginella)
Clear Heat Clean Toxin
Sweet, Acrid, Bitter, slightly Astringent[1669]
Warm[1670] to Neutral to Cold
Liver

Huang Shui Qie (Herba Solani, Solanum)
Clear Heat Clean Toxin
Acrid, Bitter
Cold
Liver

Guan Ye Lian Qiao, Guan Ye Jin Si Tao (Herba Hypericum, St. John's Wort)
Clear Heat Clean Toxin
Bitter, Acrid, Astringent
Neutral
Liver

Clear Deficient Heat

Bai Wei (Radix Cynanchi Atrati, Black Swallow-Wort Root)
Clear Deficient Heat
Bitter, Salty
Cold
Stomach, **Liver**, Kidney,[1671] Lung,[1672] Ren and Chong[1673]
Clock Neighbor (Liver/Lung), Branch (You/Chicken, Lung/Kidney, 5PM-6:59PM) + Stomach, Ren, Chong

Di Gu Pi (Cortex Lycii, Wolfberry Root Cortex)
Clear Deficient Heat
Sweet, Bland, Bitter[1674]
Cold
Lung, Kidney, **Liver**[1675]
Clock Neighbor (Liver/Lung), Branch (You/Chicken, Lung/Kidney, 5PM-6:59PM)

Hu Huang Lian, Hu Lian (Rhizoma Picrorhizae, Picrorhiza, Figwort Rhizome)
Clear Deficient Heat
Bitter
Cold
Heart, **Liver**, Stomach, Large Intestine
Name (Yang Ming, Large Intestine, Stomach), Bie Jing (Jue Yin/Yang Ming, Liver/Large Intestine), Clock Neighbor (Large Intestine, Stomach), Branch (Mao/Rabbit, Liver/Large Intestine, 5AM-6:59AM) + Heart

Qing Hao (Herba Artemesiae Annuae, Sweet Wormwood)
Clear Deficient Heat
Bitter, Acrid, Aromatic
Cold
Liver, Gall Bladder, Stomach,[1676] Kidney[1677]
Biao/Li (Gall Bladder/Liver), Branch (Zi/Rat, Kidney/Gall Bladder, 11PM-12:59AM) + Stomach

Yin Chai Hu, Niu Dan Gen (Radix Stellariae, Stellaria Root, Starwort Root)
Clear Deficient Heat
Sweet, Bitter[1678]
Cool to slightly Cold
Liver, Stomach

Purgative

Da Huang (Radix et Rhizoma Rhei, Rhubarb Root and Rhizome)
Purgative
Bitter to very Bitter[1679] to purely Bitter,[1680] Aromatic[1681]
Cold to very Cold[1682]
Spleen, Stomach, Large Intestine, **Liver**, Heart, Du[1683]
Name (Yang Ming, Large Intestine/Stomach), Bie Jing (Jue Yin/Yang Ming, Liver/Large Intestine), Biao/Li (Stomach/Spleen), Clock Neighbor (Spleen/Heart, Large Intestine/Stomach), Branch (Chou/Ox, Spleen/Liver, 1AM-2:59AM and Mao/Rabbit, Liver/Large Intestine, 5AM-6:59AM) + Du

Lu Hui, Xiang Dan (Aloe, Dried Aloe Leaf Juice)
Purgative
Very Bitter
Very Cold
Liver, Large Intestine, Stomach[1684]
Name (Yang Ming, Large Intestine/Stomach), Bie Jing (Jue Yin/Yang Ming, Liver/Large Intestine), Clock Neighbor (Large Intestine/Stomach), Branch (Mao/Rabbit, Liver/Large Intestine, 5AM-6:59AM)

Moist Laxative

Song Zi Ren (Semen Pini, Pine Nut)
Moist Laxative
Sweet
Warm
Lung, **Liver**, Large Intestine
Bie Jing (Jue Yin/Yang Ming, Liver/Large Intestine), Biao/Li (Large Intestine, Lung), Clock Neighbor (Liver/Lung), Branch (Mao/Rabbit, Liver/Large Intestine, 5AM-6:59AM)

Cathartic

Da Ji (Radix Euphorbiae seu Knoxiae)
Cathartic
Bitter, Acrid
Cold, extremely Toxic*
Spleen,[1685] Lung,[1686] Kidney, Large Intestine, **Liver**,[1687] Gall Bladder[1688]
Name (Tai Yin, Lung/Spleen), Bie Jing (Jue Yin/Yang Ming, Liver/Large Intestine), Biao/Li (Large Intestine/Lung, Gall Bladder/Liver), Clock Opposite (Kidney/Large Intestine), Clock Neighbor (Liver/Lung), Branch (Zi/Rat, Kidney/Gall Bladder, 11PM-12:59AM, Chou/Ox, Spleen/Liver, 1AM-2:59AM, Mao/Rabbit, Liver/Large Intestine, 5AM-6:59AM, and You/Chicken, Lung/Kidney, 5PM-6:59PM)

Dispel Wind Dampness, Open Channels and Luo-Network Vessels and Relieve Pain

Hong Gu She (Radix Kadsura Japonicae, Kadsura)
Dispel Wind Dampness, Open Channels and Luo-Network Vessels and Relieve Pain
Acrid, Bitter
Cool
Lung, **Liver**, Stomach
Clock Neighbor (Liver/Lung) + Stomach

Mu Gua (Fructus Chaenomelis, Japanese Quince)
Dispel Wind Dampness, Open Channels and Luo-Network Vessels and Relieve Pain
Sour, not Astringent,[1689] Aromatic[1690]
Warm
Liver, Spleen, Lung[1691]
Name (Tai Yin, Spleen/Lung), Clock Neighbor (Liver/Lung), Branch (Chou/Ox, Spleen/Liver, 1AM-2:59AM)

Chuan Shan Long, Huang Jiang, Chuan Di Long (Rhizoma Dioscoriae Nipponicae, Japanese Dioscoriae Rhizome)
Dispel Wind Dampness, Open Channels and Luo-Network Vessels and Relieve Pain
Bitter
Neutral[1692] to Cool, slightly Toxic*[1693]
Liver, Lung
Clock Neighbor (Liver/Lung)

Lao Guan Cao (Herba Erodi seu Geranii, Geranium, Common Heron's Bill Herb)
Dispel Wind Dampness, Open Channels and Luo-Network Vessels and Relieve Pain
Acrid, Bitter
Neutral
Liver, Large Intestine, Kidney,[1694] Spleen[1695]
Bie Jing (Jue Yin/Yang Ming, Liver/Large Intestine), Clock Opposite (Kidney/Large Intestine), Branch (Mao/Rabbit, Liver/Large Intestine, 5AM-6:59AM, Chou/Ox, Spleen/Liver, 1AM-2:59AM)

Ma An Teng (Herba Ipomoea Pes-caprae, Beach Morning Glory)
Dispel Wind Dampness, Open Channels and Luo-Network Vessels and Relieve Pain
Acrid, Bitter
Neutral
Liver, Kidney, Large Intestine
Bie Jing (Jue Yin/Yang Ming, Liver/Large Intestine), Clock Opposite (Kidney/Large Intestine), Branch (Mao/Rabbit, Liver/Large Intestine, 5AM-6:59AM)

Qin Jiao (Radix Gentianae Macrophyllae, Gentiana)
Dispel Wind Dampness, Open Channels and Luo-Network Vessels and Relieve Pain
Bitter, Acrid, Aromatic[1696]
Neutral[1697] to Cool to slightly Cold
Stomach, **Liver**, Gall Bladder, Spleen[1698]
Biao/Li (Gall Bladder/Liver, Stomach/Spleen), Branch (Chou/Ox, Spleen/Liver, 1AM-2:59AM)

Can Sha, Can Shi (Excrementum Bombycis Mori, Silkworm Feces)
Dispel Wind Dampness, Open Channels and Luo-Network Vessels and Relieve Pain
Sweet,[1699] Acrid
Warm
Liver, Spleen, Stomach
Biao/Li (Stomach/Spleen), Branch (Chou/Ox, Spleen/Liver, 1AM-2:59AM)

Xu Chang Qing, Liao Diao Zhu (Radix Cynanchi Paniculati, Paniculate Swallow-Wort Root)
Dispel Wind Dampness, Open Channels and Luo-Network Vessels and Relieve Pain
Acrid, Aromatic
Warm
Liver, Stomach

Tou Gu Cao (Caulis Impatientis, Garden Balsam)
Dispel Wind Dampness, Open Channels and Luo-Network Vessels and Relieve Pain
Bitter, slightly Sweet, Acrid
Cool
Liver, Spleen, Kidney
Branch (Chou/Ox, Spleen/Liver, 1AM-2:59AM) + Kidney

Hai Tong Pi (Cortex Erythrinae, Coral Bean Bark)
Dispel Wind Dampness, Open Channels and Luo-Network Vessels and Relieve Pain
Bitter, Acrid
Neutral
Liver, Spleen,[1700] Kidney[1701]
Branch (Chou/Ox, Spleen/Liver, 1AM-2:59AM) + Kidney

Shen Jin Cao, Shi Song, Shi Wu Gong (Herba Lycopodii, Ground Pine, Staghorn Moss, Wolf's Claw Club Moss)
Dispel Wind Dampness, Open Channels and Luo-Network Vessels and Relieve Pain
Bitter, Acrid
Warm
Liver, Spleen,[1702] Kidney[1703]
Branch (Chou/Ox, Spleen/Liver, 1AM-2:59AM) + Kidney

Zhe Tong Pi (Cortex Zanthoxyli, Zanthoxylum Bark)
Dispel Wind Dampness, Open Channels and Luo-Network Vessels and Relieve Pain
Acrid, slightly Bitter
Neutral, slightly Toxic*
Liver, Spleen
Branch (Chou/Ox, Spleen/Liver, 1AM-2:59AM)

Qing Feng Teng (Caulis Sinomenii, Orient Vine)
Dispel Wind Dampness, Open Channels and Luo-Network Vessels and Relieve Pain
Bitter, Acrid
Neutral, Toxic*[1704]
Liver, Spleen
Branch (Chou/Ox, Spleen/Liver, 1AM-2:59AM)

Wu Shao She (Zaocys, Black Striped Snake)
Dispel Wind Dampness, Open Channels and Luo-Network Vessels and Relieve Pain
Sweet, Salty
Neutral
Spleen,[1705] **Liver**
Branch (Chou/Ox, Spleen/Liver, 1AM-2:59AM)

Hai Feng Teng (Caulis Piperis Kadsurae, Kadsura Pepper Stem, Futokadsura Stem)
Dispel Wind Dampness, Open Channels and Luo-Network Vessels and Relieve Pain
Acrid, Bitter, Aromatic
Slightly Warm
Liver, Heart,[1706] Kidney[1707]
Name (Shao Yin, Heart/Kidney) + Liver

Luo Shi Teng, Luo Shi, Bai Hua Teng (Caulis Trachelospermi, Star Jasmine Stem)
Dispel Wind Dampness, Open Channels and Luo-Network Vessels and Relieve Pain
Bitter
Cool to slightly Cold[1708]
Heart, **Liver**

Du Huo, Da Huo, Rou Du Huo (Radix Angelicae Pubescentis, Angelica Root)
Dispel Wind Dampness, Open Channels and Luo-Network Vessels and Relieve Pain
Acrid, Bitter, Aromatic
Slightly Warm to very Warm[1709]
Liver, Kidney,[1710] Urinary Bladder, Du[1711]
Biao/Li (Urinary Bladder/Kidney) + Liver, Du

Hai Fu Rong (Herba Limonium Wrightii, Limonium)
Dispel Wind Dampness, Open Channels and Luo-Network Vessels and Relieve Pain
Acrid, Bitter
Cold
Liver, Kidney

Xi Xian Cao (Herba Siegesbeckiae, Siegesbeckia, Common St. Paul's Wort)
Dispel Wind Dampness, Open Channels and Luo-Network Vessels and Relieve Pain
Bitter, Acrid[1712]
Cold, slightly Toxic*[1713]
Kidney, **Liver**

Song Jie (Lignum Pini Nodi, Knotty Pine Wood)
Dispel Wind Dampness, Open Channels and Luo-Network Vessels and Relieve Pain
Bitter, Acrid[1714]
Warm
Liver, Kidney[1715]

Qian Nian Jian (Rhizoma Homalomenae, Homalomena)
Dispel Wind Dampness, Open Channels and Luo-Network Vessels and Relieve Pain/Dispel Wind-Dampness Strengthen Sinew/Tendon and Bone
Bitter, Acrid, Aromatic[1716]
Warm, Toxic*[1717]
Kidney, **Liver**

Yi Tiao Gen (Radix Moghaniae, Moghania)
Dispel Wind Dampness, Open Channels and Luo-Network Vessels and Relieve Pain
Acrid
Warm
Liver, Kidney

Kuan Jin Teng (Caulis Tinosporae Sinensis)
Dispel Wind Dampness, Open Channels and Luo-Network Vessels and Relieve Pain
Bitter
Slightly Cold
Liver

Sang Zhi, Sang Tiao (Ramulus Mori, Mulberry Twig)
Dispel Wind Dampness, Open Channels and Luo-Network Vessels and Relieve Pain
Bitter
Neutral to slightly Cool[1718]
Liver

Chou Wu Tong (Clerodendri Folium, Clerodenron leaf, Harlequin Glory-Bower leaf)
Dispel Wind Dampness, Open Channels and Luo-Network Vessels and Relieve Pain
Sweet, Acrid, Bitter
Cool, slightly Toxic*[1719]
Liver

Lei Gong Teng (Radix Tripterygii Wilfordii)
Dispel Wind Dampness, Open Channels and Luo-Network Vessels and Relieve Pain
Bitter, Acrid
Cool, Toxic*
Liver

Xia Tian Wu (Rhizoma Corydalis Decumbentis, Decumbent Corydalis Rhizome)
Dispel Wind Dampness, Open Channels and Luo-Network Vessels and Relieve Pain
Acrid, Bitter
Warm
Liver

Qi Ye Lian (Radix Schefflerae, Schefflera, Scandent Schefflera Root)
Dispel Wind Dampness, Open Channels and Luo-Network Vessels and Relieve Pain
Bitter, Acrid
Warm
Liver

She Tui, She Pi, Long Yi (Periostracum Serpentis, Snake Sloughing)
Dispel Wind Dampness, Open Channels and Luo-Network Vessels and Relieve Pain
Sweet, Salty
Neutral
Liver

Bai Hua She, Qi She, Jin Qian Bai Hua She (Bungarus Parvus/Agkistrodon, Bungarus/Agkistrodon Snake)
Dispel Wind Dampness, Open Channels and Luo-Network Vessels and Relieve Pain
Sweet, Salty
Warm, Toxic*
Liver

Dispel Wind-Dampness Strengthen Sinew/Tendon and Bone

Shi Nan Teng (Ramulus Piper, Piper Vine)
Dispel Wind-Dampness Strengthen Sinew/Tendon and Bone
Acrid
Warm
Liver, Lung, Kidney
Clock Neighbor (Liver/Lung), Branch (You/Chicken, Lung/Kidney, 5PM-6:59PM)

Xiang Jia Pi (Cortex Periplocae, Chinese Silkvine Root Bark)
Dispel Wind-Dampness Strengthen Sinew/Tendon and Bone
Acrid, Bitter
Warm, Toxic*
Liver, Kidney, Heart
Name (Shao Yin, Kidney/Heart) + Liver

Sang Ji Sheng (Herba Taxilli, Taxillus, Mulberry Mistletoe Stem, Mistletoe)
Dispel Wind-Dampness Strengthen Sinew/Tendon and Bone
Bitter, Sweet,[1720] Sour[1721]
Neutral
Liver, Kidney

Hu Ji Sheng, Bei Ji Sheng (Herba Visci, Colored Mistletoe)
Dispel Wind-Dampness Strengthen Sinew/Tendon and Bone
Bitter
Neutral, slightly Toxic*[1722]
Liver, Kidney

Lu Han Cao, Lu Xian Cao, Lu Ti Cao (Herba Pyrolae, Pyrola)
Dispel Wind-Dampness Strengthen Sinew/Tendon and Bone
Sweet, Bitter
Warm
Liver, Kidney

Wu Jia Pi (Cortex Acanthopanacis/Eleutherococcus, Eleutherococcus Root Bark, Acanthopanax Root Bark)
Dispel Wind-Dampness Strengthen Sinew/Tendon and Bone
Acrid, Bitter
Warm
Kidney, **Liver**

Qian Nian Jian (Rhizoma Homalomenae, Homalomena)
Dispel Wind Dampness, Open Channels and Luo-Network Vessels and Relieve Pain/Dispel Wind-Dampness Strengthen Sinew/Tendon and Bone
Bitter, Acrid, Aromatic[1723]
Warm, Toxic*[1724]
Kidney, **Liver**

Regulate Water Resolve Dampness

Che Qian Zi (Semen Plantaginis, Plantago Seed, Plantain Seed)
Regulate Water Resolve Dampness
Sweet, Bland[1725]
Cold
Kidney, Urinary Bladder, **Liver**, Lung, Small Intestine[1726]
Name (Tai Yang, Small Intestine/Urinary Bladder), Bie Jing (Tai Yin/Tai Yang, Lung/Urinary Bladder), Biao/Li (Urinary Bladder/Kidney), Clock Opposite (Lung/Urinary Bladder, Liver/Small Intestine), Clock Neighbor (Small Intestine/Urinary Bladder, Liver/Lung), Branch (You/Chicken, Lung/Kidney, 5PM-6:59PM)

Che Qian Cao (Herba Plantaginis)
Regulate Water Resolve Dampness
Sweet
Cold
Liver, Kidney, Lung, Small Intestine
Clock Opposite (Liver/Small Intestine), Clock Neighbor (Liver/Lung), Branch (You/Chicken, Lung/Kidney, 5PM-6:59PM)

Bai Long Chuan Hua Tou (Radix Clerodendron Paniculatum, Clerodendron, Scarlet Glory Bower)
Regulate Water Resolve Dampness
Slightly Bitter
Warm
Lung, **Liver**, Kidney
Clock Neighbor (Liver/Lung), Branch (You/Chicken, Lung/Kidney, 5PM-6:59PM)

Liu Zhi Huang (Herba Solidaginis, Solidago)
Regulate Water Resolve Dampness
Bitter, Sweet
Cold
Lung, **Liver**, Kidney
Clock Neighbor (Liver/Lung), Branch (You/Chicken, Lung/Kidney, 5PM-6:59PM)

Shan Pu Tao (Radix Vitis Amurensis, Viticis)
Regulate Water Resolve Dampness
Sweet
Cold
Lung, **Liver**, Kidney
Clock Neighbor (Liver/Lung), Branch (You/Chicken, Lung/Kidney, 5PM-6:59PM)

Ma Ti Jin (Herba Dichondrae Repentis, Dichondra)
Regulate Water Resolve Dampness
Bitter, Acrid
Cool
Liver, Lung
Clock Neighbor (Liver/Lung)

Qing Ma Zi, Bai Ma Zi, Kui Zi (Semen Abutili, Abutilon Seed, Indian Mallow Seed)
Regulate Water Resolve Dampness
Bitter
Neutral
Urinary Bladder, Large Intestine, **Liver**
Bie Jing (Yang Ming/Jue Yin, Large Intestine/Liver), Branch (Shen/Monkey, Large Intestine/Urinary Bladder, 3PM-4:59PM and Mao/Rabbit, Liver/Large Intestine, 5AM-6:59AM)

Ding Shu Xiu (Herba Elephantopus Scaber, Elephantopi)
Regulate Water Resolve Dampness
Sweet, Bitter
Cold
Liver, Kidney, Large Intestine
Bie Jing (Jue Yin/Yang Ming, Liver/Large Intestine), Clock Opposite (Kidney/Large Intestine), Branch (Mao/Rabbit, Liver/Large Intestine, 5AM-6:59AM)

Yin Chen Hao, Yin Chen (Herba Artemesia Scopariae, Virgate Wormwood, Capillary Wormwood)
Regulate Water Resolve Dampness
Bitter, Aromatic
Cool to Cold[1727]
Liver, Spleen, Gall Bladder, Stomach
Biao/Li (Gall Bladder/Liver, Stomach/Spleen), Branch (Chou/Ox, Spleen/Liver, 1AM-2:59AM)

Bi Xie (Rhizoma Dioscoriae Hypoglaucae, Fish Poison Yam, Tokoro)
Regulate Water Resolve Dampness
Bitter
Neutral
Urinary Bladder, **Liver**, Stomach
Qian/Hou (Front/Back, Stomach/Urinary Bladder) + Liver

Yu Mi Xu, Yu Mai Xu (Stigma Maydis, Corn Stigma, Corn Silk)
Regulate Water Resolve Dampness
Sweet, Bland
Neutral
Urinary Bladder, Kidney, **Liver**, Gall Bladder[1728]
Biao/Li (Urinary Bladder/Kidney, Gall Bladder/Liver), Branch (Zi/Rat, Kidney/Gall Bladder, 11PM-12:59AM)

Jin Qian Cao (Herba Lysimachiae, Lysimachia, Loose Strife Herb)
Regulate Water Resolve Dampness
Sweet, Salty, Bland[1729]
Cool to slightly Cold[1730]
Urinary Bladder, Gall Bladder, Kidney, **Liver**
Biao/Li (Urinary Bladder/Kidney, Gall Bladder/Liver), Branch (Zi/Rat, Kidney/Gall Bladder, 11PM-12:59AM)

Hua Shi Cao (Herba Orthosiphon Aristatus, Orthosiphon, Cat's Whiskers)
Regulate Water Resolve Dampness
Bitter
Cold
Liver, Kidney, Urinary Bladder
Biao/Li (Urinary Bladder/Kidney) + Liver

Guang Jin Qian Cao (Herba Desmodii Styracifolii, Desmodium, Snowbell Leaf Tick Clover)
Regulate Water Resolve Dampness
Sweet, Bland
Cool
Liver, Kidney, Urinary Bladder
Biao/Li (Urinary Bladder/Kidney) + Liver

Mo Gu Xiao (Caulis Hyptis Capitatae, Hyptis)
Regulate Water Resolve Dampness
Bland
Cold
Liver, Kidney

Huang Jin Gui (Caulis Vanieriae, Vanieria)
Regulate Water Resolve Dampness
Bland
Cool
Liver, Kidney

Warm Interior

Dou Chi Jiang (Rhizoma et Radix Litsae, Cubeb Rhizome and Root)
Warm Interior
Acrid, Aromatic
Warm
Liver, Lung
Clock Neighbor (Liver/Lung)

Wu Zhu Yu, Wu Yu (Fructus Evodiae, Evodia Fruit)
Warm Interior
Acrid, Bitter, Aromatic
Hot, slightly Toxic*
Liver, Spleen, Stomach, Kidney[1731]
Biao/Li (Stomach/Spleen), Branch (Chou/Ox, Spleen/Liver, 1AM-2:59AM) + Kidney

Xiao Hui Xiang, Gui Hui Xiang (Fructus Foeniculi, Fennel Seed)
Warm Interior
Acrid, Aromatic
Warm
Liver, Kidney, Spleen, Stomach
Biao/Li (Stomach/Spleen), Branch (Chou/Ox, Spleen/Liver, 1AM-2:59AM) + Kidney

Zhi Cao Wu (Radix Aconiti Kusnezoffii, Wild Aconite Root)
Warm Interior
Acrid, Bitter
Hot, extremely Toxic**
Heart, **Liver**, Spleen, Kidney[1732]
Name (Shao Yin, Kidney/Heart), Clock Neighbor (Spleen/Heart), Branch (Chou/Ox, Spleen/Liver, 1AM-2:59AM)

Rou Gui (Cortex Cinnamomi, Cinnamon Bark, Cassia Bark)
Warm Interior
Acrid to highly Acrid,[1733] Sweet, Aromatic
Greatly Warming[1734] to Hot
Heart, Kidney, **Liver**, Spleen
Name (Shao Yin, Heart/Kidney), Clock Neighbor (Spleen/Heart), Branch (Chou/Ox, Spleen/Liver, 1AM-2:59AM)

Zhi Chuan Wu (Radix Aconiti Preparata, Prepared Aconite Main Root, Mother Root of Common Monk's Hood)
Warm Interior
Acrid, Bitter
Hot, extremely Toxic**
Heart, **Liver**, Spleen, Du[1735]
Clock Neighbor (Spleen/Heart), Branch (Chou/Ox, Spleen/Liver, 1AM-2:59AM) + Du

Da Hui Xiang, Ba Jiao Hui, Ba Jiao Hui Xiang (Fructus Anisi Stellati, Star Anis)
Warm Interior
Acrid, Sweet, Aromatic
Warm
Liver, Kidney, Spleen
Branch (Chou/Ox, Spleen/Liver, 1AM-2:59AM) + Kidney

Regulate and Rectify Qi

Fo Shou (Fructus Citri Sarcodactylis, Finger Citron Fruit, Buddha's Hand Citron)
Regulate and Rectify Qi
Acrid, Bitter, Aromatic
Warm
Liver, Lung, Stomach, Spleen
Name (Tai Yin, Lung/Spleen), Biao/Li (Stomach/Spleen), Clock Neighbor (Liver/Lung), Branch (Chou/Ox, Spleen/Liver, 1AM-2:59AM)

Xiang Yuan (Fructus Citri, Citron)
Regulate and Rectify Qi
Acrid, slightly Bitter, Sour, Aromatic
Warm
Liver, Spleen, Lung
Name (Tai Yin, Spleen/Lung), Clock Neighbor (Liver/Lung), Branch (Chou/Ox, Spleen/Liver, 1AM-2:59AM)

Tu Mu Xiang, Qi Mu Xiang (Radix Inulae)
Regulate and Rectify Qi
Acrid, Bitter
Warm
Lung, **Liver**, Spleen
Name (Tai Yin, Lung/Spleen), Clock Neighbor (Liver/Lung) Branch (Chou/Ox, Spleen/Liver, 1AM-2:59AM)

Ju Luo, Ju Si, Ju Jin (Citri Reticulatae Fructus Fasciculus Vascularis, Tangerine Pith, White Vein Network of Orange Peel)
Regulate and Rectify Qi
Sweet, Bitter
Neutral
Liver, Lung
Clock Neighbor (Liver/Lung)

Chuan Lian Zi, Jin Ling Zi (Fructus Toosendan, Sichuan Pagoda Tree Fruit, Sichuan Chinaberry)
Regulate and Rectify Qi
Bitter, slightly Sour[1736]
Cold, slightly Toxic*
Liver, Small Intestine, Stomach, Urinary Bladder
Name (Tai Yang, Small Intestine/Urinary Bladder), Clock Opposite (Liver/Small Intestine), Clock Neighbor (Small Intestine/Urinary Bladder), Qian/Hou (Front/Back, Stomach/Urinary Bladder)

Po Bu Zi Ye (Folium Cordia Dichotoma, Sebastan Plum Cordia Leaf)
Regulate and Rectify Qi
Bitter, slightly Astringent
Cool
Liver, Kidney, Stomach

Jiu Ceng Ta (Herba Ocimi Basilici, Basil)
Regulate and Rectify Qi
Acrid
Warm
Stomach, **Liver**, Kidney

Qing Pi, Qing Ju Pi (Pericarpium Citri Reticulatae Viride, Green or Unripened Tangerine Peel)
Regulate and Rectify Qi
Acrid, Bitter, slightly Sour,[1737] Aromatic
Warm
Liver, Gall Bladder, Stomach, San Jiao[1738]
Name (Shao Yang, San Jiao/Gall Bladder), Biao/Li (Gall Bladder/Liver), Clock Neighbor (San Jiao/Gall Bladder) + Stomach

Ba Yue Zha, Yu Zhi Zi (Fructus Akebiae, Akebia Fruit)
Regulate and Rectify Qi
Bitter, Sweet[1739]
Neutral to slightly Cool[1740]
Liver, Stomach

Li Zhi He, Li He, Li Ren (Semen Litchi, Litchee Nut)
Regulate and Rectify Qi
Acrid,[1741] slightly Bitter,[1742] Sweet, Astringent
Warm
Liver, Stomach

Qing Mu Xiang, Ma Dou Ling Gen (Radix Aristolochiae, Aristolochia Root, Slender Dutchman's Pipe Root)
Regulate and Rectify Qi
Acrid, Bitter
Cool to Cold, Toxic*
Liver, Stomach

Suo Luo Zi, Kai Xin Guo (Semen Aesculi, Horse Chestnut, Chinese Buckeye Seed, Wilson's Buckeye Seed)
Regulate and Rectify Qi
Sweet
Warm
Liver, Stomach

Jiu Xiang Chong, Da Pi Chong (Aspongopus, Stinkbug)
Regulate and Rectify Qi
Salty
Warm
Spleen, **Liver**, Kidney
Branch (Chou/Ox, Spleen/Liver, 1AM-2:59AM) + Kidney

Xiang Fu (Rhizoma Cyperi, Cyperus Rhizome, Nut Grass Rhizome)
Regulate and Rectify Qi
Acrid to intensely Acrid,[1743] slightly Bitter, slightly Sweet, Aromatic
Neutral
Liver, Spleen,[1744] San Jiao, Gall Bladder,[1745] some sources indicate that it enters all channels.
Name (Shao Yang, San Jiao/Gall Bladder), Biao/Li (Gall Bladder/Liver), Clock Opposite (Spleen/San Jiao), Clock Neighbor (San Jiao/Gall Bladder), Branch (Chou/Ox, Spleen/Liver, 1AM-2:59AM)

Mei Gui Hua (Rosa Rugosae Flos, Young Flower of Chinese Rose, Rosebud)
Regulate and Rectify Qi
Sweet, slightly Bitter, Aromatic
Warm
Liver, Spleen
Branch (Chou/Ox, Spleen/Liver, 1AM-2:59AM)

Ju He, Ju Zi He, Ju Zi Ren, Ju Ren (Citri Reticulatae Semen, Tangerine/Orange Seed)
Regulate and Rectify Qi
Bitter
Neutral
Liver, Kidney,[1746] Urinary Bladder[1747]
Biao/Li (Urinary Bladder/Kidney) + Liver

Digestive

Hong Qu (Monascus, Red Yeast Rice)
Digestive
Sweet, Acrid
Warm
Spleen, **Liver**, Large Intestine
Bie Jing (Jue Yin/Yang Ming, Liver/Large Intestine), Branch (Chou/Ox, Spleen/Liver, 1AM-2:59AM and Mao/Rabbit, Liver/Large Intestine, 5AM-6:59AM)

Shan Zha (Fructus Crategi, Crategus, Hawthorn Fruit)
Digestive
Sweet, Sour
Neutral[1748] to slightly Warm
Liver, Spleen, Stomach
Biao/Li (Stomach/Spleen), Branch (Chou/Ox, Spleen/Liver, 1AM-2:59AM)

Mai Ya, Da Mai Ya (Fructus Hordei Germinatus, Barley Sprout, Malt)
Digestive
Sweet, Salty[1749]
Neutral
Liver, Spleen, Stomach
Biao/Li (Stomach/Spleen), Branch (Chou/Ox, Spleen/Liver, 1AM-2:59AM)

Expel Parasites

Chang Shan (Radix Dichroae, Dichroa Root)
Expel Parasites/Emetic
Acrid, Bitter
Cold, Toxic*
Lung, Heart, **Liver**
Clock Neighbor (Liver/Lung) + Heart

He Cao Ya (Gemma Agrimoniae, Agrimonia, Hairy-Vein Agrimonia Bud)
Expel Parasites
Bitter, Astringent
Cool
Liver, Small Intestine, Large Intestine
Bie Jing (Jue Yin/Yang Ming, Liver/Large Intestine), Clock Opposite (Liver, Small Intestine)
Branch (Mao/Rabbit, Liver/Large Intestine, 5AM-6:59AM)

Ku Lian Pi, Ku Lian Gen Pi (Cortex Meliae, Chinaberry Bark)
Expel Parasites
Bitter
Cold, Toxic*
Liver, Spleen, Stomach
Biao/Li (Stomach/Spleen), Branch (Chou/Ox, Spleen/Liver, 1AM-2:59AM)

Guan Zhong, Mian Ma Guan Zhong (Rhizoma Dryopteridis, Dryopteris Root, Shield-Fern Root)
Clear Heat Clean Toxin/Expel Parasites
Bitter
Cool to Cold,[1750] slightly Toxic*
Liver, Spleen, Stomach[1751]
Biao/Li (Stomach/Spleen), Branch (Chou/Ox, Spleen/Liver, 1AM-2:59AM)

He Shi, Bei He Shi (Fructus Carpesii, Carpesium Fruit)
Expel Parasites
Bitter, Acrid
Neutral, slightly Toxic*
Spleen, Stomach, **Liver**[1752]
Biao/Li (Stomach/Spleen), Branch (Chou/Ox, Spleen/Liver, 1AM-2:59AM)

Stop Bleeding

Zong Lu Tan (Trachycarpi Petiolus Carbonisatus, Charred Trachycarpus Petiole)
Stop Bleeding
Bitter, Astringent
Neutral
Lung, **Liver**, Large Intestine, Spleen[1753]
Name (Tai Yin, Lung/Spleen), Bie Jing (Jue Yin/Yang Ming, Liver/Large Intestine), Biao/Li (Large Intestine/Lung), Clock Neighbor (Liver/Lung), Branch (Mao/Rabbit, Liver/Large Intestine, 5AM-6:59AM)

Zong Lu Pi (Fibra Stipulae Trachicarpi, Trachycarpus Stipule Fiber)
Stop Bleeding
Bitter, Sour, Astringent[1754]
Neutral
Liver, Lung, Large Intestine
Bie Jing (Jue Yin/Yang Ming, Liver/Large Intestine), Biao/Li (Large Intestine/Lung), Clock Neighbor (Liver/Lung), Branch (Mao/Rabbit, Liver/Large Intestine, 5AM-6:59AM)

Ce Bai Ye (Cacumen Platycadi, Biota Leaves, Arborvitae Leaf)
Stop Bleeding
Bitter, Astringent
Cool[1755] to slightly Cold
Lung, **Liver**, Large Intestine
Biao/Li (Large Intestine/Lung), Bie Jing (Jue Yin/Yang Ming, Liver/Large Intestine), Branch (Mao/Rabbit, Liver/Large Intestine, 5AM-6:59AM)

Bai Ji, Bai Gen, Gan Gen (Rhizoma Bletillae, Bletilla Rhizome)
Stop Bleeding
Bitter, Sweet, Astringent
Cool to slightly Cold[1756]
Lung, Stomach, **Liver**
Clock Neighbor (Liver/Lung) + Stomach

Zi Zhu, Zi Zhu Cao (Folium Callicarpae, Callicarpa Leaf, Beauty-Berry Leaf)
Stop Bleeding
Bitter, Astringent
Cool
Liver, Lung, Stomach
Clock Neighbor (Liver/Lung) + Stomach

Ou Jie (Nodus Nelumbinis Rhizomatis, Lotus Rhizome Nodes)
Stop Bleeding
Sweet, Astringent
Neutral
Lung, Stomach, **Liver**
Clock Neighbor (Liver/Lung) + Stomach

Xian He Cao, Tuo Li Cao, Lang Ya Cao (Herba Agrimoniae, Agrimony Grass)
Stop Bleeding
Bitter, Astringent
Neutral
Lung, **Liver**, Spleen
Name (Tai Yin, Lung/Spleen), Clock Neighbor (Liver/Lung), Branch (Chou/Ox, Spleen/Liver, 1AM-2:59AM)

San Qi, Tian Qi (Radix Notoginseng, Pseudoginseng Root)
Stop Bleeding
Sweet, slightly Bitter
Warm
Liver, Stomach,[1757] Spleen,[1758] Large Intestine,[1759] Pericardium[1760]
Name (Yang Ming, Large Intestine/Stomach and Jue Yin, Liver/Pericardium), Bie Jing (Jue Yin/Yang Ming, Pericardium/Stomach and Liver/Large Intestine), Biao/Li (Stomach/Spleen), Clock Opposite (Pericardium/Stomach), Clock Neighbor (Large Intestine/Stomach), Branch (Chou/Ox, Spleen/Liver, 1AM-2:59AM, Mao/Rabbit, Liver/Large Intestine, 5AM-6:59AM and Shu/Dog, Stomach/Pericardium, 7PM-8:59PM)

Di Yu (Radix Sanguisorbae, Bloodwort Root, Burnet Root)
Stop Bleeding
Bitter, Sour, Astringent[1761]
Cool to Cold[1762]
Liver, Large Intestine, Stomach
Name (Yang Ming, Large Intestine/Stomach), Bie Jing (Jue Yin/Yang Ming, Liver/Large Intestine), Clock Neighbor (Large Intestine/Stomach), Branch (Mao/Rabbit, Liver/Large Intestine, 5AM-6:59AM)

Huai Jiao (Fructus Sophorae, Sophora Fruit)
Stop Bleeding
Bitter, Aromatic[1763]
Cold
Liver, Gall Bladder, Large Intestine
Bie Jing (Jue Yin/Yang Ming, Liver/Large Intestine), Biao/Li (Gall Bladder/Liver), Branch (Mao/Rabbit, Liver/Large Intestine, 5AM-6:59AM)

Huai Hua, Huai Mi, Huai Hua Mi (Flos Sophorae, Pagoda Tree Bud)
Stop Bleeding
Bitter
Cool to slightly Cold[1764]
Liver, Large Intestine
Bie Jing (Jue Yin/Yang Ming, Liver/Large Intestine), Branch (Mao/Rabbit, Liver/Large Intestine, 5AM-6:59AM)

Xue Yu Tan (Crinis Carbonitsatus, Charred Human Hair)
Stop Bleeding
Bitter, Astringent[1765]
Neutral
Liver, Stomach, Heart,[1766] Kidney[1767]
Name (Shao Yin, Heart/Kidney) + Liver, Stomach

Pu Huang (Pollen Typhae, Cattail Pollen, Bulrush Pollen)
Stop Bleeding
Sweet, Acrid,[1768] Astringent,[1769] Aromatic[1770]
Neutral
Liver, Pericardium,[1771] Heart,[1772] Spleen[1773]
Name (Jue Yin, Liver/Pericardium), Clock Neighbor (Spleen/Heart), Branch (Chou/Ox, Spleen/Liver, 1AM-2:59AM)

Da Ji, Da Xiao Ji (Herba seu Radix Cirsii Japonici, Japanese Thistle)
Stop Bleeding
Sweet, Bitter, slightly Acrid[1774]
Cool
Liver, Heart, Spleen[1775]
Clock Neighbor (Spleen/Heart), Branch (Chou/Ox, Spleen/Liver, 1AM-2:59AM)

Lian Fang (Receptaculum Nelumbinis, Lotus Peduncle)
Stop Bleeding
Bitter, Astringent
Warm
Liver, Spleen, Kidney
Branch (Chou/Ox, Spleen/Liver, 1AM-2:59AM) + Kidney

Ai Ye (Folium Artemisiae Argyi, Mugwort Leaf, Moxa)
Stop Bleeding
Bitter, Acrid, Aromatic
Warm
Spleen, **Liver**, Kidney, Dai[1776]
Branch (Chou/Ox, Spleen/Liver, 1AM-2:59AM) + Kidney, Dai

Pao Jiang (Zingiberis Rhizoma Praeparatum, Blast-Fried Ginger)
Stop Bleeding
Bitter, slightly Acrid, Astringent
Warm
Liver, Spleen
Branch (Chou/Ox, Spleen/Liver, 1AM-2:59AM)

Xiao Ji, Da Xiao Ji (Herba Cirisii, Cirsium, Field Thistle)
Stop Bleeding
Bitter,[1777] Sweet
Cool
Liver, Heart, Small Intestine,[1778] Urinary Bladder[1779]
Name (Tai Yang, Small Intestine/Urinary Bladder), Biao/Li (Small Intestine/Heart), Clock Opposite (Liver/Small Intestine), Clock Neighbor (Small Intestine/Urinary Bladder)

Qian Cao, Qian Cao Gen, Qian Gen (Radix Rubiae, Rubia Root)
Stop Bleeding
Bitter
Cold
Liver, Heart[1780]

Zhu Ma Gen (Boemeriae Radix, Ramie Root)
Stop Bleeding
Sweet
Cold
Heart, **Liver**

Hua Rui Shi (Ophicalcitum, Ophicalcite)
Stop Bleeding
Sour, Astringent
Neutral
Liver

Xiao Jin Ying (Fructus Rosae Cymosae)
Stop Bleeding
Bitter
Neutral
Liver

Vitalize Blood Transform Stasis

Tao Ren (Semen Persicae, Peach Kernel)
Vitalize Blood Transform Stasis
Bitter, Sweet[1781]
Neutral, slightly Toxic*
Heart, Large Intestine, **Liver**, Lung
Bie Jing (Jue Yin/Yang Ming, Liver/Large Intestine), Biao/Li (Large Intestine/Lung), Clock Neighbor (Liver/Lung), Branch (Mao/Rabbit, Liver/Large Intestine, 5AM-6:59AM) + Heart

Jin Bu Huan, Qian Ceng Ta (Herba Lycopodii Serrati, Lycopodium)
Vitalize Blood Transform Stasis
Acrid, Sweet
Neutral
Lung, **Liver**, Large Intestine
Bie Jing (Jue Yin/Yang Ming, Liver/Large Intestine), Biao/Li (Large Intestine/Lung), Clock Neighbor (Liver/Lung), Branch (Mao/Rabbit, Liver/Large Intestine, 5AM-6:59AM)

Wa Leng Zi (Concha Arcae, Cockle Shell, Ark Shell)
Vitalize Blood Transform Stasis/Transform Phlegm/External Application
Salty
Neutral
Liver, Stomach, Lung, Spleen[1782]
Name (Tai Yin, Lung/Spleen), Biao/Li (Stomach/Spleen), Clock Neighbor (Liver/Lung), Branch (Chou/Ox, Spleen/Liver, 1AM-2:59AM)

Yu Jin (Radix Curcumae, Aromatic Tumeric Tuber)
Vitalize Blood Transform Stasis
Acrid, Bitter, Aromatic
Cold
Heart, **Liver**, Gall Bladder, Lung[1783]
Bie Jing (Shao Yin/Shao Yang, Heart/Gall Bladder), Biao/Li (Gall Bladder/Liver), Clock Opposite (Heart/Gall Bladder), Clock Neighbor (Liver/Lung), Branch (Yin/Tiger, Gall Bladder/Lung, 3AM-4:59AM)

Tu Niu Xi (Radix Achyranthes Longiflora, Native Achyranthis Root)
Clear Heat Clean Toxin/Vitalize Blood Transform Stasis
Bitter, Sour, Acrid[1784]
Neutral to Cold,[1785] slightly Toxic[1786]
Lung, **Liver**, Kidney
Clock Neighbor (Liver/Lung), Branch (You/Chicken, Lung/Kidney, 5PM-6:59PM)

Hu Zhang (Rhizoma Polygoni Cuspidati, Bushy Knotweed Rhizome, Japanese Knotweed Rhizome, Giant Knotweed Rhizome)
Vitalize Blood Transform Stasis
Bitter
Cold
Liver, Gall Bladder, Lung
Biao/Li (Gall Bladder/Liver), Clock Neighbor (Liver/Lung), Branch (Yin/Tiger, Gall Bladder/Lung, 3AM-4:59AM)

Yan Hu Suo (Rhizoma Corydalis, Corydalis Rhizome)
Vitalize Blood Transform Stasis
Acrid, Bitter, Aromatic
Warm
Heart, **Liver**, Spleen, Stomach[1787]
Biao/Li (Stomach/Spleen), Clock Neighbor (Spleen/Heart), Branch (Chou/Ox, Spleen/Liver, 1AM-2:59AM)

Jiang Xiang (Lignum Dalbergiae Odoriferae, Dalbergia Heartwood, Rosewood)
Vitalize Blood Transform Stasis
Acrid, Aromatic
Warm
Liver, Spleen, Heart, Stomach[1788]
Biao/Li (Stomach/Spleen), Clock Neighbor (Spleen/Heart), Branch (Chou/Ox, Spleen/Liver, 1AM-2:59AM)

Jiang Huang (Rhizoma Curcumae Longae, Turmeric Rhizome)
Vitalize Blood Transform Stasis
Acrid, Bitter, Aromatic
Warm
Spleen, **Liver**, Stomach[1789]
Biao/Li (Stomach/Spleen), Branch (Chou/Ox, Spleen/Liver, 1AM-2:59AM)

Wang Bu Liu Xing (Semen Vaccariae, Vaccaria Seeds, Cow Soapwort Seed)
Vitalize Blood Transform Stasis
Acrid,[1790] Bitter
Neutral
Liver, Stomach, Urinary Bladder[1791]
Qian/Hou (Front/Back, Stomach/Urinary Bladder) + Liver

Lu Lu Tong, Feng Guo, Jiu Kong Zi (Fructus Liquidambaris, Sweetgum Fruit)
Vitalize Blood Transform Stasis
Bitter
Neutral
Liver, Stomach

Gan Qi (Resina Toxicodendri, Lacquer)
Vitalize Blood Transform Stasis
Acrid, Bitter
Warm, slightly Toxic
Liver, Stomach

Chuan Shan Jia (Squama Manis, Pangolin Scales)
Vitalize Blood Transform Stasis
Salty
Cool to slightly Cold[1792]
Liver, Stomach, some sources say that it enters and affects every channel and Luo-Network vessel.[1793]

Ji Xue Teng, Da Xue Teng (Caulis Spatholobi, Spatholobus, Millettia Vine)
Vitalize Blood Transform Stasis
Bitter, slightly Sweet, Acrid[1794]
Warm
Heart,[1795] **Liver**, Spleen[1796]
Clock Neighbor (Spleen/Heart), Branch (Chou/Ox, Spleen/Liver, 1AM-2:59AM)

Mo Yao (Commiphora Myrrha, Myrrh)
Vitalize Blood Transform Stasis
Acrid,[1797] Bitter, Aromatic
Neutral
Heart, **Liver**, Spleen
Clock Neighbor (Spleen/Heart), Branch (Chou/Ox, Spleen/Liver, 1AM-2:59AM)

Ru Xiang (Boswelia Carterii, Gummi Olibanum, Frankincense)
Vitalize Blood Transform Stasis
Acrid, Bitter, Aromatic
Warm
Heart, **Liver**, Spleen
Clock Neighbor (Spleen/Heart), Branch (Chou/Ox, Spleen/Liver, 1AM-2:59AM)

Su Mu (Lignum Sappan, Sappan Wood, Brazilwood)
Vitalize Blood Transform Stasis
Sweet, Salty, slightly Acrid to Acrid[1798]
Neutral to slightly Cooling[1799]
Heart, **Liver**, Spleen[1800]
Clock Neighbor (Spleen/Heart), Branch (Chou/Ox, Spleen/Liver, 1AM-2:59AM)

Di Bie Chong, Tu Bie Chong, Zhe Chong (Eupolyphagia, Wingless Cockroach, Ground Beetle)
Vitalize Blood Transform Stasis
Salty
Cold, slightly Toxic*
Liver, Heart, Spleen
Clock Neighbor (Spleen/Heart), Branch (Chou/Ox, Spleen/Liver, 1AM-2:59AM)

Chi Shao (Radix Paeoniae Rubrae, Red Peony Root)
Clear Heat Cool Blood/Vitalize Blood Transform Stasis
Bitter, Sour[1801]
Cool to slightly Cold
Liver, Spleen[1802]
Branch (Chou/Ox, Spleen/Liver, 1AM-2:59AM)

Ma Bian Cao, Tie Ma Bian, Feng Jing Cao (Herba Verbena, Verbena, Iron Herb)
Vitalize Blood Transform Stasis
Bitter
Cool to slightly Cold[1803]
Liver, Spleen
Branch (Chou/Ox, Spleen/Liver, 1AM-2:59AM)

Mei Gui Hua (Flos Rugosae)
Vitalize Blood Transform Stasis
Sweet, slightly Bitter
Warm
Liver, Spleen
Branch (Chou/Ox, Spleen/Liver,1AM-2:59AM)

San Leng (Rhizoma Sparganii, Scirpus Rhizome, Burr Reed Rhizome)
Vitalize Blood Transform Stasis
Bitter, Acrid[1804]
Neutral to Warm[1805]
Liver, Spleen
Branch (Chou/Ox, Spleen/Liver, 1AM-2:59AM)

Ze Lan (Herba Lycopi, Bugleweed, Water Horehound)
Vitalize Blood Transform Stasis
Bitter, Acrid, Aromatic
Slightly Warm
Liver, Spleen
Branch (Chou/Ox, Spleen/Liver, 1AM-2:59AM)

E Zhu (Rhizoma Curcumae, Zedoaria Rhizome)
Vitalize Blood Transform Stasis
Bitter, Acrid, Aromatic
Warm
Spleen, **Liver**
Branch (Chou/Ox, Spleen/Liver, 1AM-2:59AM)

Chong Wei Zi (Fructus Leonuri, Leonurus Fruit)
Vitalize Blood Transform Stasis
Sweet
Cool[1806] to slightly Cold
Liver, Spleen
Branch (Chou/Ox, Spleen/Liver, 1AM-2:59AM)

Yi Mu Cao (Herba Leonuri, Chinese Motherwort)
Vitalize Blood Transform Stasis
Acrid, Bitter
Cool to slightly Cold[1807]
Heart, **Liver**, Urinary Bladder

Mu Dan Pi, Mu Shao Yao (Cortex Moutan, Peony Tree Root Cortex)
Clear Heat Cool Blood/Vitalize Blood Transform Stasis
Bitter, Acrid, Aromatic
Cool to slightly Cold
Heart, **Liver**, Kidney, Pericardium[1808]
Name (Shao Yin, Heart/Kidney, Jue Yin, Liver/Pericardium), Clock Neighbor (Kidney/Pericardium)

Dan Shen (Radix Salviae Miltiorrhizae, Salvia Root)
Vitalize Blood Transform Stasis
Bitter
Cool to slightly Cold[1809] to Warm[1810]
Heart, Pericardium,[1811] **Liver**
Name (Jue Yin, Pericardium/Liver) + Heart

Hong Hua (Flos Carthami, Safflower Flower)
Vitalize Blood Transform Stasis
Acrid, Bitter,[1812] Sweet[1813]
Slightly Cool[1814] to Warm
Heart, **Liver**

Xi Hong Hua, Fan Hong Hua, Zhang Hong Hua (Flos Crocus Sativus, Crocus Stigma, Saffron)
Vitalize Blood Transform Stasis
Sweet
Cool to slightly Cold[1815] to Cold[1816]
Heart, **Liver**

Xue Jie (Daemonoropis Resina, Sanguis Draconis, Dragon's Blood)
Vitalize Blood Transform Stasis/External Application
Sweet, Acrid,[1817] Salty,[1818] Aromatic
Neutral
Heart, **Liver**

Shui Zhi (Hirudo, Leech)
Vitalize Blood Transform Stasis
Salty, Bitter
Neutral, slightly Toxic*
Liver, Urinary Bladder[1819]

Huai Niu Xi (Radix Achyranthis Bidentatae, Achyranthes Root)
Vitalize Blood Transform Stasis
Bitter, Sour
Neutral
Liver, Kidney

Chuan Niu Xi (Radix Cyathulae, Cyathula)
Vitalize Blood Transform Stasis
Bitter, Sour, Sweet[1820]
Neutral
Liver, Kidney

Ding Jing Cao (Herba Linderniae)
Vitalize Blood Transform Stasis
Sweet, slightly Bitter
Neutral
Liver, Kidney

Niao Bu Su (Ramus Kalopanax Pictus, Kalopanacis)
Vitalize Blood Transform Stasis
Acrid, Bitter
Warm, slightly Toxic*
Liver, Kidney

Ling Xiao Hua, Ling Xiao, Zi Wei (Flos Campsis, Campsis Flower, Trumpet Creeper)
Vitalize Blood Transform Stasis
Sweet, Sour, Salty[1821]
Slightly Cold
Liver, Pericardium
Name (Jue Yin, Liver/Pericardium)

Chuan Xiong, Xiong Qiong, Fu Xiong (Rhizoma Ligustici Chuanxiong, Szechuan Lovage Root)
Vitalize Blood Transform Stasis
Acrid, Bitter,[1822] Aromatic
Warm
Liver, Gall Bladder, Pericardium, San Jiao,[1823] Chong[1824]
Name (Jue Yin, Liver/Pericardium, Shao Yang, San Jiao/Gall Bladder), Biao/Li (Gall Bladder/Liver, San Jiao/Pericardium), Clock Neighbor (San Jiao/Gall Bladder) + Chong

Wu Ling Zhi (Excrementum Trogopteri Pteromi, Flying Squirrel Feces)
Vitalize Blood Transform Stasis
Bitter, Sweet, Acrid,[1825] Salty,[1826] Sour[1827]
Warm
Liver

Gui Jian Yu, Wei Mao (Ramulus Euonymi, Spindle Tree Wings)
Vitalize Blood Transform Stasis
Bitter
Cold
Liver

Zi Ran Tong (Pyritum, Pyrite)
Vitalize Blood Transform Stasis
Acrid, Bitter[1828]
Neutral
Liver

Meng Chong (Tabanus, Gadfly, Horse Fly)
Vitalize Blood Transform Stasis
Bitter, Salty[1829]
Cool to slightly Cold,[1830] slightly Toxic to Toxic*[1831]
Liver

Yue Ji Hua, Yue Yue Hong (Flos Rosae Chinensis, Partially Opened Flower of Chinese Tea Rose)
Vitalize Blood Transform Stasis
Sweet, Aromatic
Warm
Liver

Ye Ming Sha, Bian Fu Fen, Tian Fu Fen (Excrementum Vespertilionis Murini, Bat Feces)
Vitalize Blood Transform Stasis
Acrid
Cold
Liver

Transform Phlegm

Xuan Fu Hua, Jin Fei Hua, Jin Fu Hua (Flos Inulae, Inula Flower)
Transform Phlegm
Bitter, Acrid, Salty
Slightly Warm
Large Intestine, Lung, Stomach, Spleen, **Liver**[1832]
Name (Yang Ming, Large Intestine/Stomach, Tai Yin, Lung/Spleen), Bie Jing (Jue Yin/Yang Ming, Liver/Large Intestine), Biao/Li (Large Intestine/Lung, Stomach/Spleen), Clock Neighbor (Large Intestine/Stomach, Liver/Lung), Branch (Chou/Ox, Spleen/Liver, 1AM-2:59AM and Mao/Rabbit, Liver/Large Intestine, 5AM-6:59AM)

Bi Qi, Di Li, Wu Yu, Ma Ti (Rhizoma Eleocharitis, Water Chestnut)
Transform Phlegm
Sweet
Slightly Cold
Lung, **Liver**,[1833] Stomach, Large Intestine
Name (Yang Ming, Large Intestine/Stomach), Bie Jing (Jue Yin/Yang Ming, Liver/Large Intestine), Biao/Li (Large Intestine/Lung), Clock Neighbor (Large Intestine/Stomach, Liver/Lung), Branch (Mao/Rabbit, Liver/Large Intestine, 5AM-6:59AM)

Zhi Bai Fu Zi, Bai Fu Zi (Rhizoma Typhonii preparatum, Typhonium)
Transform Phlegm
Acrid, Sweet
Warm, Toxic*
Spleen, Stomach, Lung,[1834] **Liver**[1835]
Name (Tai Yin, Spleen/Lung), Biao/Li (Stomach/Spleen), Clock Neighbor (Liver/Lung), Branch (Chou/Ox, Spleen/Liver, 1AM-2:59AM)

Wa Leng Zi (Concha Arcae, Cockle Shell, Ark Shell)
Vitalize Blood Transform Stasis/Transform Phlegm/External Application
Salty
Neutral
Liver, Stomach, Lung, Spleen[1836]
Name (Tai Yin, Lung/Spleen), Biao/Li (Stomach/Spleen), Clock Neighbor (Liver/Lung), Branch (Chou/Ox, Spleen/Liver, 1AM-2:59AM)

Zhu Li (Succus Bambusae, Dried Bamboo Sap)
Transform Phlegm
Sweet, Bitter[1837]
Cold
Heart, Lung, Stomach, **Liver**[1838]
Clock Neighbor (Liver/Lung) + Heart, Stomach

Hai Zao (Sargassum, Seaweed, Gulfweed)
Transform Phlegm
Bitter,[1839] Salty
Cold
Liver, Kidney, Stomach,[1840] Lung[1841]
Clock Neighbor (Liver/Lung), Branch (You/Chicken, Lung/Kidney, 5PM-6:59PM) + Stomach

Si Gua Luo (Retinervus Luffae Fructus, Dried Vegetable Sponge)
Transform Phlegm/External Application
Sweet
Neutral to Cold[1842]
Lung, Stomach, **Liver**
Clock Neighbor (Liver/Lung) + Stomach

Jin Meng Shi (Micae Lapis Aureus, Vermiculite Schist)
Transform Phlegm
Sweet, Salty
Neutral
Liver, Lung, Stomach
Clock Neighbor (Liver/Lung) + Stomach

Zao Jiao Ci, Tian Ding, Zao Ci, Zao Ding (Spina Gleditsiae, Spine of Honeylocust Plant)
Transform Phlegm
Acrid
Warm
Liver, Stomach, Lung[1843]
Clock Neighbor (Liver/Lung) + Stomach

Dan Nan Xing, Dan Xing (Arisaema cum Bile)
Transform Phlegm
Bitter, slightly Acrid[1844]
Cool, slightly Toxic*
Liver, Lung,[1845] Spleen,[1846] Gall Bladder[1847]
Name (Tai Yin, Spleen/Lung), Biao/Li (Gall Bladder/Liver), Clock Neighbor (Liver/Lung), Branch (Chou/Ox, Spleen/Liver, 1AM-2:59AM and Yin/Tiger, Gall Bladder/Lung, 3AM-4:59AM)

Zhi Tian Nan Xing, Tian Nan Xing (Rhizoma Arisaematis preparatum, prepared Arisaema, Jack in the Pulpit)
Transform Phlegm
Bitter, very Acrid
Warm, Toxic*
Liver, Lung, Spleen
Name (Tai Yin, Spleen/Lung), Clock Neighbor (Liver/Lung), Branch (Chou/Ox, Spleen/Liver, 1AM-2:59AM)

Qian Hu (Radix Peucedani, Hogfennel Root)
Transform Phlegm
Bitter, Acrid
Cool to slightly Cold[1848]
Lung, **Liver**,[1849] Gall Bladder[1850]
Biao/Li (Gall Bladder/Liver), Clock Neighbor (Liver/Lung), Branch (Yin/Tiger, Gall Bladder/Lung, 3AM-4:59AM)

Ming Dang Shen, Ming Shen (Radix Changii, Changium root)
Transform Phlegm
Sweet, slightly Bitter
Cool
Lung, **Liver**
Clock Neighbor (Liver/Lung)

Huang Yao Zi (Herba Dioscoriae Bulbiferae)
Transform Phlegm
Bitter, Sweet[1851]
Neutral[1852] to Cold, Toxic*
Lung, **Liver**
Clock Neighbor (Liver/Lung)

Qing Meng Shi, Meng Shi (Lapis Micae seu Chloriti, Chlorite Schist, Mica Schist)
Transform Phlegm
Salty, Sweet
Neutral
Lung, **Liver**
Clock Neighbor (Liver/Lung)

Kun Bu (Thallus Laminariae seu Eckloniae, Kelp)
Transform Phlegm
Salty
Cold
Liver, Stomach, Kidney

Tian Zhu Huang (Concretio Silicea Bambusae, Siliceous Secretions of Bamboo, Bamboo Sugar, Tabasheer)
Transform Phlegm
Sweet, Bitter[1853]
Cold
Gall Bladder, Heart, **Liver**
Bie Jing (Shao Yin/Shao Yang, Heart/Gall Bladder), Biao/Li (Gall Bladder/Liver), Clock Opposite (Heart/Gall Bladder)

Relieve Cough and Wheezing/Panting

Li Lu (Radix et Rhizoma Veratri, Lack False Hellebore, Vanity Grass)
Relieve Cough and Wheezing/Panting/Emetic
Acrid, Bitter
Cold, extremely Toxic*
Lung, **Liver**, Stomach
Clock Neighbor (Liver/Lung) + Stomach

Yang Jin Hua (Flos Daturae, Datura Flower)
Relieve Cough and Wheezing/Panting
Acrid
Warm, Toxic*
Lung, **Liver**, Heart, Spleen
Name (Tai Yin, Lung/Spleen), Clock Neighbor (Liver/Lung, Spleen/Heart), Branch (Chou/Ox, Spleen/Liver, 1AM-2:59AM)

Kuan Dong Hua, Dong Hua, Jiu Jiu Hua (Flos Farfarae, Coltsfoot Flower)
Relieve Cough and Wheezing/Panting
Acrid, slightly Bitter,[1854] Sweet[1855]
Warm
Lung, Heart,[1856] **Liver**[1857]
Clock Neighbor (Liver/Lung) + Heart

Zi Jin Niu, Ai Di Cha, Ping Di Mu (Herba Ardisiae Japonicae, Japanese Ardisia)
Relieve Cough and Wheezing/Panting
Bitter, Acrid
Neutral
Lung, **Liver**
Clock Neighbor (Liver/Lung)

Mu Hu Die, Yu Hu Die, Gu Zhi Hua (Semen Oroxyli, Oroxylum Seeds)
Relieve Cough and Wheezing/Panting
Sweet, Bland
Cool
Liver, Lung
Clock Neighbor (Liver/Lung)

Nourish and Calm Shen

He Huan Hua, Ye He Hua, Ye He Mi (Flos Albiziae, Mimosa Flower)
Nourish and Calm Shen
Sweet
Neutral
Liver, Stomach, Spleen,[1858] Heart,[1859] Lung[1860]
Name (Tai Yin, Lung/Spleen), Biao/Li (Stomach/Spleen), Clock Neighbor (Spleen/Heart, Liver/Lung), Branch (Chou/Ox, Spleen/Liver, 1AM-2:59AM)

Ling Zhi, Zhi, Ling Zhi Cao (Ganoderma, Reishi Mushroom)
Nourish and Calm Shen
Sweet
Neutral
Heart, **Liver**, Lung
Clock Neighbor (Liver/Lung) + Heart

Suan Zao Ren, Dong Zao (Semen Zizyphi Spinosae, Sour Jujube Seed)
Nourish and Calm Shen
Sweet, Sour[1861]
Neutral
Heart, **Liver**, Gall Bladder,[1862] Spleen[1863]
Bie Jing (Shao Yin/Shao Yang, Heart/Gall Bladder), Biao/Li (Gall Bladder/Liver), Clock Opposite (Heart/Gall Bladder), Clock Neighbor (Spleen/Heart), Branch (Chou/Ox, Spleen/Liver, 1AM-2:59AM)

Ye Jiao Teng, Shou Wu Teng (Caulis Polygoni Multiflori, Polygonum Vine, Fleeceflower Vine, Flowery Knotweed Stem)
Nourish and Calm Shen
Sweet, slightly Bitter
Neutral
Heart, **Liver**

Xie Cao, Jie Cao (Radix et Rhizoma Valerianae, Valerian Root)
Nourish and Calm Shen
Bitter, Sweet, Acrid[1864]
Neutral to Warm[1865]
Heart, **Liver**

He Huan Pi (Cortex Albiziae, Mimosa Tree Bark)
Nourish and Calm Shen
Sweet
Neutral
Heart, **Liver**

Ye He Hua (Flos Magnoliae Cocinis, Magnolia Flower)
Nourish and Calm Shen
Acrid, Aromatic
Warm
Liver, Heart

Calm Shen Sedative

Long Chi (Fossilia Mastodi Dentis, fossilized teeth)
Calm Shen Sedative
Sweet, Astringent
Cool
Heart, **Liver**, Lung[1866]
Clock Neighbor (Liver/Lung) + Heart

Zi Bei Chi, Bei Zi, Zi Bei, Bao Bei (Concha Mauritiae/Cypraeae, Cowry Shell)
Calm Shen Sedative
Salty
Neutral
Spleen, **Liver**
Branch (Chou/Ox, Spleen/Liver, 1AM-2:59AM)

Hu Po (Succinum, Amber)
Calm Shen Sedative
Sweet, Bland[1867]
Neutral
Heart, **Liver**, Urinary Bladder[1868]

Ci Shi (Magnetitum, Magnetite, Loadstone)
Calm Shen Sedative
Acrid,[1869] Salty
Cold
Liver, Kidney, Heart
Name (Shao Yin, Kidney/Heart) + Liver

Long Gu (Os Draconis, Fossilia Mastodi Ossis, Fossilized Bones)
Calm Shen Sedative
Sweet, slightly Acrid,[1870] Astringent[1871]
Neutral[1872] to Cool to slightly Cold[1873]
Heart, **Liver**, Kidney,[1874] Dai[1875]
Name (Shao Yin, Heart/Kidney) + Liver, Dai

Zhen Zhu (Margarita, Pearl)
Calm Shen Sedative/Calm Liver Extinguish Wind
Sweet, Salty, Bland,[1876] Astringent[1877]
Cold
Heart, **Liver**

Zhen Zhu Mu (Concha Margaritaferae, Mother of Pearl)
Calm Shen Sedative/Calm Liver Extinguish Wind
Salty, Sweet[1878]
Cool[1879] to Cold
Heart, **Liver**

Sheng Tie Luo, Tie Luo (Frusta Ferri, Oxidized Iron Filings)
Calm Shen Sedative
Acrid
Cool
Heart, **Liver**

Zi Shi Ying (Floritum, Flourite)
Calm Shen Sedative/Calm Liver Extinguish Wind
Sweet, Acrid
Warm
Heart, **Liver**, Chong and Ren[1880]

Mu Li, Mu Li Ke (Concha Ostreae, Oyster Shell)
Calm Shen Sedative/Calm Liver Extinguish Wind
Salty, Astringent
Cool to slightly Cold[1881]
Liver, Kidney

Calm Liver Extinguish Wind

Di Long, Qiu Yin (Pheretima, Earthworm)
Calm Liver Extinguish Wind
Salty
Cold
Liver, Spleen, Kidney,[1882] Urinary Bladder, Lung[1883]
Name (Tai Yin, Spleen/Lung), Bie Jing (Tai Yin/Tai Yang, Lung/Urinary Bladder), Biao/Li (Urinary Bladder/Kidney), Clock Opposite (Lung/Urinary Bladder), Clock Neighbor (Liver/Lung), Branch (Chou/Ox, Spleen/Liver, 1AM-2:59AM)

Jiang Can, Bai Jiang Can, Tian Cong (Bombyx Batryticatus, Mummified Silkworm)
Calm Liver Extinguish Wind
Salty, Acrid
Neutral to slightly Warm[1884]
Liver, Lung
Clock Neighbor (Liver/Lung)

Jue Ming Zi, Cao Jue Ming (Semen Cassiae, Cassia Seeds, Foetid Cassia Seeds)
Clear Heat Purge Fire/Calm Liver Extinguish Wind
Sweet, Bitter, Salty[1885]
Cool to slightly Cold
Liver, Large Intestine, Kidney[1886]
Bie Jing (Jue Yin/Yang Ming, Liver/Large Intestine), Clock Opposite (Kidney/Large Intestine), Branch (Mao/Rabbit, Liver/Large Intestine, 5AM-6:59AM)

Dai Zhe Shi, Zhe Shi (Haematitum, Hematite)
Calm Liver Extinguish Wind
Bitter
Cold
Heart, **Liver**, Pericardium[1887]
Name (Jue Yin, Liver/Pericardium) + Heart

Gou Teng (Ramulus Uncariae cum Uncis, Gambir Vine Stems and Thorns)
Calm Liver Extinguish Wind
Sweet
Cool to slightly Cold[1888]
Liver, Pericardium, Heart[1889]
Name (Jue Yin, Liver/Pericardium) + Heart

Zhen Zhu (Margarita, Pearl)
Calm Shen Sedative/Calm Liver Extinguish Wind
Sweet, Salty, Bland,[1890] Astringent[1891]
Cold
Heart, **Liver**

Zhen Zhu Mu (Concha Margaritaferae, Mother of Pearl)
Calm Shen Sedative/Calm Liver Extinguish Wind
Salty, Sweet[1892]
Cool[1893] to Cold
Heart, **Liver**

Ling Yang Jiao (Cornu Saigae Tataricae, Antelope Horn)
Calm Liver Extinguish Wind
Salty
Cold
Liver, Heart

Zi Shi Ying (Floritum, Flourite)
Calm Shen Sedative/Calm Liver Extinguish Wind
Sweet, Acrid
Warm
Heart, **Liver**, Chong and Ren[1894]

Mu Li, Mu Li Ke (Concha Ostreae, Oyster Shell)
Calm Shen Sedative/Calm Liver Extinguish Wind
Salty, Astringent
Cool to slightly Cold[1895]
Liver, Kidney

Shi Jue Ming, Qian Li Guang (Concha Haliotidis, Abalone Shell)
Calm Liver Extinguish Wind
Salty
Cold
Liver, Kidney[1896]

Luo Bu Ma Ye, Ze Qi Cao, Ji Ji Ma, Hong Hua Cao (Folium Apocni Veneti, Dogbane Leaf)
Calm Liver Extinguish Wind
Sweet, Bitter, Bland[1897]
Cool to slightly Cold[1898]
Liver

Bai Ji Li, Ci Ji Li, Ji Li (Fructus Tribuli, Caltrop Fruit, Puncture Vine Fruit)
Calm Liver Extinguish Wind
Bitter, Acrid
Neutral to Warm,[1899] slightly Toxic*
Liver

Gou Qi Gen (Radix Lycii, Lycium Root)
Calm Liver Extinguish Wind
Sweet
Cold
Liver

Hei Dou Pi, Lu Dou Yi (Testa Glycinis, Soybean Skin)
Calm Liver Extinguish Wind
Sweet
Neutral
Liver

Tian Ma, Ding Feng Cao (Rhizoma Gastrodiae, Gastrodia Rhizome)
Calm Liver Extinguish Wind
Sweet, slightly Acrid[1900]
Neutral to slightly Warm[1901]
Liver

Wu Gong (Scolopendra, Centipede)
Calm Liver Extinguish Wind
Acrid to highly Acrid[1902]
Warm, Toxic*
Liver

Quan Xie (Scorpio, Scorpion)
Calm Liver Extinguish Wind
Acrid, Salty[1903]
Neutral, Toxic*
Liver

Shan Yang Jiao (Cornu Naemorhedis, Mountain Goat Horn)
Calm Liver Extinguish Wind
Salty
Cold
Liver

Open Orifices

Shui Chang Pu, Bai Chang Pu (Rhizoma Acori Calami, Calamus, Sweetflag Rhizome)
Open Orifices
Bitter, Acrid, slightly Toxic*
Warm
Heart, **Liver**, Stomach, Spleen,[1904] Large Intestine[1905]
Name (Yang Ming, Large Intestine/Stomach), Bie Jing (Jue Yin/Yang Ming, Liver/Large Intestine), Biao/Li (Stomach/Spleen), Clock Neighbor (Spleen/Heart, Large Intestine/Stomach), Branch (Chou/Ox, Spleen/Liver, 1AM-2:59AM and Mao/Rabbit, Liver/Large Intestine, 5AM-6:59AM)

An Xi Xiang (Benzoinum, Benzoin)
Open Orifices
Acrid, Bitter, Aromatic
Neutral
Heart, **Liver**, Spleen
Clock Neighbor (Spleen/Heart), Branch (Chou/Ox, Spleen/Liver, 1AM-2:59AM)

Jiu Jie Chang Pu, Jing Chang Pu (Rhizoma Anemones Altaicae)
Open Orifices
Acrid
Warm, slightly Toxic*
Heart, **Liver**, Spleen
Clock Neighbor (Spleen/Heart), Branch (Chou/Ox, Spleen/Liver, 1AM-2:59AM)

She Xiang (Moschus, Musk, Navel Gland Secretions of Musk Deer)
Open Orifices
Acrid, Aromatic
Warm
Heart, **Liver**, Spleen, some sources say all channels.
Clock Neighbor (Spleen/Heart), Branch (Chou/Ox, Spleen/Liver, 1AM-2:59AM)

Niu Huang (Calculus Bovis, Cattle Bezoar, Cattle Gallstone)
Clear Heat Clean Toxin/Open Orifices
Bitter, Aromatic
Cool to Cold[1906]
Liver, Heart, Gall Bladder[1907]
Bie Jing (Shao Yin/Shao Yang, Heart/Gall Bladder), Biao/Li (Gall Bladder/Liver), Clock Opposite (Heart/Gall Bladder)

Tonify Qi

Sha Ji, Cu Liu Guo (Fructus Hippophae, Sea Buckthorn Fruit, Swallow Thorn Fruit)
Tonify Qi
Sour, slightly Sweet, Astringent
Warm
Lung, Spleen, Stomach, Large Intestine, **Liver**, Small Intestine[1908]
Name (Tai Yin, Lung/Spleen, Yang Ming, Large Intestine/Stomach), Bie Jing (Jue Yin/Yang Ming, Liver/Large Intestine, Tai Yin/Tai Yang, Spleen/Small Intestine), Biao/Li (Large Intestine/Lung, Stomach/Spleen), Clock Opposite (Liver/Small Intestine), Clock Neighbor (Liver/Lung, Large Intestine/Stomach), Branch (Chou/Ox, Spleen/Liver, 1AM-2:59AM, Mao/Rabbit, Liver/Large Intestine, 5AM-6:59AM, Si/Snake, Small Intestine/Spleen, 9AM-10:59AM, Wei/Sheep, Spleen/Small Intestine, 1PM-2:59PM)

Tonify Yang

Zi He Che (Placenta Hominis, Human Placenta)
Tonify Yang
Sweet, Salty
Warm
Kidney, Lung, **Liver**
Clock Neighbor (Liver/Lung), Branch (You/Chicken, Lung/Kidney, 5PM-6:59PM)

Yin Yang Huo, Xian Ling Pi (Herba Epimedii, Arial Parts of Epimedium, Horny Goat Weed)
Tonify Yang
Acrid, Sweet, Aromatic[1909]
Warm
Kidney, **Liver**, and possibly Large Intestine, Stomach and San Jiao[1910]
Possibly Name (Yang Ming, Large Intestine/Stomach), Bie Jing (Jue Yin/Yang Ming, Liver/Large Intestine, Shao Yin/Shao Yang, Kidney/San Jiao), Clock Opposite (Kidney/Large Intestine), Clock Neighbor (Large Intestine/Stomach), Branch (Mao/Rabbit, Liver/Large Intestine, 5AM-6:59AM)

Suo Yang, Di Mao Qiu (Herba Cynomorii, Fleshy Stem of Cynomorium)
Tonify Yang
Sweet
Warm
Liver, Kidney, Large Intestine
Bie Jing (Jue Yin/Yang Ming, Liver/Large Intestine), Clock Opposite (Kidney/Large Intestine), Branch (Mao/Rabbit, Liver/Large Intestine, 5AM-6:59AM)

Xian Mao (Rhizoma Curculiginis, Golden Eye Grass Rhizome)
Tonify Yang
Acrid
Warm[1911] to Hot, Toxic*
Kidney, **Liver**,[1912] Spleen[1913] and possibly San Jiao[1914]
Branch (Chou/Ox, Spleen/Liver, 1AM-2:59AM) + Kidney
and possibly Bie Jing (Shao Yin/Shao Yang, Kidney/San Jiao), Clock Opposite (Spleen/San Jiao)

Tu Si Zi (Semen Cuscutae, Chinese Dodder Seeds)
Tonify Yang
Acrid, Sweet, Astringent[1915]
Neutral to Warm[1916]
Liver, Kidney, Spleen[1917]
Branch (Chou/Ox, Spleen/Liver, 1AM-2:59AM) + Kidney

Lu Jiao Shuang (Cornu Cervi Degelatinatium)
Tonify Yang
Sweet, Salty, Astringent[1918]
Slightly Warm
Kidney, **Liver**, Heart, Pericardium
Name (Shao Yin, Kidney/Heart, Jue Yin, Liver/Pericardium), Clock Neighbor (Kidney/Pericardium)

Jiu Cai Zi, Jiu Zi, Jiu Cai Ren (Semen Alli Tuberosi, Chinese Leek Seed, Allium Seed)
Tonify Yang
Acrid, Sweet, Sour,[1919] Astringent[1920]
Warm
Liver, Kidney

Gu Sui Bu, Hou Jiang, Mao Jiang, Shen Jiang (Rhizoma Drynariae, Drynaria Rhizome)
Tonify Yang
Bitter
Warm
Liver, Kidney

Hu Lu Ba (Semen Trigonellae, Fenugreek seed)
Tonify Yang
Bitter, Aromatic
Warm to very Warm[1921]
Kidney, **Liver**[1922]

Gou Ji, Jin Gou Ji (Rhizoma Cibotii, Lamb of Tartary Rhizome, Scythian Lamb Rhizome, Chain Fern Rhizome)
Tonify Yang
Sweet, Bitter, Astringent[1923]
Neutral[1924] to Warm
Liver, Kidney

Du Zhong, Si Mian Pi, Yu Zi Pi, Mu Mian (Cortex Eucommiae, Eucommia Bark)
Tonify Yang
Sweet, slightly Acrid[1925]
Warm
Kidney, **Liver**

Sha Yuan Zi, Sha Yuan Ji Li (Semen Astragali Complanati, Milkvetch Seed, Astragalus Seed)
Tonify Yang
Sweet, Astringent[1926]
Warm
Kidney, **Liver**

Hai Ma (Hippocampus, Sea Horse)
Tonify Yang
Sweet, Salty
Warm
Kidney, **Liver**

Lu Jiao Jiao, Bai Jiao (Gelatinum Cornu Cervi, Deer Antler Glue)
Tonify Yang
Sweet, Salty
Warm
Liver, Kidney

Lu Jiao (Cornu Cervi, Deer Antler)
Tonify Yang
Salty
Warm
Kidney, **Liver**

Hai Gou Shen, Wa Na Qi (Testes et Penis Otariae, Seal Testicles and Penis)
Tonify Yang
Salty
Hot
Kidney, **Liver**

Ba Ji Tian, Ba Ji, Ji Yan Teng (Radix Morindae Officinalis, Morinda Root)
Tonify Yang
Acrid, Sweet, Bitter[1927]
Slightly Warm
Kidney, **Liver**,[1928] Chong[1929]

Lu Rong (Cornu Cervi Pantotrichum, Elk/Deer Horn Velvet)
Tonify Yang
Sweet, Salty
Warm
Kidney, **Liver**, Du[1930]

Xu Duan, Chuan Duan (Radix Dipsaci, Japanese Teasel Root)
Tonify Yang
Bitter, Sweet, Acrid, Astringent
Slightly Warm
Liver, Kidney, Dai[1931]

Tonify Blood

Gou Qi Zi, Di Gu Zi (Fructus Lycii, Chinese Wolfberry Fruit, Matrimony Vine Fruit, Boxthorn Fruit)
Tonify Blood/Tonify Yin
Sweet
Neutral
Liver, Kidney, Lung
Clock Neighbor (Liver/Lung), Branch (You/Chicken, Lung/Kidney, 5PM-6:59PM)

E Jiao, Lu Pi Jiao (Colla Corii Asini, Donkey-Hide Glue, Gelatin)
Tonify Blood
Sweet
Neutral
Lung, **Liver**, Kidney
Clock Neighbor (Liver/Lung), Branch (You/Chicken, Lung/Kidney, 5PM-6:59PM)

Sheng He Shou Wu (Radix Polygoni Multiflori Recens, Fresh Fleeceflower Root)
Tonify Blood
Bitter, Sweet, Astringent, not Astringent[1932]
Neutral to Cold[1933]
Liver, Heart, Large Intestine
Bie Jing (Jue Yin/Yang Ming, Liver/Large Intestine), Branch (Mao/Rabbit, Liver/Large Intestine, 5AM-6:59AM) + Heart

Dang Gui (Radix Angelica Sinensis, Chinese Angelica Root)
Tonify Blood
Sweet, Acrid, Bitter,[1934] Aromatic
Warm
Heart, **Liver**, Spleen, Dai[1935]
Clock Neighbor (Spleen/Heart), Branch (Chou/Ox, Spleen/Liver, 1AM-2:59AM) + Dai

Bai Shao (Radix Paeoniae Alba, White Peony Root)
Tonify Blood
Bitter, Sour, Sweet,[1936] slightly Astringent
Cool to slightly Cold[1937]
Liver, Spleen, Dai[1938]
Branch (Chou/Ox, Spleen/Liver, 1AM-2:59AM) + Dai

Sang Shen Zi, Sang Shen, Sang Guo (Fructus Mori, Mulberry Fruit, White Mulberry Fruit)
Tonify Blood/Tonify Yin
Sweet
Cold
Heart,[1939] **Liver**, Kidney
Name (Shao Yin, Heart/Kidney) + Liver

Shu Di Huang (Radix Rehmanniae Preparata, Cooked and Cured Rehmannia, Cooked and Cured Chinese Foxglove Root)
Tonify Blood
Sweet
Slightly Warm
Liver, Kidney, Heart[1940]
Name (Shao Yin, Heart/Kidney) + Liver

He Shou Wu, Zhi He Shou Wu (Radix Polygoni Multiflori Preparata, Prepared Polygonum, Prepared Fleeceflower Root)
Tonify Blood
Sweet, Bitter, Astringent
Neutral to slightly Warm
Kidney, **Liver**

Tonify Yin

Gou Qi Zi, Di Gu Zi (Fructus Lycii, Chinese Wolfberry Fruit, Matrimony Vine Fruit, Boxthorn Fruit)
Tonify Blood/Tonify Yin
Sweet
Neutral
Liver, Kidney, Lung
Clock Neighbor (Liver/Lung), Branch (You/Chicken, Lung/Kidney, 5PM-6:59PM)

Hei Zhi Ma, Hu Ma Zi, Hu Ma Ren, Zhi Ma (Semen Sesame Nigrum, Black Sesame Seed)
Tonify Yin
Sweet, Aromatic[1941]
Neutral
Liver, Kidney, Large Intestine[1942]
Bie Jing (Jue Yin/Yang Ming, Liver/Large Intestine), Clock Opposite (Kidney/Large Intestine), Branch (Mao/Rabbit, Liver/Large Intestine, 5AM-6:59AM)

Chu Shi Zi, Chu Shi, Chu Shi Mi (Fructus Broussonetiae, Paper Mulberry Fruit)
Tonify Yin
Sweet
Cold
Kidney, **Liver**, Spleen[1943]
Branch (Chou/Ox, Spleen/Liver, 1AM-2:59AM) + Kidney

Bie Jia (Carapax Trionycis, Chinese Soft Shell Turtle Shell)
Tonify Yin
Salty
Slightly Cold[1944] to Cold
Liver, Kidney,[1945] Spleen,[1946] Chong[1947]
Branch (Chou/Ox, Spleen/Liver, 1AM-2:59AM) + Kidney, Chong

Sang Shen Zi, Sang Shen, Sang Guo (Fructus Mori, Mulberry Fruit, White Mulberry Fruit)
Tonify Blood/Tonify Yin
Sweet
Cold
Heart,[1948] **Liver**, Kidney
Name (Shao Yin, Heart/Kidney) + Liver

Gui Ban (Plastrum Testudinis, Tortoise Plastron)
Tonify Yin
Salty, Sweet
Cold
Liver, Kidney, Heart, Ren[1949]
Name (Shao Yin, Kidney/Heart) + Liver, Ren

Han Lian Cao, Mo Han Lian (Herba Ecliptae)
Tonify Yin
Sweet, Sour, Aromatic[1950]
Cool[1951] to Cold
Liver, Kidney

Nu Zhen Zi (Fructus Ligustri Lucidi, Japanese Privet Fruit, Wax Tree Fruit)
Tonify Yin
Sweet, Bitter
Cool
Liver, Kidney

Astringe, Stabilize and Bind

Chun Gen Pi, Chun Pi (Cortex Ailanthi, Ailanthus Bark, Tree of Heaven Bark, Chinese Sumac Bark)
Astringe, Stabilize and Bind
Bitter, Astringent
Cold
Large Intestine, Stomach,[1952] **Liver**, Lung[1953]
Name (Yang Ming, Large Intestine/Stomach), Bie Jing (Jue Yin/Yang Ming, Liver/Large Intestine), Biao/Li (Large Intestine/Lung), Clock Neighbor (Large Intestine/Stomach, Liver/Lung), Branch (Mao/Rabbit, Liver/Large Intestine, 5AM-6:59AM)

Wu Mei (Fructus Mume, Mume Fruit, Smoked Plum)
Astringe, Stabilize and Bind
Sour, Astringent
Neutral to Warm[1954]
Liver, Spleen, Lung, Large Intestine
Name (Tai Yin, Spleen/Lung), Bie Jing (Jue Yin/Yang Ming, Liver/Large Intestine), Biao/Li (Large Intestine/Lung), Clock Neighbor (Liver/Lung), Branch (Chou/Ox, Spleen/Liver, 1AM-2:59AM, Mao/Rabbit, Liver/Large Intestine, 5AM-6:59AM)

Ou Jie (Nodus Nelumbinis Rhizomatis, Lotus Rhizome Nodes)
Stop Bleeding/Astringe, Stabilize and Bind
Sweet, Astringent
Neutral
Lung, Stomach, **Liver**
Clock Neighbor (Liver/Lung) + Stomach

Nuo Dao Gen, Nuo Dao Gen Xu (Radix Oryzae Glutinosae, Glutinous Rice Root)
Astringe, Stabilize and Bind
Sweet, Acrid[1955]
Neutral
Lung, **Liver**, Kidney[1956]
Clock Neighbor (Liver/Lung), Branch (You/Chicken, Lung/Kidney, 5PM-6:59PM)

Ji Guan Hua (Flos Celosiae Cristatae, Cock's Comb Flower)
Clear Heat Cool Blood/Astringe, Stabilize and Bind
Sweet, Astringent[1957]
Cool
Large Intestine, **Liver**, Kidney[1958]
Bie Jing (Jue Yin/Yang Ming, Liver/Large Intestine), Clock Opposite (Kidney/Large Intestine), Branch (Mao/Rabbit, Liver/Large Intestine, 5AM-6:59AM)

Hai Piao Xiao, Wu Zei Gu (Endoconcha Sepiae, Cuttlefish Bone)
Astringe, Stabilize and Bind
Salty, Astringent
Slightly Warm
Liver, Kidney, Stomach[1959]

He Ye (Folium Nelumbinis, Lotus Leaf)
Clear Heat Clean Toxin/Astringe, Stabilize and Bind
Bitter, slightly Sweet,[1960] Astringent, Aromatic
Neutral
Heart, **Liver**, Spleen
Clock Neighbor (Spleen/Heart), Branch (Chou/Ox, Spleen/Liver, 1AM-2:59AM)

Lian Xu (Stamen Nelumbinis, Lotus Stamen)
Astringe, Stabilize and Bind
Sweet, Astringent
Neutral
Heart, Kidney, **Liver**[1961]
Name (Shao Yin, Heart/Kidney) + Liver

Shan Zhu Yu, Shan Yu Rou (Fructus Corni, Asiatic Cornelian Cherry Fruit)
Astringe, Stabilize and Bind
Sour, Acrid,[1962] Astringent
Slightly Warm
Kidney, **Liver**

Fu Pen Zi (Fructus Rubi, Chinese Raspberry)
Astringe, Stabilize and Bind
Sweet, Sour, Astringent
Neutral[1963] to slightly Warm
Kidney, **Liver**, Dai[1964]

Sang Piao Xiao, Sang Xiao (Ootheca Mantidis, Praying Mantis Egg Case)
Astringe, Stabilize and Bind
Sweet, Salty, Astringent[1965]
Neutral
Liver, Kidney, Dai[1966]

Emetic

Li Lu (Radix et Rhizoma Veratri, Lack False Hellebore, Vanity Grass)
Relieve Cough and Wheezing/Panting/Emetic
Acrid, Bitter
Cold, extremely Toxic*
Lung, **Liver**, Stomach
Clock Neighbor (Liver/Lung) + Stomach

Chang Shan (Radix Dichroae, Dichroa Root)
Expel Parasites/Emetic
Acrid, Bitter
Cold, Toxic*
Lung, Heart, **Liver**
Clock Neighbor (Liver/Lung) + Heart

Shu Qi (Folium Dichroae, Dichroa Leaves)
Emetic
Acrid, Bitter
Cold to Warm,[1967] Toxic*
Lung, Heart, **Liver**
Clock Neighbor (Liver/Lung) + Heart

External Application

Ming Fan, Bai Fan, Ku Fan (Alumen, Alum)
External Application
Sour, Bitter,[1968] Astringent
Cold, Toxic*
Lung, **Liver**, Spleen, Stomach,[1969] Large Intestine[1970]
Name (Tai Yin, Spleen/Lung, Yang Ming, Large Intestine/Stomach), Bie Jing (Jue Yin/Yang Ming, Liver/Large Intestine), Clock Neighbor (Liver/Lung, Large Intestine/Stomach), Biao/Li (Stomach/Spleen, Large Intestine/Lung), Branch (Chou/Ox, Spleen/Liver, 1AM-2:59AM, Mao/Rabbit, Liver/Large Intestine, 5AM-6:59AM)

Xiong Huang (Realgar)
External Application
Acrid, Bitter
Neutral to Warm, Toxic*
Heart, **Liver**, Kidney,[1971] Stomach,[1972] Lung,[1973] Large Intestine[1974]
Name (Shao Yin, Heart/Kidney, Yang Ming, Large Intestine/Stomach), Bie Jing (Jue Yin/Yang Ming, Liver/Large Intestine), Biao/Li (Large Intestine/Lung), Clock Opposite (Kidney/Large Intestine), Clock Neighbor (Large Intestine/Stomach, Liver/Lung), Branch (Mao/Rabbit, Liver/Large Intestine, 5AM-6:59AM, You/Chicken, Lung, Kidney, 5PM-6:59PM)

Wa Leng Zi (Concha Arcae, Cockle Shell, Ark Shell)
Vitalize Blood Transform Stasis/Transform Phlegm/External Application
Salty
Neutral
Liver, Stomach, Lung, Spleen[1975]
Name (Tai Yin, Lung/Spleen), Biao/Li (Stomach/Spleen), Clock Neighbor (Liver/Lung), Branch (Chou/Ox, Spleen/Liver, 1AM-2:59AM)

Si Gua Luo (Retinervus Luffae Fructus, Dried Vegetable Sponge)
Transform Phlegm/External Application
Sweet
Neutral to Cold[1976]
Lung, Stomach, **Liver**
Clock Neighbor (Liver/Lung) + Stomach

Lu Feng Fang, Feng Fang (Nidus Vespae, Wasp Nest)
External Application
Sweet
Neutral, Toxic*
Stomach, Lung,[1977] **Liver**[1978]
Clock Neighbor (Liver/Lung) + Stomach

Mu Bie Zi (Semen Momordicae, Momordica Seed)
External Application
Bitter, slightly Sweet
Warm, Toxic*
Large Intestine, **Liver**, Stomach
Name (Yang Ming, Large Intestine/Stomach), Bie Jing (Jue Yin/Yang Ming, Liver/Large Intestine), Clock Neighbor (Large Intestine/Stomach), Branch (Mao/Rabbit, Liver/Large Intestine, 5AM-6:59AM)

Qing Fen (Calomelas, Calomel)
External Application
Acrid, Bland[1979]
Cold, very Toxic*
Liver, Kidney, Large Intestine,[1980] Small Intestine[1981]
Bie Jing (Jue Yin/Yang Ming, Liver/Large Intestine), Clock Opposite (Liver/Small Intestine, Kidney/Large Intestine), Branch (Mao/Rabbit, Liver/Large Intestine, 5AM-6:59AM)

Lu Gan Shi (Galamina, Calomine, Hydrozincite, Smithsonite)
External Application
Sweet
Neutral, Non-toxic[1982] to Toxic*
Liver, Stomach

Qian Dan, Huang Dan (Minium, Lead Oxide)
External Application
Bitter, Acrid[1983]
Cool to slightly Cold,[1984] Toxic*
Heart, **Liver**, Spleen[1985]
Clock Neighbor (Spleen, Heart), Branch (Chou/Ox, Spleen/Liver, 1AM-2:59AM)

Da Feng Zi (Semen Hydnocarpi, Hydnocarpus Seed, Chaulmoogra Seed)
External Application
Acrid, Bitter[1986]
Hot, extremely Toxic*
Liver, Spleen, Kidney
Branch (Chou/Ox, Spleen/Liver,1AM-2:59AM) + Kidney

Ma Qian Zi (Semen Strychni, Nux Vomica)
External Application
Bitter, Acrid[1987]
Cold, extremely Toxic*
Liver, Spleen
Branch (Chou/Ox, Spleen/Liver, 1AM-2:59AMs)

Mi Tuo Seng (Lithargyum)
External Application
Salty, Acrid
Neutral, Toxic*
Liver, Spleen
Branch (Chou/Ox, Spleen/Liver, 1AM-2:59AM)

Xue Jie (Daemonoropis Resina, Sanguis Draconis, Dragon's Blood)
Vitalize Blood Transform Stasis/External Application
Sweet, Acrid,[1988] Salty,[1989] Aromatic
Neutral
Heart, **Liver**

Wu Ming Yi (Pyrolusitum, Pyrolusite)
External Application
Sweet
Neutral
Liver, Kidney

Chong Mai-Vessel Herbs

Clear Deficient Heat

Bai Wei (Radix Cynanchi Atrati, Black Swallow-Wort Root)
Clear Deficient Heat
Bitter, Salty
Cold
Stomach, Liver, Kidney,[1990] Lung,[1991] Ren and **Chong**[1992]
Clock Neighbor (Liver/Lung), Branch (You/Chicken, Lung/Kidney, 5PM-6:59PM) + Stomach, Ren, Chong

Vitalize Blood Transform Stasis

Chuan Xiong, Xiong Qiong, Fu Xiong (Rhizoma Ligustici Chuanxiong, Szechuan Lovage Root)
Vitalize Blood Transform Stasis
Acrid, Bitter,[1993] Aromatic
Warm
Liver, Gall Bladder, Pericardium, San Jiao,[1994] **Chong**[1995]
Name (Jue Yin, Liver/Pericardium, Shao Yang, San Jiao/Gall Bladder), Biao/Li (Gall Bladder/Liver, San Jiao/Pericardium), Clock Neighbor (San Jiao/Gall Bladder) + Chong

Calm Shen Sedative

Zi Shi Ying (Floritum, Flourite)
Calm Shen Sedative/Calm Liver Extinguish Wind
Sweet, Acrid
Warm
Heart, Liver, **Chong** and Ren[1996]

Calm Liver Extinguish Wind

Zi Shi Ying (Floritum, Flourite)
Calm Shen Sedative/Calm Liver Extinguish Wind
Sweet, Acrid
Warm
Heart, Liver, **Chong** and Ren[1997]

Tonify Yang

Ba Ji Tian, Ba Ji, Ji Yan Teng (Radix Morindae Officinalis, Morinda Root)
Tonify Yang
Acrid, Sweet, Bitter[1998]
Slightly Warm
Kidney, Liver,[1999] **Chong**[2000]

Tonify Yin

Bie Jia (Carapax Trionycis, Chinese Soft Shell Turtle Shell)
Tonify Yin
Salty
Slightly Cold[2001] to Cold
Liver, Kidney,[2002] Spleen,[2003] **Chong**[2004]
Branch (Chou/Ox, Spleen/Liver, 1AM-2:59AM) + Kidney, Chong

Du Mai-Vessel Herbs

Acrid Warm Exterior Releasing

Xi Xin (Radix et Rhizoma Asari, Asarum, Chinese Wild Ginger)
Acrid Warm Exterior Releasing/Warm Interior
Acrid to extremely Acrid,[2005] Aromatic
Warm, slightly Toxic*
Lung, Heart, Kidney, **Du**,[2006] all channels[2007]
Name (Shao Yin, Heart/Kidney), Branch (You/Chicken, Lung/Kidney, 5PM-6:59PM) + Du

Jing Jie (Herba Schizonepitae, Schizonepeta)
Acrid Warm Exterior Releasing
Acrid, Aromatic
Slightly Warm
Lung, Liver, Gall Bladder,[2008] San Jiao,[2009] **Du**[2010]
Name (Shao Yang, Gall Bladder/San Jiao), Biao/Li (Gall Bladder/Liver), Clock Neighbor (San Jiao/Gall Bladder, Liver/Lung), Branch (Yin/Tiger, Gall Bladder/Lung, 3AM-4:59AM) + Du

Cang Er Zi (Fructus Xanthii, Cocklebur Fruit, Xanthium Fruit)
Acrid Warm Exterior Releasing
Sweet,[2011] Bitter, Acrid
Warm, slightly Toxic*
Lung, Liver,[2012] **Du**[2013]
Clock Neighbor (Liver/Lung) + Du

Fang Feng, Pang Feng (Radix Saposhnikoviae, and sometimes Ledebouriella Root as a substitute)
Acrid Warm Exterior Releasing
Acrid, Sweet, Aromatic
Slightly Warm
Urinary Bladder, Liver, Spleen, **Du**,[2014] Yang Qiao[2015]
Branch (Chou/Ox, Spleen/Liver,1AM-2:59AM) + Urinary Bladder, Du, Yang Qiao

Qiang Huo, Can Qiang, Zhu Jie Qiang (Rhizoma et Radix Notopterygii)
Acrid Warm Exterior Releasing
Acrid, Bitter, Aromatic
Warm to very Warm[2016]
Urinary Bladder, Tai Yang,[2017] Kidney, Liver,[2018] **Du**[2019]
Biao/Li (Urinary Bladder/Kidney), and possibly Name (Small Intestine/Urinary Bladder), Clock Opposite (Liver/Small Intestine) and Clock Neighbor (Small Intestine/Urinary Bladder) if Tai Yang[2020] really means Tai Yang. If Tai Yang only means the Foot Tai Yang Urinary Bladder Jing-channel, then + Liver, Du

Gao Ben (Rhizoma Ligustici, Chinese Lovage Root)
Acrid Warm Exterior Releasing
Acrid, Aromatic
Warm
Urinary Bladder, **Du**[2021]

Clear Heat Dry Dampness

Huang Lian (Rhizoma Coptidis, Goldthread Rhizome, Coptis Root)
Clear Heat Dry Dampness
Very Bitter, purely Bitter[2022]
Very Cold
Heart, Liver, Stomach, Large Intestine, **Du**[2023]
Name (Yang Ming, Large Intestine/Stomach), Bie Jing (Jue Yin/Yang Ming, Liver/Large Intestine), Clock Neighbor (Large Intestine/Stomach), Branch (Mao/Rabbit, Liver/Large Intestine, 5AM-6:59AM) + Heart, Du

Purgative

Da Huang (Radix et Rhizoma Rhei, Rhubarb Root and Rhizome)
Purgative
Bitter to very Bitter[2024] to purely Bitter,[2025] Aromatic[2026]
Cold to very Cold[2027]
Spleen, Stomach, Large Intestine, Liver, Heart, **Du**[2028]
Name (Yang Ming, Large Intestine/Stomach), Bie Jing (Jue Yin/Yang Ming, Liver/Large Intestine), Biao/Li (Stomach/Spleen), Clock Neighbor (Spleen/Heart, Large Intestine/Stomach), Branch (Chou/Ox, Spleen/Liver, 1AM-2:59AM and Mao/Rabbit, Liver/Large Intestine, 5AM-6:59AM) + Du

Dispel Wind Dampness, Open Channels and Luo-Network Vessels and Relieve Pain

Du Huo, Da Huo, Rou Du Huo (Radix Angelicae Pubescentis, Angelica Root)
Dispel Wind Dampness, Open Channels and Luo-Network Vessels and Relieve Pain
Acrid, Bitter, Aromatic
Slightly Warm to very Warm[2029]
Liver, Kidney,[2030] Urinary Bladder, **Du**[2031]
Biao/Li (Urinary Bladder/Kidney) + Liver, Du

Warm Interior

Xi Xin (Radix et Rhizoma Asari, Asarum, Chinese Wild Ginger)
Acrid Warm Exterior Releasing/Warm Interior
Acrid to extremely Acrid,[2032] Aromatic
Warm, slightly Toxic*
Lung, Heart, Kidney, **Du**,[2033] all channels[2034]
Name (Shao Yin, Heart/Kidney), Branch (You/Chicken, Lung/Kidney, 5PM-6:59PM) + Du

Zhi Fu Zi, Tian Xiong (Radix Aconiti Lateralis Praeparata, Aconite, Prepared/Processed Aconite Accessory Root)
Warm Interior
Acrid to extremely Acrid,[2035] Sweet[2036]
Hot to very Hot,[2037] Toxic*
Heart, Kidney, Spleen, **Du**[2038]
Name (Shao Yin, Heart/Kidney), Clock Neighbor (Spleen/Heart) + Du

Zhi Chuan Wu (Radix Aconiti Preparata, Prepared Aconite Main Root, Mother Root of Common Monk's Hood)
Warm Interior
Acrid, Bitter
Hot, extremely Toxic**
Heart, Liver, Spleen, **Du**[2039]
Clock Neighbor (Spleen/Heart), Branch (Chou/Ox, Spleen/Liver, 1AM-2:59AM) + Du

Tonify Yang

Lu Rong (Cornu Cervi Pantotrichum, Elk/Deer Horn Velvet)
Tonify Yang
Sweet, Salty
Warm
Kidney, Liver, **Du**[2040]

Ren Mai-Vessel Herbs

Clear Deficient Heat

Bai Wei (Radix Cynanchi Atrati, Black Swallow-Wort Root)
Clear Deficient Heat
Bitter, Salty
Cold
Stomach, Liver, Kidney,[2041] Lung,[2042] **Ren** and Chong[2043]
Clock Neighbor (Liver/Lung), Branch (You/Chicken, Lung/Kidney, 5PM-6:59PM) + Stomach, Ren, Chong

Calm Shen Sedative

Zi Shi Ying (Floritum, Flourite)
Calm Shen Sedative/Calm Liver Extinguish Wind
Sweet, Acrid
Warm
Heart, Liver, Chong and **Ren**[2044]

Calm Liver Extinguish Wind

Zi Shi Ying (Floritum, Flourite)
Calm Shen Sedative/Calm Liver Extinguish Wind
Sweet, Acrid
Warm
Heart, Liver, Chong and **Ren**[2045]

Tonify Yin

Gui Ban (Plastrum Testudinis, Tortoise Plastron)
Tonify Yin
Salty, Sweet
Cold
Liver, Kidney, Heart, **Ren**[2046]
Name (Shao Yin, Kidney/Heart) + Liver, Ren

Dai Mai-Vessel Herbs

Stop Bleeding

Ai Ye (Folium Artemisiae Argyi, Mugwort Leaf, Moxa)
Stop Bleeding
Bitter, Acrid, Aromatic
Warm
Spleen, Liver, Kidney, **Dai**[2047]
Branch (Chou/Ox, Spleen/Liver, 1AM-2:59AM) + Kidney, Dai

Calm Shen Sedative

Long Gu (Os Draconis, Fossilia Mastodi Ossis, Fossilized Bones)
Calm Shen Sedative
Sweet, slightly Acrid,[2048] Astringent[2049]
Neutral[2050] to Cool to slightly Cold[2051]
Heart, Liver, Kidney,[2052] **Dai**[2053]
Name (Shao Yin, Heart/Kidney) + Liver , Dai

Tonify Qi

Gan Cao (Radix Glycyrrhizae, Licorice Root)
Tonify Qi
Sweet
Neutral
Spleen, Stomach, Lung, Heart, **Dai**,[2054] some sources indicate that it enters all channels.
Name (Tai Yin, Spleen/Lung), Biao/Li (Stomach/Spleen), Clock Neighbor (Spleen/Heart) + Dai, some sources indicate that Gan Cao enters all channels and therefore creates every relationship.

Shan Yao, Huai Shan Yao, Huai Shan, Shan Shu (Rhizoma Dioscoriae, Chinese Yam)
Tonify Qi
Sweet, Sour,[2055] slightly Astringent
Neutral
Kidney, Lung, Spleen, **Dai**[2056]
Name (Tai Yin, Lung/Spleen), Branch (You/Chicken, Lung/Kidney, 5PM-6:59PM) + Dai

Tonify Yang

Xu Duan, Chuan Duan (Radix Dipsaci, Japanese Teasel Root)
Tonify Yang
Bitter, Sweet, Acrid, Astringent
Slightly Warm
Liver, Kidney, **Dai**[2057]

Tonify Blood

Dang Gui (Radix Angelica Sinensis, Chinese Angelica Root)
Tonify Blood
Sweet, Acrid, Bitter,[2058] Aromatic
Warm
Heart, Liver, Spleen, **Dai**[2059]
Clock Neighbor (Spleen/Heart), Branch (Chou/Ox, Spleen/Liver, 1AM-2:59AM) + Dai

Bai Shao (Radix Paeoniae Alba, White Peony Root)
Tonify Blood
Bitter, Sour, Sweet,[2060] slightly Astringent
Cool to slightly Cold[2061]
Liver, Spleen, **Dai**[2062]
Branch (Chou/Ox, Spleen/Liver, 1AM-2:59AM) + Dai

Astringe, Stabilize and Bind

Wu Wei Zi (Fructus Schisandrae Chinensis, Schizandra Fruit)
Astringe, Stabilize and Bind
Sour, Sweet,[2063] Acrid,[2064] Bitter,[2065] Salty,[2066] Astringent
Warm
Kidney, Lung, Heart, **Dai**[2067]
Name (Shao Yin, Kidney/Heart), Branch (You/Chicken, Lung/Kidney, 5PM-6:59PM) + Dai

Qian Shi (Semen Euryales, Euryale Seed)
Astringe, Stabilize and Bind
Sweet, Astringent
Neutral
Kidney, Spleen, **Dai**[2068]

Fu Pen Zi (Fructus Rubi, Chinese Raspberry)
Astringe, Stabilize and Bind
Sweet, Sour, Astringent
Neutral[2069] to slightly Warm
Kidney, Liver, **Dai**[2070]

Sang Piao Xiao, Sang Xiao (Ootheca Mantidis, Praying Mantis Egg Case)
Astringe, Stabilize and Bind
Sweet, Salty, Astringent[2071]
Neutral
Liver, Kidney, **Dai**[2072]

Yang Qiao Mai-Vessel Herbs

Acrid Warm Exterior Releasing

Ma Huang, Ma Huang Cao (Herba Ephedrae, Ephedra Stem, Mormon Tea)
Acrid Warm Exterior Releasing
Acrid, slightly Bitter[2073] to Bitter, no big taste[2074]
Warm
Lung, Urinary Bladder, **Yang Qiao**[2075]
Bie Jing (Tai Yin/Tai Yang, Lung/Urinary Bladder), Clock Opposite (Lung/Urinary Bladder) + Yang Qiao

Fang Feng, Pang Feng (Radix Saposhnikoviae, and sometimes Ledebouriella Root as a substitute)
Acrid Warm Exterior Releasing
Acrid, Sweet, Aromatic[2076]
Slightly Warm
Urinary Bladder, Liver, Spleen, Du,[2077] **Yang Qiao**[2078]
Branch (Chou/Ox, Spleen/Liver,1AM-2:59AM) + Urinary Bladder, Du, Yang Qiao

Dispel Wind Dampness, Open Channels and Luo-Network Vessels and Relieve Pain

Han Fang Ji/Fen Fang Ji (Radix Stephaniae Tetandrae, Stephania Root)
Dispel Wind Dampness, Open Channels and Luo-Network Vessels and Relieve Pain
Acrid, Bitter to very Bitter[2079]
Cold to very Cold[2080]
Urinary Bladder, Lung,[2081] Spleen,[2082] Kidney, **Yang Qiao**,[2083] and possibly San Jiao[2084]
Name (Tai Yin, Spleen/Lung), Bie Jing (Tai Yin/Tai Yang, Lung/Urinary Bladder), Biao/Li (Urinary Bladder/Kidney), Clock Opposite (Lung/Urinary Bladder), Branch (You/Chicken, Lung/Kidney, 5PM-6:59PM) and possibly Bie Jing (Shao Yin/Shao Yang, Kidney/San Jiao), Clock Opposite (San Jiao/Spleen), Branch (Hai/Pig, Urinary Bladder/San Jiao, 9PM-10:59PM) + Yang Qiao

Guang Fang Ji (Radix Aristolochiae Fangchi)
Dispel Wind Dampness, Open Channels and Luo-Network Vessels and Relieve Pain
Acrid, Bitter
Cold, Toxic*
Urinary Bladder, Lung, **Yang Qiao**[2085]
Bie Jing (Tai Yin/Tai Yang, Lung/Urinary Bladder), Clock Opposite (Lung/Urinary Bladder) + Yang Qiao

Aromatic Dissolve Dampness

Cang Zhu (Rhizoma Atractylodis, Atractylodis)
Aromatic Dissolve Dampness
Acrid, Bitter, Sweet,[2086] Aromatic
Warm
Spleen, Stomach, **Yang Qiao**[2087]
Biao/Li (Stomach/Spleen) + Yang Qiao

INDEX

A

B

D

E

F

G

H

I

J

K

L

M

N

O

P

Q

R

S

X

Y

Z

FOOTNOTES

---

[1] Wang Feng Yi, *Discussion on Transforming Character*, Personal Unpublished Translation, 2018

[2] Chen, JK & TT, Chinese Medical Herbology and Pharmacology, City of Industry, Art of Medicine Press, 2001/2004, P 59

[3] Tang Rong Chuan (Tang Zonghai), Ben Cao Wen Da, Personal Unpublished Translation, 2015, 1.4.6

[4] Brand, E & Wiseman, N, Concise Chinese Materia Medica, Taos, Paradigm Publications, 2008, P 44

[5] Chen Shi Duo, via Bensky, D, Clavey, S, Stöger, E & Gamble, A, Chinese Herbal Medicine Materia Medica, 3rd Edition, Seattle, Eastland Press, 1986, 1993, 2004, P 37

[6] Chen, JK & TT, Chinese Medical Herbology and Pharmacology, City of Industry, Art of Medicine Press, 2001/2004, P 455

[77] Tang Rong Chuan (Tang Zonghai), Ben Cao Wen Da, Personal Unpublished Translation, 2015, 2.2.2

[8] Bensky, D, Clavey, S, Stöger, E & Gamble, A, Chinese Herbal Medicine Materia Medica, 3rd Edition, Seattle, Eastland Press, 1986, 1993, 2004, P 83

[9] Bensky, D, Clavey, S, Stöger, E & Gamble, A, Chinese Herbal Medicine Materia Medica, 3rd Edition, Seattle, Eastland Press, 1986, 1993, 2004, P 4

[10] Tang Rong Chuan (Tang Zonghai), Ben Cao Wen Da, Personal Unpublished Translation, 2015, 1.4.6

[11] Maciocia, G, The Channels of Acupuncture, Philadelphia, Elsevier, 2006, P 585

[12] Tang Rong Chuan (Tang Zonghai), Ben Cao Wen Da, Personal Unpublished Translation, 2015, 2.2.2

[13] Tang Rong Chuan (Tang Zonghai), Ben Cao Wen Da, Personal Unpublished Translation, 2015, 2.2.2

[14] Maciocia, G, The Channels of Acupuncture, Philadelphia, Elsevier, 2006, P 446

[15] Chen, JK & TT, Chinese Medical Herbology and Pharmacology, City of Industry, Art of Medicine Press, 2001/2004, P 57

[16] Bensky, D, Clavey, S, Stöger, E & Gamble, A, Chinese Herbal Medicine Materia Medica, 3rd Edition, Seattle, Eastland Press, 1986, 1993, 2004, P 44

[17] Bensky, D, Clavey, S, Stöger, E & Gamble, A, Chinese Herbal Medicine Materia Medica, 3rd Edition, Seattle, Eastland Press, 1986, 1993, 2004, P 39

[18] Chen, JK & TT, Chinese Medical Herbology and Pharmacology, City of Industry, Art of Medicine Press, 2001/2004, P 62, Tang Rong Chuan (Tang Zonghai), Ben Cao Wen Da, Personal Unpublished Translation, 2015, 2.1.6

[19] Maciocia, G, The Channels of Acupuncture, Philadelphia, Elsevier, 2006, P 446

[20] Bensky, D, Clavey, S, Stöger, E & Gamble, A, Chinese Herbal Medicine Materia Medica, 3rd Edition, Seattle, Eastland Press, 1986, 1993, 2004, P 78

[21] Brand, E & Wiseman, N, Concise Chinese Materia Medica, Taos, Paradigm Publications, 2008, P 56

[22] Li Shi Zhen, *Grand Materia Medica*, via Bensky, D, Clavey, S, Stöger, E & Gamble, A, Chinese Herbal Medicine Materia Medica, 3rd Edition, Seattle, Eastland Press, 1986, 1993, 2004, P 56

[23] Li Shi Zhen, *Grand Materia Medica*, via Bensky, D, Clavey, S, Stöger, E & Gamble, A, Chinese Herbal Medicine Materia Medica, 3rd Edition, Seattle, Eastland Press, 1986, 1993, 2004, P 56

[24] Zhou Yan, *Thoughtful Differention of Materia Medica*, via Bensky, D, Clavey, S, Stöger, E & Gamble, A, Chinese Herbal Medicine Materia Medica, 3rd Edition, Seattle, Eastland Press, 1986, 1993, 2004, P 62

[25] Brand, E & Wiseman, N, Concise Chinese Materia Medica, Taos, Paradigm Publications, 2008, P 58

[26] Chen, JK & TT, Chinese Medical Herbology and Pharmacology, City of Industry, Art of Medicine Press, 2001/2004, P 77

[27] Tang Rong Chuan (Tang Zonghai), Ben Cao Wen Da, Personal Unpublished Translation, 2015, 2.1.6

[28] Tang Rong Chuan (Tang Zonghai), Ben Cao Wen Da, Personal Unpublished Translation, 2015, 2.1.6

[29] Chen, JK & TT, Chinese Medical Herbology and Pharmacology, City of Industry, Art of Medicine Press, 2001/2004, P 79, and Bensky, D, Clavey, S, Stöger, E & Gamble, A, Chinese Herbal Medicine Materia Medica, 3rd Edition, Seattle, Eastland Press, 1986, 1993, 2004, P 69

[30] Brand, E & Wiseman, N, Concise Chinese Materia Medica, Taos, Paradigm Publications, 2008, P 56, Chen, JK & TT, Chinese Medical Herbology and Pharmacology, City of Industry, Art of Medicine Press, 2001/2004, P 75

[31] Bensky, D, Clavey, S, Stöger, E & Gamble, A, Chinese Herbal Medicine Materia Medica, 3rd Edition, Seattle, Eastland Press, 1986, 1993, 2004, P 58

[32] Bensky, D, Clavey, S, Stöger, E & Gamble, A, Chinese Herbal Medicine Materia Medica, 3rd Edition, Seattle, Eastland Press, 1986, 1993, 2004, P 58

[33] Bensky, D, Clavey, S, Stöger, E & Gamble, A, Chinese Herbal Medicine Materia Medica, 3rd Edition, Seattle, Eastland Press, 1986, 1993, 2004, P 166

[34] Zhang Xi Chun, *Essays on Medicine Esteeming the Chinese and Respecting the Western*, via Bensky, D, Clavey, S, Stöger, E & Gamble, A, Chinese Herbal Medicine Materia Medica, 3rd Edition, Seattle, Eastland Press, 1986, 1993, 2004, P 53

[35] Bensky, D, Clavey, S, Stöger, E & Gamble, A, Chinese Herbal Medicine Materia Medica, 3rd Edition, Seattle, Eastland Press, 1986, 1993, 2004, P 52

[36] Miao Xi Yong, *Commentary on the Divine Husbandman's Classic of Materia Medica*, via Bensky, D, Clavey, S, Stöger, E & Gamble, A, Chinese Herbal Medicine Materia Medica, 3rd Edition, Seattle, Eastland Press, 1986, 1993, 2004, P 211

[37] Tang Rong Chuan (Tang Zonghai), Ben Cao Wen Da, Personal Unpublished Translation, 2015, 1.5.14

[38] Wang Ang, via Bensky, D, Clavey, S, Stöger, E & Gamble, A, Chinese Herbal Medicine Materia Medica, 3rd Edition, Seattle, Eastland Press, 1986, 1993, 2004, P 107

[39] Bensky, D, Clavey, S, Stöger, E & Gamble, A, Chinese Herbal Medicine Materia Medica, 3rd Edition, Seattle, Eastland Press, 1986, 1993, 2004, P 101

[40] Zhou Yan, *Records of Thoughtful Differentiation of Materia Medica*, via Bensky, D, Clavey, S, Stöger, E & Gamble, A, Chinese Herbal Medicine Materia Medica, 3rd Edition, Seattle, Eastland Press, 1986, 1993, 2004, P 96

[41] Tang Rong Chuan (Tang Zonghai), Ben Cao Wen Da, Personal Unpublished Translation, 2015, 1.3.4 Although this text indicates that Huang Qin enters the San Jiao, the author is also quite specific in distinguishing between the organs and their Jing-channels. Here he does not indicate the Jing-channel, so I do not indicate otherwise.

[42] *Encountering the Sources of the Classic of Materia Medica*, via Bensky, D, Clavey, S, Stöger, E & Gamble, A, Chinese Herbal Medicine Materia Medica, 3rd Edition, Seattle, Eastland Press, 1986, 1993, 2004, P 212

[43] Bensky, D, Clavey, S, Stöger, E & Gamble, A, Chinese Herbal Medicine Materia Medica, 3rd Edition, Seattle, Eastland Press, 1986, 1993, 2004, P 177

[44] Wang, Hao Gu, *Harm and Benefit in the Materia Medica*, via Bensky, D, Clavey, S, Stöger, E & Gamble, A, Chinese Herbal Medicine Materia Medica, 3rd Edition, Seattle, Eastland Press, 1986, 1993, 2004, P 152

[45] Bensky, D, Clavey, S, Stöger, E & Gamble, A, Chinese Herbal Medicine Materia Medica, 3rd Edition, Seattle, Eastland Press, 1986, 1993, 2004, P 151

[46] Wang, Hao Gu, *Harm and Benefit in the Materia Medica*, via Bensky, D, Clavey, S, Stöger, E & Gamble, A, Chinese Herbal Medicine Materia Medica, 3rd Edition, Seattle, Eastland Press, 1986, 1993, 2004, P 152

[47] Bensky, D, Clavey, S, Stöger, E & Gamble, A, Chinese Herbal Medicine Materia Medica, 3rd Edition, Seattle, Eastland Press, 1986, 1993, 2004, P 207

[48] Brand, E & Wiseman, N, Concise Chinese Materia Medica, Taos, Paradigm Publications, 2008, P 112

[49] Bensky, D, Clavey, S, Stöger, E & Gamble, A, Chinese Herbal Medicine Materia Medica, 3rd Edition, Seattle, Eastland Press, 1986, 1993, 2004, P 207

[50] Bensky, D, Clavey, S, Stöger, E & Gamble, A, Chinese Herbal Medicine Materia Medica, 3rd Edition, Seattle, Eastland Press, 1986, 1993, 2004, P 206

[51] Brand, E & Wiseman, N, Concise Chinese Materia Medica, Taos, Paradigm Publications, 2008, P 99

[52] Brand, E & Wiseman, N, Concise Chinese Materia Medica, Taos, Paradigm Publications, 2008, P 107

[53] Bensky, D, Clavey, S, Stöger, E & Gamble, A, Chinese Herbal Medicine Materia Medica, 3rd Edition, Seattle, Eastland Press, 1986, 1993, 2004, P 205

[54] Bensky, D, Clavey, S, Stöger, E & Gamble, A, Chinese Herbal Medicine Materia Medica, 3rd Edition, Seattle, Eastland Press, 1986, 1993, 2004, P 159

[55] Brand, E & Wiseman, N, Concise Chinese Materia Medica, Taos, Paradigm Publications, 2008, P 108

[56] Zhang Bing Cheng, *Convenient Reader of Materia Medica*, via Bensky, D, Clavey, S, Stöger, E & Gamble, A, Chinese Herbal Medicine Materia Medica, 3rd Edition, Seattle, Eastland Press, 1986, 1993, 2004, P 156

[57] *Encountering the Sources of the Classic of Materia Medica*, via Bensky, D, Clavey, S, Stöger, E & Gamble, A, Chinese Herbal Medicine Materia Medica, 3rd Edition, Seattle, Eastland Press, 1986, 1993, 2004, P172

[58] *Encountering the Sources of the Classic of Materia Medica*, via Bensky, D, Clavey, S, Stöger, E & Gamble, A, Chinese Herbal Medicine Materia Medica, 3rd Edition, Seattle, Eastland Press, 1986, 1993, 2004, P172

[59] Bensky, D, Clavey, S, Stöger, E & Gamble, A, Chinese Herbal Medicine Materia Medica, 3rd Edition, Seattle, Eastland Press, 1986, 1993, 2004, P 171

[60] Bensky, D, Clavey, S, Stöger, E & Gamble, A, Chinese Herbal Medicine Materia Medica, 3rd Edition, Seattle, Eastland Press, 1986, 1993, 2004, P 161

[61] Bensky, D, Clavey, S, Stöger, E & Gamble, A, Chinese Herbal Medicine Materia Medica, 3rd Edition, Seattle, Eastland Press, 1986, 1993, 2004, P 317
[62] Bensky, D, Clavey, S, Stöger, E & Gamble, A, Chinese Herbal Medicine Materia Medica, 3rd Edition, Seattle, Eastland Press, 1986, 1993, 2004, P317
[63] Bensky, D, Clavey, S, Stöger, E & Gamble, A, Chinese Herbal Medicine Materia Medica, 3rd Edition, Seattle, Eastland Press, 1986, 1993, 2004, P 317
[64] Bensky, D, Clavey, S, Stöger, E & Gamble, A, Chinese Herbal Medicine Materia Medica, 3rd Edition, Seattle, Eastland Press, 1986, 1993, 2004, P 317
[65] Bensky, D, Clavey, S, Stöger, E & Gamble, A, Chinese Herbal Medicine Materia Medica, 3rd Edition, Seattle, Eastland Press, 1986, 1993, 2004, P 153
[66] Bensky, D, Clavey, S, Stöger, E & Gamble, A, Chinese Herbal Medicine Materia Medica, 3rd Edition, Seattle, Eastland Press, 1986, 1993, 2004, P 153
[67] *Convenient Reader of Materia Medica*, Bensky, D, Clavey, S, Stöger, E & Gamble, A, Chinese Herbal Medicine Materia Medica, 3rd Edition, Seattle, Eastland Press, 1986, 1993, 2004, P 214
[68] *Convenient Reader of Materia Medica*, Bensky, D, Clavey, S, Stöger, E & Gamble, A, Chinese Herbal Medicine Materia Medica, 3rd Edition, Seattle, Eastland Press, 1986, 1993, 2004, P 214
[69] Zhang Bing Chen, *Convenient Reader of Materia Medica*, via Bensky, D, Clavey, S, Stöger, E & Gamble, A, Chinese Herbal Medicine Materia Medica, 3rd Edition, Seattle, Eastland Press, 1986, 1993, 2004, P 214
[70] Bensky, D, Clavey, S, Stöger, E & Gamble, A, Chinese Herbal Medicine Materia Medica, 3rd Edition, Seattle, Eastland Press, 1986, 1993, 2004, P 166
[71] Brand, E & Wiseman, N, Concise Chinese Materia Medica, Taos, Paradigm Publications, 2008, P 120, Bensky, D, Clavey, S, Stöger, E & Gamble, A, Chinese Herbal Medicine Materia Medica, 3rd Edition, Seattle, Eastland Press, 1986, 1993, 2004, P 224
[72] Bensky, D, Clavey, S, Stöger, E & Gamble, A, Chinese Herbal Medicine Materia Medica, 3rd Edition, Seattle, Eastland Press, 1986, 1993, 2004, P 224
[73] Chen, JK & TT, Chinese Medical Herbology and Pharmacology, City of Industry, Art of Medicine Press, 2001/2004, P 247
[74] Tang Rong Chuan (Tang Zonghai), Ben Cao Wen Da, Personal Unpublished Translation, 2015, 2.3.5
[75] Brand, E & Wiseman, N, Concise Chinese Materia Medica, Taos, Paradigm Publications, 2008, P 121, Bensky, D, Clavey, S, Stöger, E & Gamble, A, Chinese Herbal Medicine Materia Medica, 3rd Edition, Seattle, Eastland Press, 1986, 1993, 2004, P 222
[76] Bensky, D, Clavey, S, Stöger, E & Gamble, A, Chinese Herbal Medicine Materia Medica, 3rd Edition, Seattle, Eastland Press, 1986, 1993, 2004, P 240
[77] Chen, JK & TT, Chinese Medical Herbology and Pharmacology, City of Industry, Art of Medicine Press, 2001/2004, P 274
[78] Brand, E & Wiseman, N, Concise Chinese Materia Medica, Taos, Paradigm Publications, 2008, P 142
[79] Brand, E & Wiseman, N, Concise Chinese Materia Medica, Taos, Paradigm Publications, 2008, P 142
[80] Brand, E & Wiseman, N, Concise Chinese Materia Medica, Taos, Paradigm Publications, 2008, P 143, Bensky, D, Clavey, S, Stöger, E & Gamble, A, Chinese Herbal Medicine Materia Medica, 3rd Edition, Seattle, Eastland Press, 1986, 1993, 2004, P 261

[81] Bensky, D, Clavey, S, Stöger, E & Gamble, A, Chinese Herbal Medicine Materia Medica, 3rd Edition, Seattle, Eastland Press, 1986, 1993, 2004, P 261
[82] Chen, JK & TT, Chinese Medical Herbology and Pharmacology, City of Industry, Art of Medicine Press, 2001/2004, P 287
[83] Brand, E & Wiseman, N, Concise Chinese Materia Medica, Taos, Paradigm Publications, 2008, P 139
[84] *Seeking Accuracy in the Materia Medica*, via Bensky, D, Clavey, S, Stöger, E & Gamble, A, Chinese Herbal Medicine Materia Medica, 3rd Edition, Seattle, Eastland Press, 1986, 1993, 2004, P 254
[85] *Seeking Accuracy in the Materia Medica*, via Bensky, D, Clavey, S, Stöger, E & Gamble, A, Chinese Herbal Medicine Materia Medica, 3rd Edition, Seattle, Eastland Press, 1986, 1993, 2004, P 254
[86] Chen, JK & TT, Chinese Medical Herbology and Pharmacology, City of Industry, Art of Medicine Press, 2001/2004, P 290
[87] Bensky, D, Clavey, S, Stöger, E & Gamble, A, Chinese Herbal Medicine Materia Medica, 3rd Edition, Seattle, Eastland Press, 1986, 1993, 2004, P 249
[88] Bensky, D, Clavey, S, Stöger, E & Gamble, A, Chinese Herbal Medicine Materia Medica, 3rd Edition, Seattle, Eastland Press, 1986, 1993, 2004, P 313
[89] Bensky, D, Clavey, S, Stöger, E & Gamble, A, Chinese Herbal Medicine Materia Medica, 3rd Edition, Seattle, Eastland Press, 1986, 1993, 2004, P 313
[90] Chen, JK & TT, Chinese Medical Herbology and Pharmacology, City of Industry, Art of Medicine Press, 2001/2004, P 308
[91] Brand, E & Wiseman, N, Concise Chinese Materia Medica, Taos, Paradigm Publications, 2008, P 158
[92] Maciocia, G, The Channels of Acupuncture, Philadelphia, Elsevier, 2006, P 585
[93] '…circulates the Còu Lǐ-interstices and the Sān Jiāo.' Tang Rong Chuan (Tang Zonghai), Ben Cao Wen Da, Personal Unpublished Translation, 2015, 2.2.5
[94] Bensky, D, Clavey, S, Stöger, E & Gamble, A, Chinese Herbal Medicine Materia Medica, 3rd Edition, Seattle, Eastland Press, 1986, 1993, 2004, P 332
[95] Bensky, D, Clavey, S, Stöger, E & Gamble, A, Chinese Herbal Medicine Materia Medica, 3rd Edition, Seattle, Eastland Press, 1986, 1993, 2004, P 332
[96] Li Gao, via Bensky, D, Clavey, S, Stöger, E & Gamble, A, Chinese Herbal Medicine Materia Medica, 3rd Edition, Seattle, Eastland Press, 1986, 1993, 2004, P 332
[97] Maciocia, G, The Channels of Acupuncture, Philadelphia, Elsevier, 2006, P 585
[98] Bensky, D, Clavey, S, Stöger, E & Gamble, A, Chinese Herbal Medicine Materia Medica, 3rd Edition, Seattle, Eastland Press, 1986, 1993, 2004, P 347
[99] Bensky, D, Clavey, S, Stöger, E & Gamble, A, Chinese Herbal Medicine Materia Medica, 3rd Edition, Seattle, Eastland Press, 1986, 1993, 2004, P 347
[100] Tang Rong Chuan (Tang Zonghai), Ben Cao Wen Da, Personal Unpublished Translation, 2015, 1.5.14
[101] Chen, JK & TT, Chinese Medical Herbology and Pharmacology, City of Industry, Art of Medicine Press, 2001/2004, P 461
[102] Zhang, Shan Lei, *Rectification of the Meaning of Materia Medica,* via Bensky, D, Clavey, S, Stöger, E & Gamble, A, Chinese Herbal Medicine Materia Medica, 3rd Edition, Seattle, Eastland Press, 1986, 1993, 2004, P 482

[103] Zhang, Shan Lei, *Rectification of the Meaning of Materia Medica,* via Bensky, D, Clavey, S, Stöger, E & Gamble, A, Chinese Herbal Medicine Materia Medica, 3rd Edition, Seattle, Eastland Press, 1986, 1993, 2004, P 482

[104] Huang Gong Xiu, *Seeking Accuracy in the Materia Medica*, and, *Harm and Benefit in the Materia Medica*, both via Bensky, D, Clavey, S, Stöger, E & Gamble, A, Chinese Herbal Medicine Materia Medica, 3rd Edition, Seattle, Eastland Press, 1986, 1993, 2004, P 482

[105] Brand, E & Wiseman, N, Concise Chinese Materia Medica, Taos, Paradigm Publications, 2008, P 188

[106] Bensky, D, Clavey, S, Stöger, E & Gamble, A, Chinese Herbal Medicine Materia Medica, 3rd Edition, Seattle, Eastland Press, 1986, 1993, 2004, P 407

[107] Bensky, D, Clavey, S, Stöger, E & Gamble, A, Chinese Herbal Medicine Materia Medica, 3rd Edition, Seattle, Eastland Press, 1986, 1993, 2004, P 407

[108] Brand, E & Wiseman, N, Concise Chinese Materia Medica, Taos, Paradigm Publications, 2008, P 194

[109] Brand, E & Wiseman, N, Concise Chinese Materia Medica, Taos, Paradigm Publications, 2008, P186

[110] Bensky, D, Clavey, S, Stöger, E & Gamble, A, Chinese Herbal Medicine Materia Medica, 3rd Edition, Seattle, Eastland Press, 1986, 1993, 2004, P 267

[111] Brand, E & Wiseman, N, Concise Chinese Materia Medica, Taos, Paradigm Publications, 2008, P 198

[112] Bensky, D, Clavey, S, Stöger, E & Gamble, A, Chinese Herbal Medicine Materia Medica, 3rd Edition, Seattle, Eastland Press, 1986, 1993, 2004, P 317

[113] Bensky, D, Clavey, S, Stöger, E & Gamble, A, Chinese Herbal Medicine Materia Medica, 3rd Edition, Seattle, Eastland Press, 1986, 1993, 2004, P317

[114] Bensky, D, Clavey, S, Stöger, E & Gamble, A, Chinese Herbal Medicine Materia Medica, 3rd Edition, Seattle, Eastland Press, 1986, 1993, 2004, P 317

[115] Bensky, D, Clavey, S, Stöger, E & Gamble, A, Chinese Herbal Medicine Materia Medica, 3rd Edition, Seattle, Eastland Press, 1986, 1993, 2004, P 317

[116] Bensky, D, Clavey, S, Stöger, E & Gamble, A, Chinese Herbal Medicine Materia Medica, 3rd Edition, Seattle, Eastland Press, 1986, 1993, 2004, P 285

[117] Brand, E & Wiseman, N, Concise Chinese Materia Medica, Taos, Paradigm Publications, 2008, P 194

[118] Bensky, D, Clavey, S, Stöger, E & Gamble, A, Chinese Herbal Medicine Materia Medica, 3rd Edition, Seattle, Eastland Press, 1986, 1993, 2004, P 297

[119] Bensky, D, Clavey, S, Stöger, E & Gamble, A, Chinese Herbal Medicine Materia Medica, 3rd Edition, Seattle, Eastland Press, 1986, 1993, 2004, P 278

[120] Brand, E & Wiseman, N, Concise Chinese Materia Medica, Taos, Paradigm Publications, 2008, P 191

[121] Brand, E & Wiseman, N, Concise Chinese Materia Medica, Taos, Paradigm Publications, 2008, P 197

[122] Chen, JK & TT, Chinese Medical Herbology and Pharmacology, City of Industry, Art of Medicine Press, 2001/2004, P 461

[123] Chen, JK & TT, Chinese Medical Herbology and Pharmacology, City of Industry, Art of Medicine Press, 2001/2004, P 461

[124] Chen, JK & TT, Chinese Medical Herbology and Pharmacology, City of Industry, Art of Medicine Press, 2001/2004, P 455
[125] Tang Rong Chuan (Tang Zonghai), Ben Cao Wen Da, Personal Unpublished Translation, 2015, 2.2.2
[126] Bensky, D, Clavey, S, Stöger, E & Gamble, A, Chinese Herbal Medicine Materia Medica, 3rd Edition, Seattle, Eastland Press, 1986, 1993, 2004, P 83
[127] Brand, E & Wiseman, N, Concise Chinese Materia Medica, Taos, Paradigm Publications, 2008, P 234
[128] Huang Gong Xiu, *Seeking Accuracy in the Materia Medica*, via Bensky, D, Clavey, S, Stöger, E & Gamble, A, Chinese Herbal Medicine Materia Medica, 3rd Edition, Seattle, Eastland Press, 1986, 1993, 2004, P 548
[129] Bensky, D, Clavey, S, Stöger, E & Gamble, A, Chinese Herbal Medicine Materia Medica, 3rd Edition, Seattle, Eastland Press, 1986, 1993, 2004, P 510
[130] Li Shi Zhen, via Bensky, D, Clavey, S, Stöger, E & Gamble, A, Chinese Herbal Medicine Materia Medica, 3rd Edition, Seattle, Eastland Press, 1986, 1993, 2004, P 534
[131] Bensky, D, Clavey, S, Stöger, E & Gamble, A, Chinese Herbal Medicine Materia Medica, 3rd Edition, Seattle, Eastland Press, 1986, 1993, 2004, P 1001
[132] Bensky, D, Clavey, S, Stöger, E & Gamble, A, Chinese Herbal Medicine Materia Medica, 3rd Edition, Seattle, Eastland Press, 1986, 1993, 2004, P 1001
[133] Bensky, D, Clavey, S, Stöger, E & Gamble, A, Chinese Herbal Medicine Materia Medica, 3rd Edition, Seattle, Eastland Press, 1986, 1993, 2004, P 1001
[134] Brand, E & Wiseman, N, Concise Chinese Materia Medica, Taos, Paradigm Publications, 2008, P 489
[135] Bensky, D, Clavey, S, Stöger, E & Gamble, A, Chinese Herbal Medicine Materia Medica, 3rd Edition, Seattle, Eastland Press, 1986, 1993, 2004, P 1014
[136] Bensky, D, Clavey, S, Stöger, E & Gamble, A, Chinese Herbal Medicine Materia Medica, 3rd Edition, Seattle, Eastland Press, 1986, 1993, 2004, P 590
[137] Bensky, D, Clavey, S, Stöger, E & Gamble, A, Chinese Herbal Medicine Materia Medica, 3rd Edition, Seattle, Eastland Press, 1986, 1993, 2004, P 589
[138] Chen, JK & TT, Chinese Medical Herbology and Pharmacology, City of Industry, Art of Medicine Press, 2001/2004, P 574
[139] Bensky, D, Clavey, S, Stöger, E & Gamble, A, Chinese Herbal Medicine Materia Medica, 3rd Edition, Seattle, Eastland Press, 1986, 1993, 2004, P 579
[140] Brand, E & Wiseman, N, Concise Chinese Materia Medica, Taos, Paradigm Publications, 2008, P 267
[141] Brand, E & Wiseman, N, Concise Chinese Materia Medica, Taos, Paradigm Publications, 2008, P 288, Bensky, D, Clavey, S, Stöger, E & Gamble, A, Chinese Herbal Medicine Materia Medica, 3rd Edition, Seattle, Eastland Press, 1986, 1993, 2004, P 624
[142] Bensky, D, Clavey, S, Stöger, E & Gamble, A, Chinese Herbal Medicine Materia Medica, 3rd Edition, Seattle, Eastland Press, 1986, 1993, 2004, P 655
[143] Bensky, D, Clavey, S, Stöger, E & Gamble, A, Chinese Herbal Medicine Materia Medica, 3rd Edition, Seattle, Eastland Press, 1986, 1993, 2004, P 610
[144] *Convenient Reader of Materia Medica*, Bensky, D, Clavey, S, Stöger, E & Gamble, A, Chinese Herbal Medicine Materia Medica, 3rd Edition, Seattle, Eastland Press, 1986, 1993, 2004, P 214

[145] *Convenient Reader of Materia Medica*, Bensky, D, Clavey, S, Stöger, E & Gamble, A, Chinese Herbal Medicine Materia Medica, 3rd Edition, Seattle, Eastland Press, 1986, 1993, 2004, P 214
[146] Zhang Bing Chen, *Convenient Reader of Materia Medica*, via Bensky, D, Clavey, S, Stöger, E & Gamble, A, Chinese Herbal Medicine Materia Medica, 3rd Edition, Seattle, Eastland Press, 1986, 1993, 2004, P 214
[147] Bensky, D, Clavey, S, Stöger, E & Gamble, A, Chinese Herbal Medicine Materia Medica, 3rd Edition, Seattle, Eastland Press, 1986, 1993, 2004, P 435
[148] Brand, E & Wiseman, N, Concise Chinese Materia Medica, Taos, Paradigm Publications, 2008, P 316
[149] Bensky, D, Clavey, S, Stöger, E & Gamble, A, Chinese Herbal Medicine Materia Medica, 3rd Edition, Seattle, Eastland Press, 1986, 1993, 2004, P 426
[150] Brand, E & Wiseman, N, Concise Chinese Materia Medica, Taos, Paradigm Publications, 2008, P 320
[151] Bensky, D, Clavey, S, Stöger, E & Gamble, A, Chinese Herbal Medicine Materia Medica, 3rd Edition, Seattle, Eastland Press, 1986, 1993, 2004, P 432
[152] Bensky, D, Clavey, S, Stöger, E & Gamble, A, Chinese Herbal Medicine Materia Medica, 3rd Edition, Seattle, Eastland Press, 1986, 1993, 2004, P 412
[153] Bensky, D, Clavey, S, Stöger, E & Gamble, A, Chinese Herbal Medicine Materia Medica, 3rd Edition, Seattle, Eastland Press, 1986, 1993, 2004, P 458
[154] Bensky, D, Clavey, S, Stöger, E & Gamble, A, Chinese Herbal Medicine Materia Medica, 3rd Edition, Seattle, Eastland Press, 1986, 1993, 2004, P 407
[155] Bensky, D, Clavey, S, Stöger, E & Gamble, A, Chinese Herbal Medicine Materia Medica, 3rd Edition, Seattle, Eastland Press, 1986, 1993, 2004, P 407
[156] Chen, JK & TT, Chinese Medical Herbology and Pharmacology, City of Industry, Art of Medicine Press, 2001/2004, P 713
[157] Bensky, D, Clavey, S, Stöger, E & Gamble, A, Chinese Herbal Medicine Materia Medica, 3rd Edition, Seattle, Eastland Press, 1986, 1993, 2004, P 401
[158] Brand, E & Wiseman, N, Concise Chinese Materia Medica, Taos, Paradigm Publications, 2008, P 313
[159] Brand, E & Wiseman, N, Concise Chinese Materia Medica, Taos, Paradigm Publications, 2008, P 313
[160] Brand, E & Wiseman, N, Concise Chinese Materia Medica, Taos, Paradigm Publications, 2008, P 312
[161] Brand, E & Wiseman, N, Concise Chinese Materia Medica, Taos, Paradigm Publications, 2008, P 312, Bensky, D, Clavey, S, Stöger, E & Gamble, A, Chinese Herbal Medicine Materia Medica, 3rd Edition, Seattle, Eastland Press, 1986, 1993, 2004, P 421
[162] Bensky, D, Clavey, S, Stöger, E & Gamble, A, Chinese Herbal Medicine Materia Medica, 3rd Edition, Seattle, Eastland Press, 1986, 1993, 2004, P 655
[163] Brand, E & Wiseman, N, Concise Chinese Materia Medica, Taos, Paradigm Publications, 2008, P 322
[164] Brand, E & Wiseman, N, Concise Chinese Materia Medica, Taos, Paradigm Publications, 2008, P 322
[165] Chen, JK & TT, Chinese Medical Herbology and Pharmacology, City of Industry, Art of Medicine Press, 2001/2004, P 715

[166] Chen, JK & TT, Chinese Medical Herbology and Pharmacology, City of Industry, Art of Medicine Press, 2001/2004, P 715
[167] Bensky, D, Clavey, S, Stöger, E & Gamble, A, Chinese Herbal Medicine Materia Medica, 3rd Edition, Seattle, Eastland Press, 1986, 1993, 2004, P 404
[168] Brand, E & Wiseman, N, Concise Chinese Materia Medica, Taos, Paradigm Publications, 2008, P 321
[169] Brand, E & Wiseman, N, Concise Chinese Materia Medica, Taos, Paradigm Publications, 2008, P 321
[170] Brand, E & Wiseman, N, Concise Chinese Materia Medica, Taos, Paradigm Publications, 2008, P 162
[171] Bensky, D, Clavey, S, Stöger, E & Gamble, A, Chinese Herbal Medicine Materia Medica, 3rd Edition, Seattle, Eastland Press, 1986, 1993, 2004, P 428
[172] Chen, JK & TT, Chinese Medical Herbology and Pharmacology, City of Industry, Art of Medicine Press, 2001/2004, P 688
[173] Chen, JK & TT, Chinese Medical Herbology and Pharmacology, City of Industry, Art of Medicine Press, 2001/2004, P 688
[174] Brand, E & Wiseman, N, Concise Chinese Materia Medica, Taos, Paradigm Publications, 2008, P 311
[175] Brand, E & Wiseman, N, Concise Chinese Materia Medica, Taos, Paradigm Publications, 2008, P 318
[176] Brand, E & Wiseman, N, Concise Chinese Materia Medica, Taos, Paradigm Publications, 2008, P 326
[177] Brand, E & Wiseman, N, Concise Chinese Materia Medica, Taos, Paradigm Publications, 2008, P 316
[178] Bensky, D, Clavey, S, Stöger, E & Gamble, A, Chinese Herbal Medicine Materia Medica, 3rd Edition, Seattle, Eastland Press, 1986, 1993, 2004, P 377
[179] Bensky, D, Clavey, S, Stöger, E & Gamble, A, Chinese Herbal Medicine Materia Medica, 3rd Edition, Seattle, Eastland Press, 1986, 1993, 2004, P 377
[180] *Detailed Materia Medica*, via Bensky, D, Clavey, S, Stöger, E & Gamble, A, Chinese Herbal Medicine Materia Medica, 3rd Edition, Seattle, Eastland Press, 1986, 1993, 2004, P 409
[181] *Detailed Materia Medica*, via Bensky, D, Clavey, S, Stöger, E & Gamble, A, Chinese Herbal Medicine Materia Medica, 3rd Edition, Seattle, Eastland Press, 1986, 1993, 2004, P 409
[182] *Illustrated Classic of Materia Medica*, via Zhang, Shan Lei, *Rectification of the Meaning of Materia Medica*, via Bensky, D, Clavey, S, Stöger, E & Gamble, A, Chinese Herbal Medicine Materia Medica, 3rd Edition, Seattle, Eastland Press, 1986, 1993, 2004, P 449
[183] Brand, E & Wiseman, N, Concise Chinese Materia Medica, Taos, Paradigm Publications, 2008, P 329, Bensky, D, Clavey, S, Stöger, E & Gamble, A, Chinese Herbal Medicine Materia Medica, 3rd Edition, Seattle, Eastland Press, 1986, 1993, 2004, P 448
[184] Brand, E & Wiseman, N, Concise Chinese Materia Medica, Taos, Paradigm Publications, 2008, P 330, Bensky, D, Clavey, S, Stöger, E & Gamble, A, Chinese Herbal Medicine Materia Medica, 3rd Edition, Seattle, Eastland Press, 1986, 1993, 2004, P 440, Brand, E & Wiseman, N, Concise Chinese Materia Medica, Taos, Paradigm Publications, 2008, P 330
[185] Chen, JK & TT, Chinese Medical Herbology and Pharmacology, City of Industry, Art of Medicine Press, 2001/2004, P 739

[186] Bensky, D, Clavey, S, Stöger, E & Gamble, A, Chinese Herbal Medicine Materia Medica, 3rd Edition, Seattle, Eastland Press, 1986, 1993, 2004, P 458
[187] Bensky, D, Clavey, S, Stöger, E & Gamble, A, Chinese Herbal Medicine Materia Medica, 3rd Edition, Seattle, Eastland Press, 1986, 1993, 2004, P 446
[188] Brand, E & Wiseman, N, Concise Chinese Materia Medica, Taos, Paradigm Publications, 2008, P 332
[189] Bensky, D, Clavey, S, Stöger, E & Gamble, A, Chinese Herbal Medicine Materia Medica, 3rd Edition, Seattle, Eastland Press, 1986, 1993, 2004, P 813
[190] Brand, E & Wiseman, N, Concise Chinese Materia Medica, Taos, Paradigm Publications, 2008, P 330
[191] Chen Shi Duo, *New Edition of Materia Medica*, via Bensky, D, Clavey, S, Stöger, E & Gamble, A, Chinese Herbal Medicine Materia Medica, 3rd Edition, Seattle, Eastland Press, 1986, 1993, 2004, P 443
[192] Chen, JK & TT, Chinese Medical Herbology and Pharmacology, City of Industry, Art of Medicine Press, 2001/2004, P 729
[193] Chen Shi Duo, *New Edition of Materia Medica*, via Bensky, D, Clavey, S, Stöger, E & Gamble, A, Chinese Herbal Medicine Materia Medica, 3rd Edition, Seattle, Eastland Press, 1986, 1993, 2004, P 443
[194] Brand, E & Wiseman, N, Concise Chinese Materia Medica, Taos, Paradigm Publications, 2008, P 332
[195] Brand, E & Wiseman, N, Concise Chinese Materia Medica, Taos, Paradigm Publications, 2008, P 333, Bensky, D, Clavey, S, Stöger, E & Gamble, A, Chinese Herbal Medicine Materia Medica, 3rd Edition, Seattle, Eastland Press, 1986, 1993, 2004, P 894
[196] *Sichuan Chinese Materia Medica*, via Bensky, D, Clavey, S, Stöger, E & Gamble, A, Chinese Herbal Medicine Materia Medica, 3rd Edition, Seattle, Eastland Press, 1986, 1993, 2004, P 939
[197] *Sichuan Chinese Materia Medica*, via Bensky, D, Clavey, S, Stöger, E & Gamble, A, Chinese Herbal Medicine Materia Medica, 3rd Edition, Seattle, Eastland Press, 1986, 1993, 2004, P 939
[198] Bensky, D, Clavey, S, Stöger, E & Gamble, A, Chinese Herbal Medicine Materia Medica, 3rd Edition, Seattle, Eastland Press, 1986, 1993, 2004, P 543
[199] Brand, E & Wiseman, N, Concise Chinese Materia Medica, Taos, Paradigm Publications, 2008, P 352
[200] Bensky, D, Clavey, S, Stöger, E & Gamble, A, Chinese Herbal Medicine Materia Medica, 3rd Edition, Seattle, Eastland Press, 1986, 1993, 2004, P 912
[201] Bensky, D, Clavey, S, Stöger, E & Gamble, A, Chinese Herbal Medicine Materia Medica, 3rd Edition, Seattle, Eastland Press, 1986, 1993, 2004, P 982
[202] Chen, JK & TT, Chinese Medical Herbology and Pharmacology, City of Industry, Art of Medicine Press, 2001/2004, P 794, Bensky, D, Clavey, S, Stöger, E & Gamble, A, Chinese Herbal Medicine Materia Medica, 3rd Edition, Seattle, Eastland Press, 1986, 1993, 2004, P 982
[203] Zhang Jie Gu via Li Shi Zhen, *Grand Materia Medica*, via Bensky, D, Clavey, S, Stöger, E & Gamble, A, Chinese Herbal Medicine Materia Medica, 3rd Edition, Seattle, Eastland Press, 1986, 1993, 2004, P 985
[204] Brand, E & Wiseman, N, Concise Chinese Materia Medica, Taos, Paradigm Publications, 2008, P 383

[205] Bensky, D, Clavey, S, Stöger, E & Gamble, A, Chinese Herbal Medicine Materia Medica, 3rd Edition, Seattle, Eastland Press, 1986, 1993, 2004, P 954
[206] *High Plateau Handbook of Treatment with Chinese Materia Medica*, via Bensky, D, Clavey, S, Stöger, E & Gamble, A, Chinese Herbal Medicine Materia Medica, 3rd Edition, Seattle, Eastland Press, 1986, 1993, 2004, P 742
[207] Bensky, D, Clavey, S, Stöger, E & Gamble, A, Chinese Herbal Medicine Materia Medica, 3rd Edition, Seattle, Eastland Press, 1986, 1993, 2004, P 742
[208] Maciocia, G, The Channels of Acupuncture, Philadelphia, Elsevier, 2006, P 545
[209] Bensky, D, Clavey, S, Stöger, E & Gamble, A, Chinese Herbal Medicine Materia Medica, 3rd Edition, Seattle, Eastland Press, 1986, 1993, 2004, P 718
[210] I think virtually anyone tasting Hong Jing Tian would immediately agree on its astringency.
[211] Brand, E & Wiseman, N, Concise Chinese Materia Medica, Taos, Paradigm Publications, 2008, P 411
[212] Brand, E & Wiseman, N, Concise Chinese Materia Medica, Taos, Paradigm Publications, 2008, P 411
[213] Chen, JK & TT, Chinese Medical Herbology and Pharmacology, City of Industry, Art of Medicine Press, 2001/2004, P 853
[214] Bensky, D, Clavey, S, Stöger, E & Gamble, A, Chinese Herbal Medicine Materia Medica, 3rd Edition, Seattle, Eastland Press, 1986, 1993, 2004, P 822
[215] Zhang, Shan Lei, *Rectification of the Meaning of Materia Medica,* via Bensky, D, Clavey, S, Stöger, E & Gamble, A, Chinese Herbal Medicine Materia Medica, 3rd Edition, Seattle, Eastland Press, 1986, 1993, 2004, P 823
[216] Brand, E & Wiseman, N, Concise Chinese Materia Medica, Taos, Paradigm Publications, 2008, P 398
[217] Brand, E & Wiseman, N, Concise Chinese Materia Medica, Taos, Paradigm Publications, 2008, P 395
[218] Brand, E & Wiseman, N, Concise Chinese Materia Medica, Taos, Paradigm Publications, 2008, P 395
[219] Brand, E & Wiseman, N, Concise Chinese Materia Medica, Taos, Paradigm Publications, 2008, P 409
[220] Tang Rong Chuan (Tang Zonghai), Ben Cao Wen Da, Personal Unpublished Translation, 2015, 1.3.3
[221] Maciocia, G, The Channels of Acupuncture, Philadelphia, Elsevier, 2006, P 545
[222] Me, on the basis of Tang Rong Chuan (Tang Zonghai), Ben Cao Wen Da, Personal Unpublished Translation, 2015, 1.2.1, etc., here contained. Although nowhere in the text does the author state that Huang Qi enters the San Jiao Jing-channel, he goes through such extensive and multiple descriptions of the structure and mechanisms of the San Jiao itself, plus his clear delineations of exactly how this herb physically enters and embodies the San Jiao, I would challenge anybody to prove that it *doesn't* enter the San Jiao Jing-channel. In addition, when we consider Huang Qi's central role in Bu Zhong Yi Qi Tang's use in treating qi deficiency with deficient heat symptoms, that is really all about the Shao Yang level of disease. I would put forth the question of why would one not use Huang Qi whenever its known set of qualities were needed to be applied to any aspect or dimension of the San Jiao Jing-channel?

[223] Brand, E & Wiseman, N, Concise Chinese Materia Medica, Taos, Paradigm Publications, 2008, P 415
[224] Bensky, D, Clavey, S, Stöger, E & Gamble, A, Chinese Herbal Medicine Materia Medica, 3rd Edition, Seattle, Eastland Press, 1986, 1993, 2004, P 813
[225] Brand, E & Wiseman, N, Concise Chinese Materia Medica, Taos, Paradigm Publications, 2008, P 435, Bensky, D, Clavey, S, Stöger, E & Gamble, A, Chinese Herbal Medicine Materia Medica, 3rd Edition, Seattle, Eastland Press, 1986, 1993, 2004, P 818
[226] Brand, E & Wiseman, N, Concise Chinese Materia Medica, Taos, Paradigm Publications, 2008, P 435, Bensky, D, Clavey, S, Stöger, E & Gamble, A, Chinese Herbal Medicine Materia Medica, 3rd Edition, Seattle, Eastland Press, 1986, 1993, 2004, P 818
[227] Zhang Xi Chun, *Essays on Medicine Esteeming the Chinese and Respecting the Western*, via Bensky, D, Clavey, S, Stöger, E & Gamble, A, Chinese Herbal Medicine Materia Medica, 3rd Edition, Seattle, Eastland Press, 1986, 1993, 2004, P 821
[228] Brand, E & Wiseman, N, Concise Chinese Materia Medica, Taos, Paradigm Publications, 2008, P 439
[229] Brand, E & Wiseman, N, Concise Chinese Materia Medica, Taos, Paradigm Publications, 2008, P 436, Bensky, D, Clavey, S, Stöger, E & Gamble, A, Chinese Herbal Medicine Materia Medica, 3rd Edition, Seattle, Eastland Press, 1986, 1993, 2004, P 825
[230] Chen, JK & TT, Chinese Medical Herbology and Pharmacology, City of Industry, Art of Medicine Press, 2001/2004, P 943
[231] Brand, E & Wiseman, N, Concise Chinese Materia Medica, Taos, Paradigm Publications, 2008, P 436, Bensky, D, Clavey, S, Stöger, E & Gamble, A, Chinese Herbal Medicine Materia Medica, 3rd Edition, Seattle, Eastland Press, 1986, 1993, 2004, P 825
[232] Brand, E & Wiseman, N, Concise Chinese Materia Medica, Taos, Paradigm Publications, 2008, P 437
[233] Bensky, D, Clavey, S, Stöger, E & Gamble, A, Chinese Herbal Medicine Materia Medica, 3rd Edition, Seattle, Eastland Press, 1986, 1993, 2004, P 822
[234] Zhang, Shan Lei, *Rectification of the Meaning of Materia Medica,* via Bensky, D, Clavey, S, Stöger, E & Gamble, A, Chinese Herbal Medicine Materia Medica, 3rd Edition, Seattle, Eastland Press, 1986, 1993, 2004, P 823
[235] Brand, E & Wiseman, N, Concise Chinese Materia Medica, Taos, Paradigm Publications, 2008, P 398
[236] Bensky, D, Clavey, S, Stöger, E & Gamble, A, Chinese Herbal Medicine Materia Medica, 3rd Edition, Seattle, Eastland Press, 1986, 1993, 2004, P 835
[237] Zhang, Shan Lei, *Rectification of the Meaning of Materia Medica,* via Bensky, D, Clavey, S, Stöger, E & Gamble, A, Chinese Herbal Medicine Materia Medica, 3rd Edition, Seattle, Eastland Press, 1986, 1993, 2004, P 836
[238] Zhang, Shan Lei, *Rectification of the Meaning of Materia Medica,* via Bensky, D, Clavey, S, Stöger, E & Gamble, A, Chinese Herbal Medicine Materia Medica, 3rd Edition, Seattle, Eastland Press, 1986, 1993, 2004, P 836
[239] Brand, E & Wiseman, N, Concise Chinese Materia Medica, Taos, Paradigm Publications, 2008, P 440, Bensky, D, Clavey, S, Stöger, E & Gamble, A, Chinese Herbal Medicine Materia Medica, 3rd Edition, Seattle, Eastland Press, 1986, 1993, 2004, P 835

[240] Tang Rong Chuan (Tang Zonghai), Ben Cao Wen Da, Personal Unpublished Translation, 2015, 1.5.17
[241] Brand, E & Wiseman, N, Concise Chinese Materia Medica, Taos, Paradigm Publications, 2008, P 461, Bensky, D, Clavey, S, Stöger, E & Gamble, A, Chinese Herbal Medicine Materia Medica, 3rd Edition, Seattle, Eastland Press, 1986, 1993, 2004, P 867
[242] Chen, JK & TT, Chinese Medical Herbology and Pharmacology, City of Industry, Art of Medicine Press, 2001/2004, P 1003, Bensky, D, Clavey, S, Stöger, E & Gamble, A, Chinese Herbal Medicine Materia Medica, 3rd Edition, Seattle, Eastland Press, 1986, 1993, 2004, P 875
[243] Bensky, D, Clavey, S, Stöger, E & Gamble, A, Chinese Herbal Medicine Materia Medica, 3rd Edition, Seattle, Eastland Press, 1986, 1993, 2004, P 875
[244] Bensky, D, Clavey, S, Stöger, E & Gamble, A, Chinese Herbal Medicine Materia Medica, 3rd Edition, Seattle, Eastland Press, 1986, 1993, 2004, P 864
[245] Bensky, D, Clavey, S, Stöger, E & Gamble, A, Chinese Herbal Medicine Materia Medica, 3rd Edition, Seattle, Eastland Press, 1986, 1993, 2004, P 893
[246] Brand, E & Wiseman, N, Concise Chinese Materia Medica, Taos, Paradigm Publications, 2008, P 457, Bensky, D, Clavey, S, Stöger, E & Gamble, A, Chinese Herbal Medicine Materia Medica, 3rd Edition, Seattle, Eastland Press, 1986, 1993, 2004, P 860
[247] Li Shi Zhen, *Grand Materia Medica*, via Bensky, D, Clavey, S, Stöger, E & Gamble, A, Chinese Herbal Medicine Materia Medica, 3rd Edition, Seattle, Eastland Press, 1986, 1993, 2004, P 861
[248] Li Shi Zhen, *Grand Materia Medica*, via Bensky, D, Clavey, S, Stöger, E & Gamble, A, Chinese Herbal Medicine Materia Medica, 3rd Edition, Seattle, Eastland Press, 1986, 1993, 2004, P 861
[249] Li Shi Zhen, *Grand Materia Medica*, via Bensky, D, Clavey, S, Stöger, E & Gamble, A, Chinese Herbal Medicine Materia Medica, 3rd Edition, Seattle, Eastland Press, 1986, 1993, 2004, P 861
[250] Maciocia, G, The Channels of Acupuncture, Philadelphia, Elsevier, 2006, P 545
[251] Brand, E & Wiseman, N, Concise Chinese Materia Medica, Taos, Paradigm Publications, 2008, P 333, Bensky, D, Clavey, S, Stöger, E & Gamble, A, Chinese Herbal Medicine Materia Medica, 3rd Edition, Seattle, Eastland Press, 1986, 1993, 2004, P 894
[252] Ye Gui, *Renewed Materia Medica*, via Bensky, D, Clavey, S, Stöger, E & Gamble, A, Chinese Herbal Medicine Materia Medica, 3rd Edition, Seattle, Eastland Press, 1986, 1993, 2004, P 900
[253] Ye Gui, *Renewed Materia Medica*, via Bensky, D, Clavey, S, Stöger, E & Gamble, A, Chinese Herbal Medicine Materia Medica, 3rd Edition, Seattle, Eastland Press, 1986, 1993, 2004, P 900
[254] Bensky, D, Clavey, S, Stöger, E & Gamble, A, Chinese Herbal Medicine Materia Medica, 3rd Edition, Seattle, Eastland Press, 1986, 1993, 2004, P 1017
[255] Bensky, D, Clavey, S, Stöger, E & Gamble, A, Chinese Herbal Medicine Materia Medica, 3rd Edition, Seattle, Eastland Press, 1986, 1993, 2004, P 1033
[256] Brand, E & Wiseman, N, Concise Chinese Materia Medica, Taos, Paradigm Publications, 2008, P 489
[257] Bensky, D, Clavey, S, Stöger, E & Gamble, A, Chinese Herbal Medicine Materia Medica, 3rd Edition, Seattle, Eastland Press, 1986, 1993, 2004, P 1014
[258] Li Shi Zhen, *Grand Materia Medica*, via Bensky, D, Clavey, S, Stöger, E & Gamble, A, Chinese Herbal Medicine Materia Medica, 3rd Edition, Seattle, Eastland Press, 1986, 1993, 2004, P 1022
[259] Chen, JK & TT, Chinese Medical Herbology and Pharmacology, City of Industry, Art of Medicine Press, 2001/2004, P 1045

[260] Li Shi Zhen, *Grand Materia Medica*, via Bensky, D, Clavey, S, Stöger, E & Gamble, A, Chinese Herbal Medicine Materia Medica, 3rd Edition, Seattle, Eastland Press, 1986, 1993, 2004, P 1022

[261] Chen, JK & TT, Chinese Medical Herbology and Pharmacology, City of Industry, Art of Medicine Press, 2001/2004, P 1039

[262] Brand, E & Wiseman, N, Concise Chinese Materia Medica, Taos, Paradigm Publications, 2008, P 484

[263] Brand, E & Wiseman, N, Concise Chinese Materia Medica, Taos, Paradigm Publications, 2008, P 484

[264] Brand, E & Wiseman, N, Concise Chinese Materia Medica, Taos, Paradigm Publications, 2008, P 484

[265] Brand, E & Wiseman, N, Concise Chinese Materia Medica, Taos, Paradigm Publications, 2008, P 493

[266] Brand, E & Wiseman, N, Concise Chinese Materia Medica, Taos, Paradigm Publications, 2008, P 493

[267] Bensky, D, Clavey, S, Stöger, E & Gamble, A, Chinese Herbal Medicine Materia Medica, 3rd Edition, Seattle, Eastland Press, 1986, 1993, 2004, P 655

[268] Brand, E & Wiseman, N, Concise Chinese Materia Medica, Taos, Paradigm Publications, 2008, P 162

[269] Chen, JK & TT, Chinese Medical Herbology and Pharmacology, City of Industry, Art of Medicine Press, 2001/2004, P 1056, Bensky, D, Clavey, S, Stöger, E & Gamble, A, Chinese Herbal Medicine Materia Medica, 3rd Edition, Seattle, Eastland Press, 1986, 1993, 2004, P 1040

[270] Brand, E & Wiseman, N, Concise Chinese Materia Medica, Taos, Paradigm Publications, 2008, P 488

[271] Bensky, D, Clavey, S, Stöger, E & Gamble, A, Chinese Herbal Medicine Materia Medica, 3rd Edition, Seattle, Eastland Press, 1986, 1993, 2004, P 1030

[272] Chen, JK & TT, Chinese Medical Herbology and Pharmacology, City of Industry, Art of Medicine Press, 2001/2004, P 59

[273] Tang Rong Chuan (Tang Zonghai), Ben Cao Wen Da, Personal Unpublished Translation, 2015, 1.4.6

[274] Bensky, D, Clavey, S, Stöger, E & Gamble, A, Chinese Herbal Medicine Materia Medica, 3rd Edition, Seattle, Eastland Press, 1986, 1993, 2004, P 78

[275] Brand, E & Wiseman, N, Concise Chinese Materia Medica, Taos, Paradigm Publications, 2008, P 56

[276] Li Shi Zhen, *Grand Materia Medica*, via Bensky, D, Clavey, S, Stöger, E & Gamble, A, Chinese Herbal Medicine Materia Medica, 3rd Edition, Seattle, Eastland Press, 1986, 1993, 2004, P 56

[277] Li Shi Zhen, *Grand Materia Medica*, via Bensky, D, Clavey, S, Stöger, E & Gamble, A, Chinese Herbal Medicine Materia Medica, 3rd Edition, Seattle, Eastland Press, 1986, 1993, 2004, P 56

[278] Tang Rong Chuan (Tang Zonghai), Ben Cao Wen Da, Personal Unpublished Translation, 2015, 1.5.10

[279] Tang Rong Chuan (Tang Zonghai), Ben Cao Wen Da, Personal Unpublished Translation, 2015, 1.4.6

[280] Tang Rong Chuan (Tang Zonghai), Ben Cao Wen Da, Personal Unpublished Translation, 2015, 1.5.9

[281] Tang Rong Chuan (Tang Zonghai), Ben Cao Wen Da, Personal Unpublished Translation, 2015, 1.5.9

[282] Tang Rong Chuan (Tang Zonghai), Ben Cao Wen Da, Personal Unpublished Translation, 2015, 1.4.6

[283] Brand, E & Wiseman, N, Concise Chinese Materia Medica, Taos, Paradigm Publications, 2008, P 84, and Huang Gong Xiu, *Seeking Accuracy in the Materia Medica*, via Bensky, D, Clavey, S, Stöger, E & Gamble, A, Chinese Herbal Medicine Materia Medica, 3rd Edition, Seattle, Eastland Press, 1986, 1993, 2004, P 112

[284] Brand, E & Wiseman, N, Concise Chinese Materia Medica, Taos, Paradigm Publications, 2008, P 84

[285] Tang Rong Chuan (Tang Zonghai), Ben Cao Wen Da, Personal Unpublished Translation, 2015, 1.3.4 Although this text indicates that Huang Qin enters the San Jiao, the author is also quite specific in distinguishing between the organs and their Jing-channels. Here he does not indicate the Jing-channel, so I do not indicate otherwise.

[286] Chen, JK & TT, Chinese Medical Herbology and Pharmacology, City of Industry, Art of Medicine Press, 2001/2004, P 151

[287] Bensky, D, Clavey, S, Stöger, E & Gamble, A, Chinese Herbal Medicine Materia Medica, 3rd Edition, Seattle, Eastland Press, 1986, 1993, 2004, P 144

[288] Tang Rong Chuan (Tang Zonghai), Ben Cao Wen Da, Personal Unpublished Translation, 2015, 1.5.3

[289] Maciocia, G, The Channels of Acupuncture, Philadelphia, Elsevier, 2006, P 446

[290] Brand, E & Wiseman, N, Concise Chinese Materia Medica, Taos, Paradigm Publications, 2008, P 114

[291] Brand, E & Wiseman, N, Concise Chinese Materia Medica, Taos, Paradigm Publications, 2008, P114, Bensky, D, Clavey, S, Stöger, E & Gamble, A, Chinese Herbal Medicine Materia Medica, 3rd Edition, Seattle, Eastland Press, 1986, 1993, 2004, P 147

[292] Bensky, D, Clavey, S, Stöger, E & Gamble, A, Chinese Herbal Medicine Materia Medica, 3rd Edition, Seattle, Eastland Press, 1986, 1993, 2004, P 147

[293] Bensky, D, Clavey, S, Stöger, E & Gamble, A, Chinese Herbal Medicine Materia Medica, 3rd Edition, Seattle, Eastland Press, 1986, 1993, 2004, P 904

[294] Bensky, D, Clavey, S, Stöger, E & Gamble, A, Chinese Herbal Medicine Materia Medica, 3rd Edition, Seattle, Eastland Press, 1986, 1993, 2004, P 905

[295] Bensky, D, Clavey, S, Stöger, E & Gamble, A, Chinese Herbal Medicine Materia Medica, 3rd Edition, Seattle, Eastland Press, 1986, 1993, 2004, P 177

[296] Wang, Hao Gu, *Harm and Benefit in the Materia Medica*, via Bensky, D, Clavey, S, Stöger, E & Gamble, A, Chinese Herbal Medicine Materia Medica, 3rd Edition, Seattle, Eastland Press, 1986, 1993, 2004, P 152

[297] Bensky, D, Clavey, S, Stöger, E & Gamble, A, Chinese Herbal Medicine Materia Medica, 3rd Edition, Seattle, Eastland Press, 1986, 1993, 2004, P 151

[298] Wang, Hao Gu, *Harm and Benefit in the Materia Medica*, via Bensky, D, Clavey, S, Stöger, E & Gamble, A, Chinese Herbal Medicine Materia Medica, 3rd Edition, Seattle, Eastland Press, 1986, 1993, 2004, P 152

[299] Bensky, D, Clavey, S, Stöger, E & Gamble, A, Chinese Herbal Medicine Materia Medica, 3rd Edition, Seattle, Eastland Press, 1986, 1993, 2004, P 207

[300] Brand, E & Wiseman, N, Concise Chinese Materia Medica, Taos, Paradigm Publications, 2008, P 112
[301] Bensky, D, Clavey, S, Stöger, E & Gamble, A, Chinese Herbal Medicine Materia Medica, 3rd Edition, Seattle, Eastland Press, 1986, 1993, 2004, P 207
[302] Bensky, D, Clavey, S, Stöger, E & Gamble, A, Chinese Herbal Medicine Materia Medica, 3rd Edition, Seattle, Eastland Press, 1986, 1993, 2004, P 206
[303] Brand, E & Wiseman, N, Concise Chinese Materia Medica, Taos, Paradigm Publications, 2008, P 99
[304] Brand, E & Wiseman, N, Concise Chinese Materia Medica, Taos, Paradigm Publications, 2008, P 107
[305] Bensky, D, Clavey, S, Stöger, E & Gamble, A, Chinese Herbal Medicine Materia Medica, 3rd Edition, Seattle, Eastland Press, 1986, 1993, 2004, P 205
[306] Brand, E & Wiseman, N, Concise Chinese Materia Medica, Taos, Paradigm Publications, 2008, P 115
[307] Bensky, D, Clavey, S, Stöger, E & Gamble, A, Chinese Herbal Medicine Materia Medica, 3rd Edition, Seattle, Eastland Press, 1986, 1993, 2004, P 216
[308] Bensky, D, Clavey, S, Stöger, E & Gamble, A, Chinese Herbal Medicine Materia Medica, 3rd Edition, Seattle, Eastland Press, 1986, 1993, 2004, P 216
[309] Bensky, D, Clavey, S, Stöger, E & Gamble, A, Chinese Herbal Medicine Materia Medica, 3rd Edition, Seattle, Eastland Press, 1986, 1993, 2004, P 183
[310] Brand, E & Wiseman, N, Concise Chinese Materia Medica, Taos, Paradigm Publications, 2008, P 114
[311] Brand, E & Wiseman, N, Concise Chinese Materia Medica, Taos, Paradigm Publications, 2008, P114, Bensky, D, Clavey, S, Stöger, E & Gamble, A, Chinese Herbal Medicine Materia Medica, 3rd Edition, Seattle, Eastland Press, 1986, 1993, 2004, P 147
[312] Bensky, D, Clavey, S, Stöger, E & Gamble, A, Chinese Herbal Medicine Materia Medica, 3rd Edition, Seattle, Eastland Press, 1986, 1993, 2004, P 147
[313] *Miscellaneous Records of Famous Physicians*, via Bensky, D, Clavey, S, Stöger, E & Gamble, A, Chinese Herbal Medicine Materia Medica, 3rd Edition, Seattle, Eastland Press, 1986, 1993, 2004, P 174
[314] Tang Rong Chuan (Tang Zonghai), Ben Cao Wen Da, Personal Unpublished Translation, 2015, 2.3.5
[315] Bensky, D, Clavey, S, Stöger, E & Gamble, A, Chinese Herbal Medicine Materia Medica, 3rd Edition, Seattle, Eastland Press, 1986, 1993, 2004, P 189
[316] Brand, E & Wiseman, N, Concise Chinese Materia Medica, Taos, Paradigm Publications, 2008, P 116, Bensky, D, Clavey, S, Stöger, E & Gamble, A, Chinese Herbal Medicine Materia Medica, 3rd Edition, Seattle, Eastland Press, 1986, 1993, 2004, P 196
[317] Tang Rong Chuan (Tang Zonghai), Ben Cao Wen Da, Personal Unpublished Translation, 2015, 1.3.4
[318] Bensky, D, Clavey, S, Stöger, E & Gamble, A, Chinese Herbal Medicine Materia Medica, 3rd Edition, Seattle, Eastland Press, 1986, 1993, 2004, P 240
[319] Chen, JK & TT, Chinese Medical Herbology and Pharmacology, City of Industry, Art of Medicine Press, 2001/2004, P 274

[320] Brand, E & Wiseman, N, Concise Chinese Materia Medica, Taos, Paradigm Publications, 2008, P 142
[321] Bensky, D, Clavey, S, Stöger, E & Gamble, A, Chinese Herbal Medicine Materia Medica, 3rd Edition, Seattle, Eastland Press, 1986, 1993, 2004, P 242
[322] Brand, E & Wiseman, N, Concise Chinese Materia Medica, Taos, Paradigm Publications, 2008, P 132
[323] Tang Rong Chuan (Tang Zonghai), Ben Cao Wen Da, Personal Unpublished Translation, 2015, 1.5.3
[324] Bensky, D, Clavey, S, Stöger, E & Gamble, A, Chinese Herbal Medicine Materia Medica, 3rd Edition, Seattle, Eastland Press, 1986, 1993, 2004, P 239
[325] Tang Rong Chuan (Tang Zonghai), Ben Cao Wen Da, Personal Unpublished Translation, 2015, 1.5.2
[326] Maciocia, G, The Channels of Acupuncture, Philadelphia, Elsevier, 2006, P 446
[327] Bensky, D, Clavey, S, Stöger, E & Gamble, A, Chinese Herbal Medicine Materia Medica, 3rd Edition, Seattle, Eastland Press, 1986, 1993, 2004, P 243
[328] Brand, E & Wiseman, N, Concise Chinese Materia Medica, Taos, Paradigm Publications, 2008, P 142
[329] Brand, E & Wiseman, N, Concise Chinese Materia Medica, Taos, Paradigm Publications, 2008, P 143, Bensky, D, Clavey, S, Stöger, E & Gamble, A, Chinese Herbal Medicine Materia Medica, 3rd Edition, Seattle, Eastland Press, 1986, 1993, 2004, P 261
[330] Bensky, D, Clavey, S, Stöger, E & Gamble, A, Chinese Herbal Medicine Materia Medica, 3rd Edition, Seattle, Eastland Press, 1986, 1993, 2004, P 261
[331] Chen, JK & TT, Chinese Medical Herbology and Pharmacology, City of Industry, Art of Medicine Press, 2001/2004, P 287
[332] Brand, E & Wiseman, N, Concise Chinese Materia Medica, Taos, Paradigm Publications, 2008, P 139
[333] *Seeking Accuracy in the Materia Medica*, via Bensky, D, Clavey, S, Stöger, E & Gamble, A, Chinese Herbal Medicine Materia Medica, 3rd Edition, Seattle, Eastland Press, 1986, 1993, 2004, P 254
[334] *Seeking Accuracy in the Materia Medica*, via Bensky, D, Clavey, S, Stöger, E & Gamble, A, Chinese Herbal Medicine Materia Medica, 3rd Edition, Seattle, Eastland Press, 1986, 1993, 2004, P 254
[335] Chen, JK & TT, Chinese Medical Herbology and Pharmacology, City of Industry, Art of Medicine Press, 2001/2004, P 290
[336] Bensky, D, Clavey, S, Stöger, E & Gamble, A, Chinese Herbal Medicine Materia Medica, 3rd Edition, Seattle, Eastland Press, 1986, 1993, 2004, P 249
[337] Bensky, D, Clavey, S, Stöger, E & Gamble, A, Chinese Herbal Medicine Materia Medica, 3rd Edition, Seattle, Eastland Press, 1986, 1993, 2004, P 342
[338] Bensky, D, Clavey, S, Stöger, E & Gamble, A, Chinese Herbal Medicine Materia Medica, 3rd Edition, Seattle, Eastland Press, 1986, 1993, 2004, P 342
[339] Brand, E & Wiseman, N, Concise Chinese Materia Medica, Taos, Paradigm Publications, 2008, P 188
[340] Bensky, D, Clavey, S, Stöger, E & Gamble, A, Chinese Herbal Medicine Materia Medica, 3rd Edition, Seattle, Eastland Press, 1986, 1993, 2004, P 407

[341] Bensky, D, Clavey, S, Stöger, E & Gamble, A, Chinese Herbal Medicine Materia Medica, 3rd Edition, Seattle, Eastland Press, 1986, 1993, 2004, P 407
[342] Zhang Bing Chen, *Convenient Reader of Materia Medica*, via Bensky, D, Clavey, S, Stöger, E & Gamble, A, Chinese Herbal Medicine Materia Medica, 3rd Edition, Seattle, Eastland Press, 1986, 1993, 2004, P 299
[343] Zhang Bing Chen, *Convenient Reader of Materia Medica*, via Bensky, D, Clavey, S, Stöger, E & Gamble, A, Chinese Herbal Medicine Materia Medica, 3rd Edition, Seattle, Eastland Press, 1986, 1993, 2004, P 299
[344] Brand, E & Wiseman, N, Concise Chinese Materia Medica, Taos, Paradigm Publications, 2008, P 216
[345] Bensky, D, Clavey, S, Stöger, E & Gamble, A, Chinese Herbal Medicine Materia Medica, 3rd Edition, Seattle, Eastland Press, 1986, 1993, 2004, P 519
[346] Brand, E & Wiseman, N, Concise Chinese Materia Medica, Taos, Paradigm Publications, 2008, P 226
[347] Brand, E & Wiseman, N, Concise Chinese Materia Medica, Taos, Paradigm Publications, 2008, P 226, Bensky, D, Clavey, S, Stöger, E & Gamble, A, Chinese Herbal Medicine Materia Medica, 3rd Edition, Seattle, Eastland Press, 1986, 1993, 2004, P 517
[348] Bensky, D, Clavey, S, Stöger, E & Gamble, A, Chinese Herbal Medicine Materia Medica, 3rd Edition, Seattle, Eastland Press, 1986, 1993, 2004, P 543
[349] Bensky, D, Clavey, S, Stöger, E & Gamble, A, Chinese Herbal Medicine Materia Medica, 3rd Edition, Seattle, Eastland Press, 1986, 1993, 2004, P 544
[350] Bensky, D, Clavey, S, Stöger, E & Gamble, A, Chinese Herbal Medicine Materia Medica, 3rd Edition, Seattle, Eastland Press, 1986, 1993, 2004, P 530
[351] Brand, E & Wiseman, N, Concise Chinese Materia Medica, Taos, Paradigm Publications, 2008, P 228, Bensky, D, Clavey, S, Stöger, E & Gamble, A, Chinese Herbal Medicine Materia Medica, 3rd Edition, Seattle, Eastland Press, 1986, 1993, 2004, P 530
[352] Bensky, D, Clavey, S, Stöger, E & Gamble, A, Chinese Herbal Medicine Materia Medica, 3rd Edition, Seattle, Eastland Press, 1986, 1993, 2004, P 1001
[353] Bensky, D, Clavey, S, Stöger, E & Gamble, A, Chinese Herbal Medicine Materia Medica, 3rd Edition, Seattle, Eastland Press, 1986, 1993, 2004, P 1001
[354] Bensky, D, Clavey, S, Stöger, E & Gamble, A, Chinese Herbal Medicine Materia Medica, 3rd Edition, Seattle, Eastland Press, 1986, 1993, 2004, P 1001
[355] Brand, E & Wiseman, N, Concise Chinese Materia Medica, Taos, Paradigm Publications, 2008, P 489
[356] Bensky, D, Clavey, S, Stöger, E & Gamble, A, Chinese Herbal Medicine Materia Medica, 3rd Edition, Seattle, Eastland Press, 1986, 1993, 2004, P 1014
[357] Even though this herb is classically reported to be slightly toxic, modern research has found no evidence of its toxicity thus far. In the probable event that modern research has missed something here, I have included the classical proscription.
[358] Bensky, D, Clavey, S, Stöger, E & Gamble, A, Chinese Herbal Medicine Materia Medica, 3rd Edition, Seattle, Eastland Press, 1986, 1993, 2004, P 590
[359] Bensky, D, Clavey, S, Stöger, E & Gamble, A, Chinese Herbal Medicine Materia Medica, 3rd Edition, Seattle, Eastland Press, 1986, 1993, 2004, P 589

[360] Chen, JK & TT, Chinese Medical Herbology and Pharmacology, City of Industry, Art of Medicine Press, 2001/2004, P 574

[361] Chen, JK & TT, Chinese Medical Herbology and Pharmacology, City of Industry, Art of Medicine Press, 2001/2004, P 587, Bensky, D, Clavey, S, Stöger, E & Gamble, A, Chinese Herbal Medicine Materia Medica, 3rd Edition, Seattle, Eastland Press, 1986, 1993, 2004, P 559

[362] Brand, E & Wiseman, N, Concise Chinese Materia Medica, Taos, Paradigm Publications, 2008, P 264

[363] Zhang Bing Chen, *Convenient Reader of Materia Medica*, via Bensky, D, Clavey, S, Stöger, E & Gamble, A, Chinese Herbal Medicine Materia Medica, 3rd Edition, Seattle, Eastland Press, 1986, 1993, 2004, P 560

[364] Zhang Bing Chen, *Convenient Reader of Materia Medica*, via Bensky, D, Clavey, S, Stöger, E & Gamble, A, Chinese Herbal Medicine Materia Medica, 3rd Edition, Seattle, Eastland Press, 1986, 1993, 2004, P 560. In this section Bensky, D, Clavey, S, Stöger, E & Gamble, A, Chinese Herbal Medicine Materia Medica, 3rd Edition, Seattle, Eastland Press, 1986, 1993, 2004, P, et al. quote Zhang as saying that San Qi enters the Yang Ming and Jue Yin channels. For some reason they only include the large intestine in their assessment, but not the pericardium. I include it here as it is at least as reasonable a conclusion, and I have used clinically San Qi as a pericardium herb for many years with excellent effects.

[365] Chen, JK & TT, Chinese Medical Herbology and Pharmacology, City of Industry, Art of Medicine Press, 2001/2004, P 568

[366] Brand, E & Wiseman, N, Concise Chinese Materia Medica, Taos, Paradigm Publications, 2008, P 261

[367] Huang Gong Xiu, *Seeking Accuracy in the Materia Medica*, via Bensky, D, Clavey, S, Stöger, E & Gamble, A, Chinese Herbal Medicine Materia Medica, 3rd Edition, Seattle, Eastland Press, 1986, 1993, 2004, P 576

[368] Brand, E & Wiseman, N, Concise Chinese Materia Medica, Taos, Paradigm Publications, 2008, P 261

[369] Brand, E & Wiseman, N, Concise Chinese Materia Medica, Taos, Paradigm Publications, 2008, P 288, Bensky, D, Clavey, S, Stöger, E & Gamble, A, Chinese Herbal Medicine Materia Medica, 3rd Edition, Seattle, Eastland Press, 1986, 1993, 2004, P 624

[370] Brand, E & Wiseman, N, Concise Chinese Materia Medica, Taos, Paradigm Publications, 2008, P 320

[371] Bensky, D, Clavey, S, Stöger, E & Gamble, A, Chinese Herbal Medicine Materia Medica, 3rd Edition, Seattle, Eastland Press, 1986, 1993, 2004, P 432

[372] Bensky, D, Clavey, S, Stöger, E & Gamble, A, Chinese Herbal Medicine Materia Medica, 3rd Edition, Seattle, Eastland Press, 1986, 1993, 2004, P 412

[373] Bensky, D, Clavey, S, Stöger, E & Gamble, A, Chinese Herbal Medicine Materia Medica, 3rd Edition, Seattle, Eastland Press, 1986, 1993, 2004, P 458

[374] Bensky, D, Clavey, S, Stöger, E & Gamble, A, Chinese Herbal Medicine Materia Medica, 3rd Edition, Seattle, Eastland Press, 1986, 1993, 2004, P 407

[375] Bensky, D, Clavey, S, Stöger, E & Gamble, A, Chinese Herbal Medicine Materia Medica, 3rd Edition, Seattle, Eastland Press, 1986, 1993, 2004, P 407

[376] Bensky, D, Clavey, S, Stöger, E & Gamble, A, Chinese Herbal Medicine Materia Medica, 3rd Edition, Seattle, Eastland Press, 1986, 1993, 2004, P 458

[377] Li Shi Zhen, *Grand Materia Medica*, via Bensky, D, Clavey, S, Stöger, E & Gamble, A, Chinese Herbal Medicine Materia Medica, 3rd Edition, Seattle, Eastland Press, 1986, 1993, 2004, P 931
[378] Zhang, Jie Bin, *Rectification of the Meaning of Materia Medica*, via Bensky, D, Clavey, S, Stöger, E & Gamble, A, Chinese Herbal Medicine Materia Medica, 3rd Edition, Seattle, Eastland Press, 1986, 1993, 2004, P 931
[379] Zhang, Jie Bin, *Rectification of the Meaning of Materia Medica*, via Bensky, D, Clavey, S, Stöger, E & Gamble, A, Chinese Herbal Medicine Materia Medica, 3rd Edition, Seattle, Eastland Press, 1986, 1993, 2004, P 931
[380] Brand, E & Wiseman, N, Concise Chinese Materia Medica, Taos, Paradigm Publications, 2008, P 84, and Huang Gong Xiu, *Seeking Accuracy in the Materia Medica*, via Bensky, D, Clavey, S, Stöger, E & Gamble, A, Chinese Herbal Medicine Materia Medica, 3rd Edition, Seattle, Eastland Press, 1986, 1993, 2004, P 112
[381] Brand, E & Wiseman, N, Concise Chinese Materia Medica, Taos, Paradigm Publications, 2008, P 84
[382] Chen, JK & TT, Chinese Medical Herbology and Pharmacology, City of Industry, Art of Medicine Press, 2001/2004, P 825
[383] Chen, JK & TT, Chinese Medical Herbology and Pharmacology, City of Industry, Art of Medicine Press, 2001/2004, P 825
[384] *High Plateau Handbook of Treatment with Chinese Materia Medica*, via Bensky, D, Clavey, S, Stöger, E & Gamble, A, Chinese Herbal Medicine Materia Medica, 3rd Edition, Seattle, Eastland Press, 1986, 1993, 2004, P 742
[385] Brand, E & Wiseman, N, Concise Chinese Materia Medica, Taos, Paradigm Publications, 2008, P 415
[386] Li Shi Zhen, *Grand Materia Medica*, via Bensky, D, Clavey, S, Stöger, E & Gamble, A, Chinese Herbal Medicine Materia Medica, 3rd Edition, Seattle, Eastland Press, 1986, 1993, 2004, P 779
[387] Li Shi Zhen says that Yin Yang Huo is an herb of the Arm and Leg Yang Ming, San Jiao and Ming Men, Li Shi Zhen, *Grand Materia Medica*, via Bensky, D, Clavey, S, Stöger, E & Gamble, A, Chinese Herbal Medicine Materia Medica, 3rd Edition, Seattle, Eastland Press, 1986, 1993, 2004, P 779
[388] Brand, E & Wiseman, N, Concise Chinese Materia Medica, Taos, Paradigm Publications, 2008, P 432
[389] Chen, JK & TT, Chinese Medical Herbology and Pharmacology, City of Industry, Art of Medicine Press, 2001/2004, P 928
[390] Brand, E & Wiseman, N, Concise Chinese Materia Medica, Taos, Paradigm Publications, 2008, P 447
[391] Brand, E & Wiseman, N, Concise Chinese Materia Medica, Taos, Paradigm Publications, 2008, P 446, Bensky, D, Clavey, S, Stöger, E & Gamble, A, Chinese Herbal Medicine Materia Medica, 3rd Edition, Seattle, Eastland Press, 1986, 1993, 2004, P 841
[392] Brand, E & Wiseman, N, Concise Chinese Materia Medica, Taos, Paradigm Publications, 2008, P 461, Bensky, D, Clavey, S, Stöger, E & Gamble, A, Chinese Herbal Medicine Materia Medica, 3rd Edition, Seattle, Eastland Press, 1986, 1993, 2004, P 867
[393] Chen, JK & TT, Chinese Medical Herbology and Pharmacology, City of Industry, Art of Medicine Press, 2001/2004, P 1003, Bensky, D, Clavey, S, Stöger, E & Gamble, A, Chinese Herbal Medicine Materia Medica, 3rd Edition, Seattle, Eastland Press, 1986, 1993, 2004, P 875

[394] Bensky, D, Clavey, S, Stöger, E & Gamble, A, Chinese Herbal Medicine Materia Medica, 3rd Edition, Seattle, Eastland Press, 1986, 1993, 2004, P 875
[395] Bensky, D, Clavey, S, Stöger, E & Gamble, A, Chinese Herbal Medicine Materia Medica, 3rd Edition, Seattle, Eastland Press, 1986, 1993, 2004, P 864
[396] Bensky, D, Clavey, S, Stöger, E & Gamble, A, Chinese Herbal Medicine Materia Medica, 3rd Edition, Seattle, Eastland Press, 1986, 1993, 2004, P 893
[397] Li Shi Zhen, *Grand Materia Medica*, via Bensky, D, Clavey, S, Stöger, E & Gamble, A, Chinese Herbal Medicine Materia Medica, 3rd Edition, Seattle, Eastland Press, 1986, 1993, 2004, P 873
[398] Zhang Xi Chun, *Essays on Medicine Esteeming the Chinese and Respecting the Western*, via Bensky, D, Clavey, S, Stöger, E & Gamble, A, Chinese Herbal Medicine Materia Medica, 3rd Edition, Seattle, Eastland Press, 1986, 1993, 2004, P 873
[399] Chen, JK & TT, Chinese Medical Herbology and Pharmacology, City of Industry, Art of Medicine Press, 2001/2004, P 1002, Bensky, D, Clavey, S, Stöger, E & Gamble, A, Chinese Herbal Medicine Materia Medica, 3rd Edition, Seattle, Eastland Press, 1986, 1993, 2004, P 872
[400] Tang Rong Chuan (Tang Zonghai), Ben Cao Wen Da, Personal Unpublished Translation, 2015, 1.3.3
[401] Bensky, D, Clavey, S, Stöger, E & Gamble, A, Chinese Herbal Medicine Materia Medica, 3rd Edition, Seattle, Eastland Press, 1986, 1993, 2004, P 880
[402] Chen, JK & TT, Chinese Medical Herbology and Pharmacology, City of Industry, Art of Medicine Press, 2001/2004, P 997, Brand, E & Wiseman, N, Concise Chinese Materia Medica, Taos, Paradigm Publications, 2008, P 463
[403] Bensky, D, Clavey, S, Stöger, E & Gamble, A, Chinese Herbal Medicine Materia Medica, 3rd Edition, Seattle, Eastland Press, 1986, 1993, 2004, P 877
[404] Miao Xi Yong, *Commentary on the Divine Husbandman's Classic of Materia Medica*, via Bensky, D, Clavey, S, Stöger, E & Gamble, A, Chinese Herbal Medicine Materia Medica, 3rd Edition, Seattle, Eastland Press, 1986, 1993, 2004, P 888
[405] Bensky, D, Clavey, S, Stöger, E & Gamble, A, Chinese Herbal Medicine Materia Medica, 3rd Edition, Seattle, Eastland Press, 1986, 1993, 2004, P 904
[406] Bensky, D, Clavey, S, Stöger, E & Gamble, A, Chinese Herbal Medicine Materia Medica, 3rd Edition, Seattle, Eastland Press, 1986, 1993, 2004, P 905
[407] Brand, E & Wiseman, N, Concise Chinese Materia Medica, Taos, Paradigm Publications, 2008, P 489
[408] Bensky, D, Clavey, S, Stöger, E & Gamble, A, Chinese Herbal Medicine Materia Medica, 3rd Edition, Seattle, Eastland Press, 1986, 1993, 2004, P 1014
[409] Li Shi Zhen, *Grand Materia Medica*, via Bensky, D, Clavey, S, Stöger, E & Gamble, A, Chinese Herbal Medicine Materia Medica, 3rd Edition, Seattle, Eastland Press, 1986, 1993, 2004, P 1022
[410] Chen, JK & TT, Chinese Medical Herbology and Pharmacology, City of Industry, Art of Medicine Press, 2001/2004, P 1045
[411] Li Shi Zhen, *Grand Materia Medica*, via Bensky, D, Clavey, S, Stöger, E & Gamble, A, Chinese Herbal Medicine Materia Medica, 3rd Edition, Seattle, Eastland Press, 1986, 1993, 2004, P 1022
[412] Chen, JK & TT, Chinese Medical Herbology and Pharmacology, City of Industry, Art of Medicine Press, 2001/2004, P 1039
[413] Brand, E & Wiseman, N, Concise Chinese Materia Medica, Taos, Paradigm Publications, 2008, P 484

[414] Brand, E & Wiseman, N, Concise Chinese Materia Medica, Taos, Paradigm Publications, 2008, P 484
[415] Brand, E & Wiseman, N, Concise Chinese Materia Medica, Taos, Paradigm Publications, 2008, P 484
[416] Brand, E & Wiseman, N, Concise Chinese Materia Medica, Taos, Paradigm Publications, 2008, P 492
[417] Brand, E & Wiseman, N, Concise Chinese Materia Medica, Taos, Paradigm Publications, 2008, P 492
[418] Brand, E & Wiseman, N, Concise Chinese Materia Medica, Taos, Paradigm Publications, 2008, P 492
[419] Brand, E & Wiseman, N, Concise Chinese Materia Medica, Taos, Paradigm Publications, 2008, P 485
[420] Bensky, D, Clavey, S, Stöger, E & Gamble, A, Chinese Herbal Medicine Materia Medica, 3rd Edition, Seattle, Eastland Press, 1986, 1993, 2004, P 1025
[421] Bensky, D, Clavey, S, Stöger, E & Gamble, A, Chinese Herbal Medicine Materia Medica, 3rd Edition, Seattle, Eastland Press, 1986, 1993, 2004, P 1025
[422] Chen, JK & TT, Chinese Medical Herbology and Pharmacology, City of Industry, Art of Medicine Press, 2001/2004, P 59
[423] Tang Rong Chuan (Tang Zonghai), Ben Cao Wen Da, Personal Unpublished Translation, 2015, 1.4.6
[424] Brand, E & Wiseman, N, Concise Chinese Materia Medica, Taos, Paradigm Publications, 2008, P 44
[425] Chen Shi Duo, via Bensky, D, Clavey, S, Stöger, E & Gamble, A, Chinese Herbal Medicine Materia Medica, 3rd Edition, Seattle, Eastland Press, 1986, 1993, 2004, P 37
[426] *Materia Medica of the Kai Bao Era*, via Bensky, D, Clavey, S, Stöger, E & Gamble, A, Chinese Herbal Medicine Materia Medica, 3rd Edition, Seattle, Eastland Press, 1986, 1993, 2004, P 46
[427] Bensky, D, Clavey, S, Stöger, E & Gamble, A, Chinese Herbal Medicine Materia Medica, 3rd Edition, Seattle, Eastland Press, 1986, 1993, 2004, P 78
[428] Brand, E & Wiseman, N, Concise Chinese Materia Medica, Taos, Paradigm Publications, 2008, P 56
[429] Li Shi Zhen, *Grand Materia Medica*, via Bensky, D, Clavey, S, Stöger, E & Gamble, A, Chinese Herbal Medicine Materia Medica, 3rd Edition, Seattle, Eastland Press, 1986, 1993, 2004, P 56
[430] Li Shi Zhen, *Grand Materia Medica*, via Bensky, D, Clavey, S, Stöger, E & Gamble, A, Chinese Herbal Medicine Materia Medica, 3rd Edition, Seattle, Eastland Press, 1986, 1993, 2004, P 56
[431] Zhou Yan, *Thoughtful Differention of Materia Medica*, via Bensky, D, Clavey, S, Stöger, E & Gamble, A, Chinese Herbal Medicine Materia Medica, 3rd Edition, Seattle, Eastland Press, 1986, 1993, 2004, P 62
[432] Brand, E & Wiseman, N, Concise Chinese Materia Medica, Taos, Paradigm Publications, 2008, P 58
[433] Chen, JK & TT, Chinese Medical Herbology and Pharmacology, City of Industry, Art of Medicine Press, 2001/2004, P 77
[434] Tang Rong Chuan (Tang Zonghai), Ben Cao Wen Da, Personal Unpublished Translation, 2015, 2.1.6

[435] Tang Rong Chuan (Tang Zonghai), Ben Cao Wen Da, Personal Unpublished Translation, 2015, 2.1.6

[436] Tang Rong Chuan (Tang Zonghai), Ben Cao Wen Da, Personal Unpublished Translation, 2015, 1.5.10

[437] Tang Rong Chuan (Tang Zonghai), Ben Cao Wen Da, Personal Unpublished Translation, 2015, 1.4.6

[438] Tang Rong Chuan (Tang Zonghai), Ben Cao Wen Da, Personal Unpublished Translation, 2015, 1.5.9

[439] Tang Rong Chuan (Tang Zonghai), Ben Cao Wen Da, Personal Unpublished Translation, 2015, 1.5.9

[440] Tang Rong Chuan (Tang Zonghai), Ben Cao Wen Da, Personal Unpublished Translation, 2015, 1.4.6

[441] Miao Xi Yong, *Commentary on the Divine Husbandman's Classic of Materia Medica*, via Bensky, D, Clavey, S, Stöger, E & Gamble, A, Chinese Herbal Medicine Materia Medica, 3rd Edition, Seattle, Eastland Press, 1986, 1993, 2004, P 211

[442] Tang Rong Chuan (Tang Zonghai), Ben Cao Wen Da, Personal Unpublished Translation, 2015, 1.5.14

[443] Wang Ang, via Bensky, D, Clavey, S, Stöger, E & Gamble, A, Chinese Herbal Medicine Materia Medica, 3rd Edition, Seattle, Eastland Press, 1986, 1993, 2004, P 107

[444] Bensky, D, Clavey, S, Stöger, E & Gamble, A, Chinese Herbal Medicine Materia Medica, 3rd Edition, Seattle, Eastland Press, 1986, 1993, 2004, P 101

[445] Zhou Yan, *Records of Thoughtful Differentiation of Materia Medica*, via Bensky, D, Clavey, S, Stöger, E & Gamble, A, Chinese Herbal Medicine Materia Medica, 3rd Edition, Seattle, Eastland Press, 1986, 1993, 2004, P 96

[446] *Grand Materia Medica*, via Bensky, D, Clavey, S, Stöger, E & Gamble, A, Chinese Herbal Medicine Materia Medica, 3rd Edition, Seattle, Eastland Press, 1986, 1993, 2004, P 104

[447] Brand, E & Wiseman, N, Concise Chinese Materia Medica, Taos, Paradigm Publications, 2008, P 85

[448] Brand, E & Wiseman, N, Concise Chinese Materia Medica, Taos, Paradigm Publications, 2008, P 85

[449] Zhang Shan Lei, via Bensky, D, Clavey, S, Stöger, E & Gamble, A, Chinese Herbal Medicine Materia Medica, 3rd Edition, Seattle, Eastland Press, 1986, 1993, 2004, P 116

[450] Tang Rong Chuan (Tang Zonghai), Ben Cao Wen Da, Personal Unpublished Translation, 2015, 1.3.4 Although this text indicates that Huang Qin enters the San Jiao, the author is also quite specific in distinguishing between the organs and their Jing-channels. Here he does not indicate the Jing-channel, so I do not indicate otherwise.

[451] Chen, JK & TT, Chinese Medical Herbology and Pharmacology, City of Industry, Art of Medicine Press, 2001/2004, P 151

[452] Bensky, D, Clavey, S, Stöger, E & Gamble, A, Chinese Herbal Medicine Materia Medica, 3rd Edition, Seattle, Eastland Press, 1986, 1993, 2004, P 144

[453] Tang Rong Chuan (Tang Zonghai), Ben Cao Wen Da, Personal Unpublished Translation, 2015, 1.5.3

[454] Maciocia, G, The Channels of Acupuncture, Philadelphia, Elsevier, 2006, P 446

[455] Brand, E & Wiseman, N, Concise Chinese Materia Medica, Taos, Paradigm Publications, 2008, P 114
[456] Brand, E & Wiseman, N, Concise Chinese Materia Medica, Taos, Paradigm Publications, 2008, P114, Bensky, D, Clavey, S, Stöger, E & Gamble, A, Chinese Herbal Medicine Materia Medica, 3rd Edition, Seattle, Eastland Press, 1986, 1993, 2004, P 147
[457] Bensky, D, Clavey, S, Stöger, E & Gamble, A, Chinese Herbal Medicine Materia Medica, 3rd Edition, Seattle, Eastland Press, 1986, 1993, 2004, P 147
[458] Tang Rong Chuan (Tang Zonghai), Ben Cao Wen Da, Personal Unpublished Translation, 2015, 1.3.4
[459] Brand, E & Wiseman, N, Concise Chinese Materia Medica, Taos, Paradigm Publications, 2008, P 90
[460] Bensky, D, Clavey, S, Stöger, E & Gamble, A, Chinese Herbal Medicine Materia Medica, 3rd Edition, Seattle, Eastland Press, 1986, 1993, 2004, P 119
[461] Wang, Hao Gu, *Harm and Benefit in the Materia Medica*, via Bensky, D, Clavey, S, Stöger, E & Gamble, A, Chinese Herbal Medicine Materia Medica, 3rd Edition, Seattle, Eastland Press, 1986, 1993, 2004, P 152
[462] Bensky, D, Clavey, S, Stöger, E & Gamble, A, Chinese Herbal Medicine Materia Medica, 3rd Edition, Seattle, Eastland Press, 1986, 1993, 2004, P 151
[463] Wang, Hao Gu, *Harm and Benefit in the Materia Medica*, via Bensky, D, Clavey, S, Stöger, E & Gamble, A, Chinese Herbal Medicine Materia Medica, 3rd Edition, Seattle, Eastland Press, 1986, 1993, 2004, P 152
[464] Bensky, D, Clavey, S, Stöger, E & Gamble, A, Chinese Herbal Medicine Materia Medica, 3rd Edition, Seattle, Eastland Press, 1986, 1993, 2004, P 207
[465] Brand, E & Wiseman, N, Concise Chinese Materia Medica, Taos, Paradigm Publications, 2008, P 112
[466] Bensky, D, Clavey, S, Stöger, E & Gamble, A, Chinese Herbal Medicine Materia Medica, 3rd Edition, Seattle, Eastland Press, 1986, 1993, 2004, P 207
[467] Bensky, D, Clavey, S, Stöger, E & Gamble, A, Chinese Herbal Medicine Materia Medica, 3rd Edition, Seattle, Eastland Press, 1986, 1993, 2004, P 206
[468] Brand, E & Wiseman, N, Concise Chinese Materia Medica, Taos, Paradigm Publications, 2008, P 99
[469] Brand, E & Wiseman, N, Concise Chinese Materia Medica, Taos, Paradigm Publications, 2008, P 107
[470] Bensky, D, Clavey, S, Stöger, E & Gamble, A, Chinese Herbal Medicine Materia Medica, 3rd Edition, Seattle, Eastland Press, 1986, 1993, 2004, P 205
[471] Bensky, D, Clavey, S, Stöger, E & Gamble, A, Chinese Herbal Medicine Materia Medica, 3rd Edition, Seattle, Eastland Press, 1986, 1993, 2004, P 159
[472] Brand, E & Wiseman, N, Concise Chinese Materia Medica, Taos, Paradigm Publications, 2008, P 108
[473] Zhang Bing Cheng, *Convenient Reader of Materia Medica*, via Bensky, D, Clavey, S, Stöger, E & Gamble, A, Chinese Herbal Medicine Materia Medica, 3rd Edition, Seattle, Eastland Press, 1986, 1993, 2004, P 156

[474] *Encountering the Sources of the Classic of Materia Medica*, via Bensky, D, Clavey, S, Stöger, E & Gamble, A, Chinese Herbal Medicine Materia Medica, 3rd Edition, Seattle, Eastland Press, 1986, 1993, 2004, P172
[475] *Encountering the Sources of the Classic of Materia Medica*, via Bensky, D, Clavey, S, Stöger, E & Gamble, A, Chinese Herbal Medicine Materia Medica, 3rd Edition, Seattle, Eastland Press, 1986, 1993, 2004, P172
[476] Bensky, D, Clavey, S, Stöger, E & Gamble, A, Chinese Herbal Medicine Materia Medica, 3rd Edition, Seattle, Eastland Press, 1986, 1993, 2004, P 171
[477] Bensky, D, Clavey, S, Stöger, E & Gamble, A, Chinese Herbal Medicine Materia Medica, 3rd Edition, Seattle, Eastland Press, 1986, 1993, 2004, P 161
[478] Brand, E & Wiseman, N, Concise Chinese Materia Medica, Taos, Paradigm Publications, 2008, P 115
[479479] Bensky, D, Clavey, S, Stöger, E & Gamble, A, Chinese Herbal Medicine Materia Medica, 3rd Edition, Seattle, Eastland Press, 1986, 1993, 2004, P 216
[480] Bensky, D, Clavey, S, Stöger, E & Gamble, A, Chinese Herbal Medicine Materia Medica, 3rd Edition, Seattle, Eastland Press, 1986, 1993, 2004, P 216
[481] Bensky, D, Clavey, S, Stöger, E & Gamble, A, Chinese Herbal Medicine Materia Medica, 3rd Edition, Seattle, Eastland Press, 1986, 1993, 2004, P 183
[482] Brand, E & Wiseman, N, Concise Chinese Materia Medica, Taos, Paradigm Publications, 2008, P 114
[483] Brand, E & Wiseman, N, Concise Chinese Materia Medica, Taos, Paradigm Publications, 2008, P114, Bensky, D, Clavey, S, Stöger, E & Gamble, A, Chinese Herbal Medicine Materia Medica, 3rd Edition, Seattle, Eastland Press, 1986, 1993, 2004, P 147
[484] Bensky, D, Clavey, S, Stöger, E & Gamble, A, Chinese Herbal Medicine Materia Medica, 3rd Edition, Seattle, Eastland Press, 1986, 1993, 2004, P 147
[485] *Miscellaneous Records of Famous Physicians*, via Bensky, D, Clavey, S, Stöger, E & Gamble, A, Chinese Herbal Medicine Materia Medica, 3rd Edition, Seattle, Eastland Press, 1986, 1993, 2004, P 174
[486] Bensky, D, Clavey, S, Stöger, E & Gamble, A, Chinese Herbal Medicine Materia Medica, 3rd Edition, Seattle, Eastland Press, 1986, 1993, 2004, P 215
[487] Bensky, D, Clavey, S, Stöger, E & Gamble, A, Chinese Herbal Medicine Materia Medica, 3rd Edition, Seattle, Eastland Press, 1986, 1993, 2004, P 215
[488] Bensky, D, Clavey, S, Stöger, E & Gamble, A, Chinese Herbal Medicine Materia Medica, 3rd Edition, Seattle, Eastland Press, 1986, 1993, 2004, P 215
[489] Bensky, D, Clavey, S, Stöger, E & Gamble, A, Chinese Herbal Medicine Materia Medica, 3rd Edition, Seattle, Eastland Press, 1986, 1993, 2004, P 1010
[490] Bensky, D, Clavey, S, Stöger, E & Gamble, A, Chinese Herbal Medicine Materia Medica, 3rd Edition, Seattle, Eastland Press, 1986, 1993, 2004, P 1010
[491] Brand, E & Wiseman, N, Concise Chinese Materia Medica, Taos, Paradigm Publications, 2008, P 102
[492] Zhang Bing Chen, *Convenient Reader of Materia Medica*, via Bensky, D, Clavey, S, Stöger, E & Gamble, A, Chinese Herbal Medicine Materia Medica, 3rd Edition, Seattle, Eastland Press, 1986, 1993, 2004, P 165

[493] *Rectification of the Meaning of Materia Medica*, via Bensky, D, Clavey, S, Stöger, E & Gamble, A, Chinese Herbal Medicine Materia Medica, 3rd Edition, Seattle, Eastland Press, 1986, 1993, 2004, P 185
[494] Brand, E & Wiseman, N, Concise Chinese Materia Medica, Taos, Paradigm Publications, 2008, P 120, Bensky, D, Clavey, S, Stöger, E & Gamble, A, Chinese Herbal Medicine Materia Medica, 3rd Edition, Seattle, Eastland Press, 1986, 1993, 2004, P 224
[495] Bensky, D, Clavey, S, Stöger, E & Gamble, A, Chinese Herbal Medicine Materia Medica, 3rd Edition, Seattle, Eastland Press, 1986, 1993, 2004, P 224
[496] Chen, JK & TT, Chinese Medical Herbology and Pharmacology, City of Industry, Art of Medicine Press, 2001/2004, P 247
[497] Tang Rong Chuan (Tang Zonghai), Ben Cao Wen Da, Personal Unpublished Translation, 2015, 1.3.4
[498] Chen, JK & TT, Chinese Medical Herbology and Pharmacology, City of Industry, Art of Medicine Press, 2001/2004, P 244
[499] Brand, E & Wiseman, N, Concise Chinese Materia Medica, Taos, Paradigm Publications, 2008, P 119
[500] Brand, E & Wiseman, N, Concise Chinese Materia Medica, Taos, Paradigm Publications, 2008, P 121
[501] Bensky, D, Clavey, S, Stöger, E & Gamble, A, Chinese Herbal Medicine Materia Medica, 3rd Edition, Seattle, Eastland Press, 1986, 1993, 2004, P 240
[502] Chen, JK & TT, Chinese Medical Herbology and Pharmacology, City of Industry, Art of Medicine Press, 2001/2004, P 274
[503] Brand, E & Wiseman, N, Concise Chinese Materia Medica, Taos, Paradigm Publications, 2008, P 142
[504] Brand, E & Wiseman, N, Concise Chinese Materia Medica, Taos, Paradigm Publications, 2008, P 132
[505] Tang Rong Chuan (Tang Zonghai), Ben Cao Wen Da, Personal Unpublished Translation, 2015, 1.5.3
[506] Bensky, D, Clavey, S, Stöger, E & Gamble, A, Chinese Herbal Medicine Materia Medica, 3rd Edition, Seattle, Eastland Press, 1986, 1993, 2004, P 239
[507] Tang Rong Chuan (Tang Zonghai), Ben Cao Wen Da, Personal Unpublished Translation, 2015, 1.5.2
[508] Maciocia, G, The Channels of Acupuncture, Philadelphia, Elsevier, 2006, P 446
[509] Bensky, D, Clavey, S, Stöger, E & Gamble, A, Chinese Herbal Medicine Materia Medica, 3rd Edition, Seattle, Eastland Press, 1986, 1993, 2004, P 243
[510] Brand, E & Wiseman, N, Concise Chinese Materia Medica, Taos, Paradigm Publications, 2008, P 142
[511] Bensky, D, Clavey, S, Stöger, E & Gamble, A, Chinese Herbal Medicine Materia Medica, 3rd Edition, Seattle, Eastland Press, 1986, 1993, 2004, P 355
[512] Bensky, D, Clavey, S, Stöger, E & Gamble, A, Chinese Herbal Medicine Materia Medica, 3rd Edition, Seattle, Eastland Press, 1986, 1993, 2004, P 354
[513] Bensky, D, Clavey, S, Stöger, E & Gamble, A, Chinese Herbal Medicine Materia Medica, 3rd Edition, Seattle, Eastland Press, 1986, 1993, 2004, P 354

[514] Brand, E & Wiseman, N, Concise Chinese Materia Medica, Taos, Paradigm Publications, 2008, P 154, Chen, JK & TT, Chinese Medical Herbology and Pharmacology, City of Industry, Art of Medicine Press, 2001/2004, P 312

[515] Tang Rong Chuan (Tang Zonghai), Ben Cao Wen Da, Personal Unpublished Translation, 2015, 1.5.14

[516] Chen, JK & TT, Chinese Medical Herbology and Pharmacology, City of Industry, Art of Medicine Press, 2001/2004, P 461

[517] Zhang, Shan Lei, *Rectification of the Meaning of Materia Medica,* via Bensky, D, Clavey, S, Stöger, E & Gamble, A, Chinese Herbal Medicine Materia Medica, 3rd Edition, Seattle, Eastland Press, 1986, 1993, 2004, P 482

[518] Zhang, Shan Lei, *Rectification of the Meaning of Materia Medica,* via Bensky, D, Clavey, S, Stöger, E & Gamble, A, Chinese Herbal Medicine Materia Medica, 3rd Edition, Seattle, Eastland Press, 1986, 1993, 2004, P 482

[519] Huang Gong Xiu, *Seeking Accuracy in the Materia Medica*, and, *Harm and Benefit in the Materia Medica*, both via Bensky, D, Clavey, S, Stöger, E & Gamble, A, Chinese Herbal Medicine Materia Medica, 3rd Edition, Seattle, Eastland Press, 1986, 1993, 2004, P 482

[520] Bensky, D, Clavey, S, Stöger, E & Gamble, A, Chinese Herbal Medicine Materia Medica, 3rd Edition, Seattle, Eastland Press, 1986, 1993, 2004, P 487

[521] Tang Rong Chuan (Tang Zonghai), Ben Cao Wen Da, Personal Unpublished Translation, 2015, 1.3.3

[522] Maciocia, G, The Channels of Acupuncture, Philadelphia, Elsevier, 2006, P 585

[523] Brand, E & Wiseman, N, Concise Chinese Materia Medica, Taos, Paradigm Publications, 2008, P 188

[524] Brand, E & Wiseman, N, Concise Chinese Materia Medica, Taos, Paradigm Publications, 2008, P 194

[525] Brand, E & Wiseman, N, Concise Chinese Materia Medica, Taos, Paradigm Publications, 2008, P186

[526] Zhang Bing Chen, *Convenient Reader of Materia Medica*, via Bensky, D, Clavey, S, Stöger, E & Gamble, A, Chinese Herbal Medicine Materia Medica, 3rd Edition, Seattle, Eastland Press, 1986, 1993, 2004, P 299

[527] Zhang Bing Chen, *Convenient Reader of Materia Medica*, via Bensky, D, Clavey, S, Stöger, E & Gamble, A, Chinese Herbal Medicine Materia Medica, 3rd Edition, Seattle, Eastland Press, 1986, 1993, 2004, P 299

[528] Brand, E & Wiseman, N, Concise Chinese Materia Medica, Taos, Paradigm Publications, 2008, P 200

[529] Chen, JK & TT, Chinese Medical Herbology and Pharmacology, City of Industry, Art of Medicine Press, 2001/2004, P 461

[530] Brand, E & Wiseman, N, Concise Chinese Materia Medica, Taos, Paradigm Publications, 2008, P 216

[531] Bensky, D, Clavey, S, Stöger, E & Gamble, A, Chinese Herbal Medicine Materia Medica, 3rd Edition, Seattle, Eastland Press, 1986, 1993, 2004, P 700

[532] Tang Rong Chuan (Tang Zonghai), Ben Cao Wen Da, Personal Unpublished Translation, 2015, 1.5.13

[533] Brand, E & Wiseman, N, Concise Chinese Materia Medica, Taos, Paradigm Publications, 2008, P 212
[534] Brand, E & Wiseman, N, Concise Chinese Materia Medica, Taos, Paradigm Publications, 2008, P 234
[535] Huang Gong Xiu, *Seeking Accuracy in the Materia Medica*, via Bensky, D, Clavey, S, Stöger, E & Gamble, A, Chinese Herbal Medicine Materia Medica, 3rd Edition, Seattle, Eastland Press, 1986, 1993, 2004, P 548
[536] Bensky, D, Clavey, S, Stöger, E & Gamble, A, Chinese Herbal Medicine Materia Medica, 3rd Edition, Seattle, Eastland Press, 1986, 1993, 2004, P 510
[537] Bensky, D, Clavey, S, Stöger, E & Gamble, A, Chinese Herbal Medicine Materia Medica, 3rd Edition, Seattle, Eastland Press, 1986, 1993, 2004, P 519
[538] Brand, E & Wiseman, N, Concise Chinese Materia Medica, Taos, Paradigm Publications, 2008, P 226
[539] Brand, E & Wiseman, N, Concise Chinese Materia Medica, Taos, Paradigm Publications, 2008, P 226, Bensky, D, Clavey, S, Stöger, E & Gamble, A, Chinese Herbal Medicine Materia Medica, 3rd Edition, Seattle, Eastland Press, 1986, 1993, 2004, P 517
[540] Bensky, D, Clavey, S, Stöger, E & Gamble, A, Chinese Herbal Medicine Materia Medica, 3rd Edition, Seattle, Eastland Press, 1986, 1993, 2004, P 543
[541] Bensky, D, Clavey, S, Stöger, E & Gamble, A, Chinese Herbal Medicine Materia Medica, 3rd Edition, Seattle, Eastland Press, 1986, 1993, 2004, P 544
[542] Bensky, D, Clavey, S, Stöger, E & Gamble, A, Chinese Herbal Medicine Materia Medica, 3rd Edition, Seattle, Eastland Press, 1986, 1993, 2004, P 530
[543] Brand, E & Wiseman, N, Concise Chinese Materia Medica, Taos, Paradigm Publications, 2008, P 228, Bensky, D, Clavey, S, Stöger, E & Gamble, A, Chinese Herbal Medicine Materia Medica, 3rd Edition, Seattle, Eastland Press, 1986, 1993, 2004, P 530
[544] Zhang Xi Chun, *Essays on Medicine Esteeming the Chinese and Respecting the Western*, via Bensky, D, Clavey, S, Stöger, E & Gamble, A, Chinese Herbal Medicine Materia Medica, 3rd Edition, Seattle, Eastland Press, 1986, 1993, 2004, P 545
[545] Zhang, Jie Bin, *Rectification of the Meaning of Materia Medica*, via Bensky, D, Clavey, S, Stöger, E & Gamble, A, Chinese Herbal Medicine Materia Medica, 3rd Edition, Seattle, Eastland Press, 1986, 1993, 2004, P 515
[546] Zhang, Jie Bin, *Rectification of the Meaning of Materia Medica*, via Bensky, D, Clavey, S, Stöger, E & Gamble, A, Chinese Herbal Medicine Materia Medica, 3rd Edition, Seattle, Eastland Press, 1986, 1993, 2004, P 515
[547] Bensky, D, Clavey, S, Stöger, E & Gamble, A, Chinese Herbal Medicine Materia Medica, 3rd Edition, Seattle, Eastland Press, 1986, 1993, 2004, P 550
[548] Bensky, D, Clavey, S, Stöger, E & Gamble, A, Chinese Herbal Medicine Materia Medica, 3rd Edition, Seattle, Eastland Press, 1986, 1993, 2004, P 550
[549] Brand, E & Wiseman, N, Concise Chinese Materia Medica, Taos, Paradigm Publications, 2008, P 233
[550] Brand, E & Wiseman, N, Concise Chinese Materia Medica, Taos, Paradigm Publications, 2008, P 233
[551] Li Shi Zhen, *Grand Materia Medica*, via Bensky, D, Clavey, S, Stöger, E & Gamble, A, Chinese Herbal Medicine Materia Medica, 3rd Edition, Seattle, Eastland Press, 1986, 1993, 2004, P 500

[552] Zhang Xi Chun, *Essays on Medicine Esteeming the Chinese and Respecting the Western*, via Bensky, D, Clavey, S, Stöger, E & Gamble, A, Chinese Herbal Medicine Materia Medica, 3rd Edition, Seattle, Eastland Press, 1986, 1993, 2004, P 494

[553] Li Shi Zhen and Huang Gong Xiu, *Seeking Accuracy in the Materia Medica*, via Bensky, D, Clavey, S, Stöger, E & Gamble, A, Chinese Herbal Medicine Materia Medica, 3rd Edition, Seattle, Eastland Press, 1986, 1993, 2004, P 498

[554] Bensky, D, Clavey, S, Stöger, E & Gamble, A, Chinese Herbal Medicine Materia Medica, 3rd Edition, Seattle, Eastland Press, 1986, 1993, 2004, P 1001

[555] Bensky, D, Clavey, S, Stöger, E & Gamble, A, Chinese Herbal Medicine Materia Medica, 3rd Edition, Seattle, Eastland Press, 1986, 1993, 2004, P 1001

[556] Bensky, D, Clavey, S, Stöger, E & Gamble, A, Chinese Herbal Medicine Materia Medica, 3rd Edition, Seattle, Eastland Press, 1986, 1993, 2004, P 1001

[557] Brand, E & Wiseman, N, Concise Chinese Materia Medica, Taos, Paradigm Publications, 2008, P 489

[558] Bensky, D, Clavey, S, Stöger, E & Gamble, A, Chinese Herbal Medicine Materia Medica, 3rd Edition, Seattle, Eastland Press, 1986, 1993, 2004, P 1014

[559] Even though this herb is classically reported to be slightly toxic, modern research has found no evidence of its toxicity thus far. In the probable event that modern research has missed something here, I have included the classical proscription.

[560] Bensky, D, Clavey, S, Stöger, E & Gamble, A, Chinese Herbal Medicine Materia Medica, 3rd Edition, Seattle, Eastland Press, 1986, 1993, 2004, P 1007

[561] *Divine Husbandman's Classic of Materia Medica*, via Bensky, D, Clavey, S, Stöger, E & Gamble, A, Chinese Herbal Medicine Materia Medica, 3rd Edition, Seattle, Eastland Press, 1986, 1993, 2004, P 1007

[562] Bensky, D, Clavey, S, Stöger, E & Gamble, A, Chinese Herbal Medicine Materia Medica, 3rd Edition, Seattle, Eastland Press, 1986, 1993, 2004, P 998

[563] Bensky, D, Clavey, S, Stöger, E & Gamble, A, Chinese Herbal Medicine Materia Medica, 3rd Edition, Seattle, Eastland Press, 1986, 1993, 2004, P 1010

[564] Bensky, D, Clavey, S, Stöger, E & Gamble, A, Chinese Herbal Medicine Materia Medica, 3rd Edition, Seattle, Eastland Press, 1986, 1993, 2004, P 1010

[565] Zhang Lu, *Encountering the Sources of the Classic of Materia Medica*, via Bensky, D, Clavey, S, Stöger, E & Gamble, A, Chinese Herbal Medicine Materia Medica, 3rd Edition, Seattle, Eastland Press, 1986, 1993, 2004, P 1003

[566] Bensky, D, Clavey, S, Stöger, E & Gamble, A, Chinese Herbal Medicine Materia Medica, 3rd Edition, Seattle, Eastland Press, 1986, 1993, 2004, P 579

[567] Brand, E & Wiseman, N, Concise Chinese Materia Medica, Taos, Paradigm Publications, 2008, P 267

[568] Chen, JK & TT, Chinese Medical Herbology and Pharmacology, City of Industry, Art of Medicine Press, 2001/2004, P 587, Bensky, D, Clavey, S, Stöger, E & Gamble, A, Chinese Herbal Medicine Materia Medica, 3rd Edition, Seattle, Eastland Press, 1986, 1993, 2004, P 559

[569] Brand, E & Wiseman, N, Concise Chinese Materia Medica, Taos, Paradigm Publications, 2008, P 264

[570] Zhang Bing Chen, *Convenient Reader of Materia Medica*, via Bensky, D, Clavey, S, Stöger, E & Gamble, A, Chinese Herbal Medicine Materia Medica, 3rd Edition, Seattle, Eastland Press, 1986, 1993, 2004, P 560

[571] Zhang Bing Chen, *Convenient Reader of Materia Medica*, via Bensky, D, Clavey, S, Stöger, E & Gamble, A, Chinese Herbal Medicine Materia Medica, 3rd Edition, Seattle, Eastland Press, 1986, 1993, 2004, P 560. In this section Bensky, D, Clavey, S, Stöger, E & Gamble, A, Chinese Herbal Medicine Materia Medica, 3rd Edition, Seattle, Eastland Press, 1986, 1993, 2004, P, et al. quote Zhang as saying that San Qi enters the Yang Ming and Jue Yin channels. For some reason they only include the large intestine in their assessment, but not the pericardium. I include it here as it is at least as reasonable a conclusion, and I have used clinically San Qi as a pericardium herb for many years with excellent effects.

[572] Chen, JK & TT, Chinese Medical Herbology and Pharmacology, City of Industry, Art of Medicine Press, 2001/2004, P 568

[573] Brand, E & Wiseman, N, Concise Chinese Materia Medica, Taos, Paradigm Publications, 2008, P 261

[574] Brand, E & Wiseman, N, Concise Chinese Materia Medica, Taos, Paradigm Publications, 2008, P 269

[575] Bensky, D, Clavey, S, Stöger, E & Gamble, A, Chinese Herbal Medicine Materia Medica, 3rd Edition, Seattle, Eastland Press, 1986, 1993, 2004, P 588

[576] Bensky, D, Clavey, S, Stöger, E & Gamble, A, Chinese Herbal Medicine Materia Medica, 3rd Edition, Seattle, Eastland Press, 1986, 1993, 2004, P 588

[577] Bensky, D, Clavey, S, Stöger, E & Gamble, A, Chinese Herbal Medicine Materia Medica, 3rd Edition, Seattle, Eastland Press, 1986, 1993, 2004, P 655

[578] Zhang Bing Chen, *Convenient Reader of Materia Medica*, via Bensky, D, Clavey, S, Stöger, E & Gamble, A, Chinese Herbal Medicine Materia Medica, 3rd Edition, Seattle, Eastland Press, 1986, 1993, 2004, P 607

[579] Bensky, D, Clavey, S, Stöger, E & Gamble, A, Chinese Herbal Medicine Materia Medica, 3rd Edition, Seattle, Eastland Press, 1986, 1993, 2004, P 653

[580] Bensky, D, Clavey, S, Stöger, E & Gamble, A, Chinese Herbal Medicine Materia Medica, 3rd Edition, Seattle, Eastland Press, 1986, 1993, 2004, P 612

[581] Brand, E & Wiseman, N, Concise Chinese Materia Medica, Taos, Paradigm Publications, 2008, P 293

[582] Brand, E & Wiseman, N, Concise Chinese Materia Medica, Taos, Paradigm Publications, 2008, P 293

[583] Brand, E & Wiseman, N, Concise Chinese Materia Medica, Taos, Paradigm Publications, 2008, P 300

[584] Chen, JK & TT, Chinese Medical Herbology and Pharmacology, City of Industry, Art of Medicine Press, 2001/2004, P 655

[585] Brand, E & Wiseman, N, Concise Chinese Materia Medica, Taos, Paradigm Publications, 2008, P 320

[586] Bensky, D, Clavey, S, Stöger, E & Gamble, A, Chinese Herbal Medicine Materia Medica, 3rd Edition, Seattle, Eastland Press, 1986, 1993, 2004, P 432

[587] Bensky, D, Clavey, S, Stöger, E & Gamble, A, Chinese Herbal Medicine Materia Medica, 3rd Edition, Seattle, Eastland Press, 1986, 1993, 2004, P 412

[588] Chen, JK & TT, Chinese Medical Herbology and Pharmacology, City of Industry, Art of Medicine Press, 2001/2004, P 713
[589] Bensky, D, Clavey, S, Stöger, E & Gamble, A, Chinese Herbal Medicine Materia Medica, 3rd Edition, Seattle, Eastland Press, 1986, 1993, 2004, P 401
[590] Brand, E & Wiseman, N, Concise Chinese Materia Medica, Taos, Paradigm Publications, 2008, P 313
[591] Brand, E & Wiseman, N, Concise Chinese Materia Medica, Taos, Paradigm Publications, 2008, P 313
[592] Brand, E & Wiseman, N, Concise Chinese Materia Medica, Taos, Paradigm Publications, 2008, P 312
[593593] Brand, E & Wiseman, N, Concise Chinese Materia Medica, Taos, Paradigm Publications, 2008, 312, Bensky, D, Clavey, S, Stöger, E & Gamble, A, Chinese Herbal Medicine Materia Medica, 3rd Edition, Seattle, Eastland Press, 1986, 1993, 2004, P 421
[594] Bensky, D, Clavey, S, Stöger, E & Gamble, A, Chinese Herbal Medicine Materia Medica, 3rd Edition, Seattle, Eastland Press, 1986, 1993, 2004, P 655
[595] Brand, E & Wiseman, N, Concise Chinese Materia Medica, Taos, Paradigm Publications, 2008, P 322
[596] Brand, E & Wiseman, N, Concise Chinese Materia Medica, Taos, Paradigm Publications, 2008, P 322
[597] Chen, JK & TT, Chinese Medical Herbology and Pharmacology, City of Industry, Art of Medicine Press, 2001/2004, P 715
[598] Chen, JK & TT, Chinese Medical Herbology and Pharmacology, City of Industry, Art of Medicine Press, 2001/2004, P 715
[599] Bensky, D, Clavey, S, Stöger, E & Gamble, A, Chinese Herbal Medicine Materia Medica, 3rd Edition, Seattle, Eastland Press, 1986, 1993, 2004, P 404
[600] Brand, E & Wiseman, N, Concise Chinese Materia Medica, Taos, Paradigm Publications, 2008, P 321
[601] Brand, E & Wiseman, N, Concise Chinese Materia Medica, Taos, Paradigm Publications, 2008, P 321
[602] Brand, E & Wiseman, N, Concise Chinese Materia Medica, Taos, Paradigm Publications, 2008, P 162
[603] Bensky, D, Clavey, S, Stöger, E & Gamble, A, Chinese Herbal Medicine Materia Medica, 3rd Edition, Seattle, Eastland Press, 1986, 1993, 2004, P 428
[604] Bensky, D, Clavey, S, Stöger, E & Gamble, A, Chinese Herbal Medicine Materia Medica, 3rd Edition, Seattle, Eastland Press, 1986, 1993, 2004, P 446
[605] Brand, E & Wiseman, N, Concise Chinese Materia Medica, Taos, Paradigm Publications, 2008, P 332
[606] Bensky, D, Clavey, S, Stöger, E & Gamble, A, Chinese Herbal Medicine Materia Medica, 3rd Edition, Seattle, Eastland Press, 1986, 1993, 2004, P 813
[607] *Sichuan Chinese Materia Medica*, via Bensky, D, Clavey, S, Stöger, E & Gamble, A, Chinese Herbal Medicine Materia Medica, 3rd Edition, Seattle, Eastland Press, 1986, 1993, 2004, P 939
[608] *Sichuan Chinese Materia Medica*, via Bensky, D, Clavey, S, Stöger, E & Gamble, A, Chinese Herbal Medicine Materia Medica, 3rd Edition, Seattle, Eastland Press, 1986, 1993, 2004, P 939

[609] Bensky, D, Clavey, S, Stöger, E & Gamble, A, Chinese Herbal Medicine Materia Medica, 3rd Edition, Seattle, Eastland Press, 1986, 1993, 2004, P 543
[610] Chen, JK & TT, Chinese Medical Herbology and Pharmacology, City of Industry, Art of Medicine Press, 2001/2004, P 825
[611] Chen, JK & TT, Chinese Medical Herbology and Pharmacology, City of Industry, Art of Medicine Press, 2001/2004, P 825
[612] Brand, E & Wiseman, N, Concise Chinese Materia Medica, Taos, Paradigm Publications, 2008, P 385, Bensky, D, Clavey, S, Stöger, E & Gamble, A, Chinese Herbal Medicine Materia Medica, 3rd Edition, Seattle, Eastland Press, 1986, 1993, 2004, P 956
[613] *High Plateau Handbook of Treatment with Chinese Materia Medica*, via Bensky, D, Clavey, S, Stöger, E & Gamble, A, Chinese Herbal Medicine Materia Medica, 3rd Edition, Seattle, Eastland Press, 1986, 1993, 2004, P 742
[614] Bensky, D, Clavey, S, Stöger, E & Gamble, A, Chinese Herbal Medicine Materia Medica, 3rd Edition, Seattle, Eastland Press, 1986, 1993, 2004, P 742
[615] Maciocia, G, The Channels of Acupuncture, Philadelphia, Elsevier, 2006, P 545
[616] Huang Gong Xiu, *Seeking Accuracy in the Materia Medica*, via Bensky, D, Clavey, S, Stöger, E & Gamble, A, Chinese Herbal Medicine Materia Medica, 3rd Edition, Seattle, Eastland Press, 1986, 1993, 2004, P 727
[617] Brand, E & Wiseman, N, Concise Chinese Materia Medica, Taos, Paradigm Publications, 2008, P 407
[618] Tang Rong Chuan (Tang Zonghai), Ben Cao Wen Da, Personal Unpublished Translation, 2015, 2.2.5
[619] Bensky, D, Clavey, S, Stöger, E & Gamble, A, Chinese Herbal Medicine Materia Medica, 3rd Edition, Seattle, Eastland Press, 1986, 1993, 2004, P 739
[620] Bensky, D, Clavey, S, Stöger, E & Gamble, A, Chinese Herbal Medicine Materia Medica, 3rd Edition, Seattle, Eastland Press, 1986, 1993, 2004, P 813
[621] Li Shi Zhen, *Grand Materia Medica*, via Bensky, D, Clavey, S, Stöger, E & Gamble, A, Chinese Herbal Medicine Materia Medica, 3rd Edition, Seattle, Eastland Press, 1986, 1993, 2004, P 779
[622] Li Shi Zhen says that Yin Yang Huo is an herb of the Arm and Leg Yang Ming, San Jiao and Ming Men, Li Shi Zhen, *Grand Materia Medica*, via Bensky, D, Clavey, S, Stöger, E & Gamble, A, Chinese Herbal Medicine Materia Medica, 3rd Edition, Seattle, Eastland Press, 1986, 1993, 2004, P 779
[623] Brand, E & Wiseman, N, Concise Chinese Materia Medica, Taos, Paradigm Publications, 2008, P 435, Bensky, D, Clavey, S, Stöger, E & Gamble, A, Chinese Herbal Medicine Materia Medica, 3rd Edition, Seattle, Eastland Press, 1986, 1993, 2004, P 818
[624] Brand, E & Wiseman, N, Concise Chinese Materia Medica, Taos, Paradigm Publications, 2008, P 435, Bensky, D, Clavey, S, Stöger, E & Gamble, A, Chinese Herbal Medicine Materia Medica, 3rd Edition, Seattle, Eastland Press, 1986, 1993, 2004, P 818
[625] Zhang Xi Chun, *Essays on Medicine Esteeming the Chinese and Respecting the Western*, via Bensky, D, Clavey, S, Stöger, E & Gamble, A, Chinese Herbal Medicine Materia Medica, 3rd Edition, Seattle, Eastland Press, 1986, 1993, 2004, P 821
[626] Brand, E & Wiseman, N, Concise Chinese Materia Medica, Taos, Paradigm Publications, 2008, P 439

[627] Brand, E & Wiseman, N, Concise Chinese Materia Medica, Taos, Paradigm Publications, 2008, P 436, Bensky, D, Clavey, S, Stöger, E & Gamble, A, Chinese Herbal Medicine Materia Medica, 3rd Edition, Seattle, Eastland Press, 1986, 1993, 2004, P 825
[628] Chen, JK & TT, Chinese Medical Herbology and Pharmacology, City of Industry, Art of Medicine Press, 2001/2004, P 943
[629] Brand, E & Wiseman, N, Concise Chinese Materia Medica, Taos, Paradigm Publications, 2008, P 436, Bensky, D, Clavey, S, Stöger, E & Gamble, A, Chinese Herbal Medicine Materia Medica, 3rd Edition, Seattle, Eastland Press, 1986, 1993, 2004, P 825
[630] Brand, E & Wiseman, N, Concise Chinese Materia Medica, Taos, Paradigm Publications, 2008, P 437
[631] Bensky, D, Clavey, S, Stöger, E & Gamble, A, Chinese Herbal Medicine Materia Medica, 3rd Edition, Seattle, Eastland Press, 1986, 1993, 2004, P 830
[632] Bensky, D, Clavey, S, Stöger, E & Gamble, A, Chinese Herbal Medicine Materia Medica, 3rd Edition, Seattle, Eastland Press, 1986, 1993, 2004, P 830
[633] Brand, E & Wiseman, N, Concise Chinese Materia Medica, Taos, Paradigm Publications, 2008, P 461, Bensky, D, Clavey, S, Stöger, E & Gamble, A, Chinese Herbal Medicine Materia Medica, 3rd Edition, Seattle, Eastland Press, 1986, 1993, 2004, P 867
[634] Chen, JK & TT, Chinese Medical Herbology and Pharmacology, City of Industry, Art of Medicine Press, 2001/2004, P 1003, Bensky, D, Clavey, S, Stöger, E & Gamble, A, Chinese Herbal Medicine Materia Medica, 3rd Edition, Seattle, Eastland Press, 1986, 1993, 2004, P 875
[635] Bensky, D, Clavey, S, Stöger, E & Gamble, A, Chinese Herbal Medicine Materia Medica, 3rd Edition, Seattle, Eastland Press, 1986, 1993, 2004, P 875
[636] Li Shi Zhen, *Grand Materia Medica*, via Bensky, D, Clavey, S, Stöger, E & Gamble, A, Chinese Herbal Medicine Materia Medica, 3rd Edition, Seattle, Eastland Press, 1986, 1993, 2004, P 873
[637] Zhang Xi Chun, *Essays on Medicine Esteeming the Chinese and Respecting the Western*, via Bensky, D, Clavey, S, Stöger, E & Gamble, A, Chinese Herbal Medicine Materia Medica, 3rd Edition, Seattle, Eastland Press, 1986, 1993, 2004, P 873
[638] Chen, JK & TT, Chinese Medical Herbology and Pharmacology, City of Industry, Art of Medicine Press, 2001/2004, P 1002, Bensky, D, Clavey, S, Stöger, E & Gamble, A, Chinese Herbal Medicine Materia Medica, 3rd Edition, Seattle, Eastland Press, 1986, 1993, 2004, P 872
[639] Tang Rong Chuan (Tang Zonghai), Ben Cao Wen Da, Personal Unpublished Translation, 2015, 1.3.3
[640] Bensky, D, Clavey, S, Stöger, E & Gamble, A, Chinese Herbal Medicine Materia Medica, 3rd Edition, Seattle, Eastland Press, 1986, 1993, 2004, P 880
[641] Chen, JK & TT, Chinese Medical Herbology and Pharmacology, City of Industry, Art of Medicine Press, 2001/2004, P 997, Brand, E & Wiseman, N, Concise Chinese Materia Medica, Taos, Paradigm Publications, 2008, P 463
[642] Bensky, D, Clavey, S, Stöger, E & Gamble, A, Chinese Herbal Medicine Materia Medica, 3rd Edition, Seattle, Eastland Press, 1986, 1993, 2004, P 877
[643] Bensky, D, Clavey, S, Stöger, E & Gamble, A, Chinese Herbal Medicine Materia Medica, 3rd Edition, Seattle, Eastland Press, 1986, 1993, 2004, P 900
[644] Brand, E & Wiseman, N, Concise Chinese Materia Medica, Taos, Paradigm Publications, 2008, P 489

[645] Bensky, D, Clavey, S, Stöger, E & Gamble, A, Chinese Herbal Medicine Materia Medica, 3rd Edition, Seattle, Eastland Press, 1986, 1993, 2004, P 1014
[646] Li Shi Zhen, *Grand Materia Medica*, via Bensky, D, Clavey, S, Stöger, E & Gamble, A, Chinese Herbal Medicine Materia Medica, 3rd Edition, Seattle, Eastland Press, 1986, 1993, 2004, P 1022
[647] Chen, JK & TT, Chinese Medical Herbology and Pharmacology, City of Industry, Art of Medicine Press, 2001/2004, P 1045
[648] Li Shi Zhen, *Grand Materia Medica*, via Bensky, D, Clavey, S, Stöger, E & Gamble, A, Chinese Herbal Medicine Materia Medica, 3rd Edition, Seattle, Eastland Press, 1986, 1993, 2004, P 1022
[649] Li Shi Zhen, *Grand Materia Medica*, via Bensky, D, Clavey, S, Stöger, E & Gamble, A, Chinese Herbal Medicine Materia Medica, 3rd Edition, Seattle, Eastland Press, 1986, 1993, 2004, P 1022
[650] Chen, JK & TT, Chinese Medical Herbology and Pharmacology, City of Industry, Art of Medicine Press, 2001/2004, P 1039
[651] Brand, E & Wiseman, N, Concise Chinese Materia Medica, Taos, Paradigm Publications, 2008, P 484
[652] Brand, E & Wiseman, N, Concise Chinese Materia Medica, Taos, Paradigm Publications, 2008, P 484
[653] Brand, E & Wiseman, N, Concise Chinese Materia Medica, Taos, Paradigm Publications, 2008, P 484
[654] Brand, E & Wiseman, N, Concise Chinese Materia Medica, Taos, Paradigm Publications, 2008, P 493
[655] Brand, E & Wiseman, N, Concise Chinese Materia Medica, Taos, Paradigm Publications, 2008, P 493
[656] Bensky, D, Clavey, S, Stöger, E & Gamble, A, Chinese Herbal Medicine Materia Medica, 3rd Edition, Seattle, Eastland Press, 1986, 1993, 2004, P 655
[657] Brand, E & Wiseman, N, Concise Chinese Materia Medica, Taos, Paradigm Publications, 2008, P 162
[658] Chen, JK & TT, Chinese Medical Herbology and Pharmacology, City of Industry, Art of Medicine Press, 2001/2004, P 1056, Bensky, D, Clavey, S, Stöger, E & Gamble, A, Chinese Herbal Medicine Materia Medica, 3rd Edition, Seattle, Eastland Press, 1986, 1993, 2004, P 1040
[659] Brand, E & Wiseman, N, Concise Chinese Materia Medica, Taos, Paradigm Publications, 2008, P 488
[660] Brand, E & Wiseman, N, Concise Chinese Materia Medica, Taos, Paradigm Publications, 2008, P 490, Bensky, D, Clavey, S, Stöger, E & Gamble, A, Chinese Herbal Medicine Materia Medica, 3rd Edition, Seattle, Eastland Press, 1986, 1993, 2004, P 1038
[661] Bensky, D, Clavey, S, Stöger, E & Gamble, A, Chinese Herbal Medicine Materia Medica, 3rd Edition, Seattle, Eastland Press, 1986, 1993, 2004, P 1023
[662] Chen, JK & TT, Chinese Medical Herbology and Pharmacology, City of Industry, Art of Medicine Press, 2001/2004, P 59
[663] Tang Rong Chuan (Tang Zonghai), Ben Cao Wen Da, Personal Unpublished Translation, 2015, 1.4.6
[664] Brand, E & Wiseman, N, Concise Chinese Materia Medica, Taos, Paradigm Publications, 2008, P 44
[665] Chen Shi Duo, via Bensky, D, Clavey, S, Stöger, E & Gamble, A, Chinese Herbal Medicine Materia Medica, 3rd Edition, Seattle, Eastland Press, 1986, 1993, 2004, P 37

[666] Maciocia, G, The Channels of Acupuncture, Philadelphia, Elsevier, 2006, P 446
[667] Maciocia, G, The Channels of Acupuncture, Philadelphia, Elsevier, 2006, P 585
[668] Bensky, D, Clavey, S, Stöger, E & Gamble, A, Chinese Herbal Medicine Materia Medica, 3rd Edition, Seattle, Eastland Press, 1986, 1993, 2004, P 78
[669] Tang Rong Chuan (Tang Zonghai), Ben Cao Wen Da, Personal Unpublished Translation, 2015, 1.5.10
[670] Tang Rong Chuan (Tang Zonghai), Ben Cao Wen Da, Personal Unpublished Translation, 2015, 1.4.6
[671] Tang Rong Chuan (Tang Zonghai), Ben Cao Wen Da, Personal Unpublished Translation, 2015, 1.5.9
[672] Tang Rong Chuan (Tang Zonghai), Ben Cao Wen Da, Personal Unpublished Translation, 2015, 1.5.9
[673] Tang Rong Chuan (Tang Zonghai), Ben Cao Wen Da, Personal Unpublished Translation, 2015, 1.4.6
[674] Miao Xi Yong, *Commentary on the Divine Husbandman's Classic of Materia Medica*, via Bensky, D, Clavey, S, Stöger, E & Gamble, A, Chinese Herbal Medicine Materia Medica, 3rd Edition, Seattle, Eastland Press, 1986, 1993, 2004, P 211
[675] Bensky, D, Clavey, S, Stöger, E & Gamble, A, Chinese Herbal Medicine Materia Medica, 3rd Edition, Seattle, Eastland Press, 1986, 1993, 2004, P 622
[676] Bensky, D, Clavey, S, Stöger, E & Gamble, A, Chinese Herbal Medicine Materia Medica, 3rd Edition, Seattle, Eastland Press, 1986, 1993, 2004, P 622
[677] Wang, Hao Gu, *Harm and Benefit in the Materia Medica*, via Bensky, D, Clavey, S, Stöger, E & Gamble, A, Chinese Herbal Medicine Materia Medica, 3rd Edition, Seattle, Eastland Press, 1986, 1993, 2004, P 152
[678] Bensky, D, Clavey, S, Stöger, E & Gamble, A, Chinese Herbal Medicine Materia Medica, 3rd Edition, Seattle, Eastland Press, 1986, 1993, 2004, P 151
[679] Wang, Hao Gu, *Harm and Benefit in the Materia Medica*, via Bensky, D, Clavey, S, Stöger, E & Gamble, A, Chinese Herbal Medicine Materia Medica, 3rd Edition, Seattle, Eastland Press, 1986, 1993, 2004, P 152
[680] Bensky, D, Clavey, S, Stöger, E & Gamble, A, Chinese Herbal Medicine Materia Medica, 3rd Edition, Seattle, Eastland Press, 1986, 1993, 2004, P 215
[681] Bensky, D, Clavey, S, Stöger, E & Gamble, A, Chinese Herbal Medicine Materia Medica, 3rd Edition, Seattle, Eastland Press, 1986, 1993, 2004, P 215
[682] Bensky, D, Clavey, S, Stöger, E & Gamble, A, Chinese Herbal Medicine Materia Medica, 3rd Edition, Seattle, Eastland Press, 1986, 1993, 2004, P 215
[683] Bensky, D, Clavey, S, Stöger, E & Gamble, A, Chinese Herbal Medicine Materia Medica, 3rd Edition, Seattle, Eastland Press, 1986, 1993, 2004, P 1010
[684] Bensky, D, Clavey, S, Stöger, E & Gamble, A, Chinese Herbal Medicine Materia Medica, 3rd Edition, Seattle, Eastland Press, 1986, 1993, 2004, P 1010
[685] Bensky, D, Clavey, S, Stöger, E & Gamble, A, Chinese Herbal Medicine Materia Medica, 3rd Edition, Seattle, Eastland Press, 1986, 1993, 2004, P 193
[686] Brand, E & Wiseman, N, Concise Chinese Materia Medica, Taos, Paradigm Publications, 2008, P 132

[687] Tang Rong Chuan (Tang Zonghai), Ben Cao Wen Da, Personal Unpublished Translation, 2015, 1.5.3
[688] Bensky, D, Clavey, S, Stöger, E & Gamble, A, Chinese Herbal Medicine Materia Medica, 3rd Edition, Seattle, Eastland Press, 1986, 1993, 2004, P 239
[689] Tang Rong Chuan (Tang Zonghai), Ben Cao Wen Da, Personal Unpublished Translation, 2015, 1.5.2
[690] Maciocia, G, The Channels of Acupuncture, Philadelphia, Elsevier, 2006, P 446
[691] Brand, E & Wiseman, N, Concise Chinese Materia Medica, Taos, Paradigm Publications, 2008, P 143, Bensky, D, Clavey, S, Stöger, E & Gamble, A, Chinese Herbal Medicine Materia Medica, 3rd Edition, Seattle, Eastland Press, 1986, 1993, 2004, P 261
[692] Bensky, D, Clavey, S, Stöger, E & Gamble, A, Chinese Herbal Medicine Materia Medica, 3rd Edition, Seattle, Eastland Press, 1986, 1993, 2004, P 261
[693] Chen, JK & TT, Chinese Medical Herbology and Pharmacology, City of Industry, Art of Medicine Press, 2001/2004, P 287
[694] Brand, E & Wiseman, N, Concise Chinese Materia Medica, Taos, Paradigm Publications, 2008, P 139
[695] *Seeking Accuracy in the Materia Medica*, via Bensky, D, Clavey, S, Stöger, E & Gamble, A, Chinese Herbal Medicine Materia Medica, 3rd Edition, Seattle, Eastland Press, 1986, 1993, 2004, P 254
[696] *Seeking Accuracy in the Materia Medica*, via Bensky, D, Clavey, S, Stöger, E & Gamble, A, Chinese Herbal Medicine Materia Medica, 3rd Edition, Seattle, Eastland Press, 1986, 1993, 2004, P 254
[697] Bensky, D, Clavey, S, Stöger, E & Gamble, A, Chinese Herbal Medicine Materia Medica, 3rd Edition, Seattle, Eastland Press, 1986, 1993, 2004, P 313
[698] Bensky, D, Clavey, S, Stöger, E & Gamble, A, Chinese Herbal Medicine Materia Medica, 3rd Edition, Seattle, Eastland Press, 1986, 1993, 2004, P 313
[699] Chen, JK & TT, Chinese Medical Herbology and Pharmacology, City of Industry, Art of Medicine Press, 2001/2004, P 308
[700] Brand, E & Wiseman, N, Concise Chinese Materia Medica, Taos, Paradigm Publications, 2008, P 158
[701] Maciocia, G, The Channels of Acupuncture, Philadelphia, Elsevier, 2006, P 585
[702] '…circulates the Còu Lǐ-interstices and the Sān Jiāo.' Tang Rong Chuan (Tang Zonghai), Ben Cao Wen Da, Personal Unpublished Translation, 2015, 2.2.5
[703] Bensky, D, Clavey, S, Stöger, E & Gamble, A, Chinese Herbal Medicine Materia Medica, 3rd Edition, Seattle, Eastland Press, 1986, 1993, 2004, P 332
[704] Bensky, D, Clavey, S, Stöger, E & Gamble, A, Chinese Herbal Medicine Materia Medica, 3rd Edition, Seattle, Eastland Press, 1986, 1993, 2004, P 332
[705] Li Gao, via Bensky, D, Clavey, S, Stöger, E & Gamble, A, Chinese Herbal Medicine Materia Medica, 3rd Edition, Seattle, Eastland Press, 1986, 1993, 2004, P 332
[706] Bensky, D, Clavey, S, Stöger, E & Gamble, A, Chinese Herbal Medicine Materia Medica, 3rd Edition, Seattle, Eastland Press, 1986, 1993, 2004, P 342
[707] Bensky, D, Clavey, S, Stöger, E & Gamble, A, Chinese Herbal Medicine Materia Medica, 3rd Edition, Seattle, Eastland Press, 1986, 1993, 2004, P 342

[708] Bensky, D, Clavey, S, Stöger, E & Gamble, A, Chinese Herbal Medicine Materia Medica, 3rd Edition, Seattle, Eastland Press, 1986, 1993, 2004, P 355
[709] Bensky, D, Clavey, S, Stöger, E & Gamble, A, Chinese Herbal Medicine Materia Medica, 3rd Edition, Seattle, Eastland Press, 1986, 1993, 2004, P 354
[710] Bensky, D, Clavey, S, Stöger, E & Gamble, A, Chinese Herbal Medicine Materia Medica, 3rd Edition, Seattle, Eastland Press, 1986, 1993, 2004, P 354
[711] Brand, E & Wiseman, N, Concise Chinese Materia Medica, Taos, Paradigm Publications, 2008, P 154, Chen, JK & TT, Chinese Medical Herbology and Pharmacology, City of Industry, Art of Medicine Press, 2001/2004, P 312
[712] Bensky, D, Clavey, S, Stöger, E & Gamble, A, Chinese Herbal Medicine Materia Medica, 3rd Edition, Seattle, Eastland Press, 1986, 1993, 2004, P 329
[713] Bensky, D, Clavey, S, Stöger, E & Gamble, A, Chinese Herbal Medicine Materia Medica, 3rd Edition, Seattle, Eastland Press, 1986, 1993, 2004, P 329
[714] Brand, E & Wiseman, N, Concise Chinese Materia Medica, Taos, Paradigm Publications, 2008, P 155
[715] Brand, E & Wiseman, N, Concise Chinese Materia Medica, Taos, Paradigm Publications, 2008, P 155
[716] Bensky, D, Clavey, S, Stöger, E & Gamble, A, Chinese Herbal Medicine Materia Medica, 3rd Edition, Seattle, Eastland Press, 1986, 1993, 2004, P 349
[717] Chen, JK & TT, Chinese Medical Herbology and Pharmacology, City of Industry, Art of Medicine Press, 2001/2004, P 333
[718] Tang Rong Chuan (Tang Zonghai), Ben Cao Wen Da, Personal Unpublished Translation, 2015, 1.5.14
[719] Chen, JK & TT, Chinese Medical Herbology and Pharmacology, City of Industry, Art of Medicine Press, 2001/2004, P 461
[720] Zhang, Shan Lei, *Rectification of the Meaning of Materia Medica,* via Bensky, D, Clavey, S, Stöger, E & Gamble, A, Chinese Herbal Medicine Materia Medica, 3rd Edition, Seattle, Eastland Press, 1986, 1993, 2004, P 482
[721] Huang Gong Xiu, *Seeking Accuracy in the Materia Medica*, and, *Harm and Benefit in the Materia Medica*, both via Bensky, D, Clavey, S, Stöger, E & Gamble, A, Chinese Herbal Medicine Materia Medica, 3rd Edition, Seattle, Eastland Press, 1986, 1993, 2004, P 482
[722] Bensky, D, Clavey, S, Stöger, E & Gamble, A, Chinese Herbal Medicine Materia Medica, 3rd Edition, Seattle, Eastland Press, 1986, 1993, 2004, P 487
[723] Tang Rong Chuan (Tang Zonghai), Ben Cao Wen Da, Personal Unpublished Translation, 2015, 1.3.3
[724] Maciocia, G, The Channels of Acupuncture, Philadelphia, Elsevier, 2006, P 585
[725] Brand, E & Wiseman, N, Concise Chinese Materia Medica, Taos, Paradigm Publications, 2008, P186
[726] Bensky, D, Clavey, S, Stöger, E & Gamble, A, Chinese Herbal Medicine Materia Medica, 3rd Edition, Seattle, Eastland Press, 1986, 1993, 2004, P 267
[727] Brand, E & Wiseman, N, Concise Chinese Materia Medica, Taos, Paradigm Publications, 2008, P 200
[728] Chen, JK & TT, Chinese Medical Herbology and Pharmacology, City of Industry, Art of Medicine Press, 2001/2004, P 461

[729] Brand, E & Wiseman, N, Concise Chinese Materia Medica, Taos, Paradigm Publications, 2008, P 216
[730] Bensky, D, Clavey, S, Stöger, E & Gamble, A, Chinese Herbal Medicine Materia Medica, 3rd Edition, Seattle, Eastland Press, 1986, 1993, 2004, P 700
[731] Tang Rong Chuan (Tang Zonghai), Ben Cao Wen Da, Personal Unpublished Translation, 2015, 1.5.13
[732] Brand, E & Wiseman, N, Concise Chinese Materia Medica, Taos, Paradigm Publications, 2008, P 212
[733] Bensky, D, Clavey, S, Stöger, E & Gamble, A, Chinese Herbal Medicine Materia Medica, 3rd Edition, Seattle, Eastland Press, 1986, 1993, 2004, P 680
[734] Tang Rong Chuan (Tang Zonghai), Ben Cao Wen Da, Personal Unpublished Translation, 2015, 1.2.4
[735] Tang Rong Chuan (Tang Zonghai), Ben Cao Wen Da, Personal Unpublished Translation, 2015, 1.2.4
[736] Chen, JK & TT, Chinese Medical Herbology and Pharmacology, City of Industry, Art of Medicine Press, 2001/2004, P 441
[737] Brand, E & Wiseman, N, Concise Chinese Materia Medica, Taos, Paradigm Publications, 2008, P 208
[738] Zhang, Shan Lei, *Rectification of the Meaning of Materia Medica,* via Bensky, D, Clavey, S, Stöger, E & Gamble, A, Chinese Herbal Medicine Materia Medica, 3rd Edition, Seattle, Eastland Press, 1986, 1993, 2004, P 675
[739] Tang Rong Chuan (Tang Zonghai), Ben Cao Wen Da, Personal Unpublished Translation, 2015, 2.2.2
[740] Maciocia, G, The Channels of Acupuncture, Philadelphia, Elsevier, 2006, P 446
[741] Bensky, D, Clavey, S, Stöger, E & Gamble, A, Chinese Herbal Medicine Materia Medica, 3rd Edition, Seattle, Eastland Press, 1986, 1993, 2004, P 510
[742] Li Shi Zhen, via Bensky, D, Clavey, S, Stöger, E & Gamble, A, Chinese Herbal Medicine Materia Medica, 3rd Edition, Seattle, Eastland Press, 1986, 1993, 2004, P 534
[743] Bensky, D, Clavey, S, Stöger, E & Gamble, A, Chinese Herbal Medicine Materia Medica, 3rd Edition, Seattle, Eastland Press, 1986, 1993, 2004, P 519
[744] Brand, E & Wiseman, N, Concise Chinese Materia Medica, Taos, Paradigm Publications, 2008, P 226
[745] Brand, E & Wiseman, N, Concise Chinese Materia Medica, Taos, Paradigm Publications, 2008, P 226, Bensky, D, Clavey, S, Stöger, E & Gamble, A, Chinese Herbal Medicine Materia Medica, 3rd Edition, Seattle, Eastland Press, 1986, 1993, 2004, P 517
[746] Bensky, D, Clavey, S, Stöger, E & Gamble, A, Chinese Herbal Medicine Materia Medica, 3rd Edition, Seattle, Eastland Press, 1986, 1993, 2004, P 543
[747] Bensky, D, Clavey, S, Stöger, E & Gamble, A, Chinese Herbal Medicine Materia Medica, 3rd Edition, Seattle, Eastland Press, 1986, 1993, 2004, P 544
[748] Bensky, D, Clavey, S, Stöger, E & Gamble, A, Chinese Herbal Medicine Materia Medica, 3rd Edition, Seattle, Eastland Press, 1986, 1993, 2004, P 530
[749] Brand, E & Wiseman, N, Concise Chinese Materia Medica, Taos, Paradigm Publications, 2008, P 228, Bensky, D, Clavey, S, Stöger, E & Gamble, A, Chinese Herbal Medicine Materia Medica, 3rd Edition, Seattle, Eastland Press, 1986, 1993, 2004, P 530

[750] Zhang, Shan Lei, *Rectification of the Meaning of Materia Medica,* via Bensky, D, Clavey, S, Stöger, E & Gamble, A, Chinese Herbal Medicine Materia Medica, 3rd Edition, Seattle, Eastland Press, 1986, 1993, 2004, P 528

[751] Brand, E & Wiseman, N, Concise Chinese Materia Medica, Taos, Paradigm Publications, 2008, P 229

[752] Bensky, D, Clavey, S, Stöger, E & Gamble, A, Chinese Herbal Medicine Materia Medica, 3rd Edition, Seattle, Eastland Press, 1986, 1993, 2004, P 527

[753] Li Shi Zhen, *Grand Materia Medica*, via Bensky, D, Clavey, S, Stöger, E & Gamble, A, Chinese Herbal Medicine Materia Medica, 3rd Edition, Seattle, Eastland Press, 1986, 1993, 2004, P 500

[754] Zhang Xi Chun, *Essays on Medicine Esteeming the Chinese and Respecting the Western*, via Bensky, D, Clavey, S, Stöger, E & Gamble, A, Chinese Herbal Medicine Materia Medica, 3rd Edition, Seattle, Eastland Press, 1986, 1993, 2004, P 494

[755] Li Shi Zhen and Huang Gong Xiu, *Seeking Accuracy in the Materia Medica*, via Bensky, D, Clavey, S, Stöger, E & Gamble, A, Chinese Herbal Medicine Materia Medica, 3rd Edition, Seattle, Eastland Press, 1986, 1993, 2004, P 498

[756] Brand, E & Wiseman, N, Concise Chinese Materia Medica, Taos, Paradigm Publications, 2008, P 489

[757] Bensky, D, Clavey, S, Stöger, E & Gamble, A, Chinese Herbal Medicine Materia Medica, 3rd Edition, Seattle, Eastland Press, 1986, 1993, 2004, P 1014

[758] Bensky, D, Clavey, S, Stöger, E & Gamble, A, Chinese Herbal Medicine Materia Medica, 3rd Edition, Seattle, Eastland Press, 1986, 1993, 2004, P 1007

[759] *Divine Husbandman's Classic of Materia Medica*, via Bensky, D, Clavey, S, Stöger, E & Gamble, A, Chinese Herbal Medicine Materia Medica, 3rd Edition, Seattle, Eastland Press, 1986, 1993, 2004, P 1007

[760] Bensky, D, Clavey, S, Stöger, E & Gamble, A, Chinese Herbal Medicine Materia Medica, 3rd Edition, Seattle, Eastland Press, 1986, 1993, 2004, P 998

[761] Bensky, D, Clavey, S, Stöger, E & Gamble, A, Chinese Herbal Medicine Materia Medica, 3rd Edition, Seattle, Eastland Press, 1986, 1993, 2004, P 1010

[762] Bensky, D, Clavey, S, Stöger, E & Gamble, A, Chinese Herbal Medicine Materia Medica, 3rd Edition, Seattle, Eastland Press, 1986, 1993, 2004, P 1010

[763] Zhang Lu, *Encountering the Sources of the Classic of Materia Medica*, via Bensky, D, Clavey, S, Stöger, E & Gamble, A, Chinese Herbal Medicine Materia Medica, 3rd Edition, Seattle, Eastland Press, 1986, 1993, 2004, P 1003

[764] Bensky, D, Clavey, S, Stöger, E & Gamble, A, Chinese Herbal Medicine Materia Medica, 3rd Edition, Seattle, Eastland Press, 1986, 1993, 2004, P 590

[765] Chen, JK & TT, Chinese Medical Herbology and Pharmacology, City of Industry, Art of Medicine Press, 2001/2004, P 587, Bensky, D, Clavey, S, Stöger, E & Gamble, A, Chinese Herbal Medicine Materia Medica, 3rd Edition, Seattle, Eastland Press, 1986, 1993, 2004, P 559

[766] Brand, E & Wiseman, N, Concise Chinese Materia Medica, Taos, Paradigm Publications, 2008, P 264

[767] Zhang Bing Chen, *Convenient Reader of Materia Medica*, via Bensky, D, Clavey, S, Stöger, E & Gamble, A, Chinese Herbal Medicine Materia Medica, 3rd Edition, Seattle, Eastland Press, 1986, 1993, 2004, P 560

[768] Zhang Bing Chen, *Convenient Reader of Materia Medica*, via Bensky, D, Clavey, S, Stöger, E & Gamble, A, Chinese Herbal Medicine Materia Medica, 3rd Edition, Seattle, Eastland Press, 1986, 1993, 2004, P 560. In this section Bensky, D, Clavey, S, Stöger, E & Gamble, A, Chinese Herbal Medicine Materia Medica, 3rd Edition, Seattle, Eastland Press, 1986, 1993, 2004, P, et al. quote Zhang as saying that San Qi enters the Yang Ming and Jue Yin channels. For some reason they only include the large intestine in their assessment, but not the pericardium. I include it here as it is at least as reasonable a conclusion, and I have used clinically San Qi as a pericardium herb for many years with excellent effects.
[769] Bensky, D, Clavey, S, Stöger, E & Gamble, A, Chinese Herbal Medicine Materia Medica, 3rd Edition, Seattle, Eastland Press, 1986, 1993, 2004, P 563
[770] Bensky, D, Clavey, S, Stöger, E & Gamble, A, Chinese Herbal Medicine Materia Medica, 3rd Edition, Seattle, Eastland Press, 1986, 1993, 2004, P 562
[771] Bensky, D, Clavey, S, Stöger, E & Gamble, A, Chinese Herbal Medicine Materia Medica, 3rd Edition, Seattle, Eastland Press, 1986, 1993, 2004, P 652
[772] Chen, JK & TT, Chinese Medical Herbology and Pharmacology, City of Industry, Art of Medicine Press, 2001/2004, P 593
[773] Brand, E & Wiseman, N, Concise Chinese Materia Medica, Taos, Paradigm Publications, 2008, P 266
[774] Bensky, D, Clavey, S, Stöger, E & Gamble, A, Chinese Herbal Medicine Materia Medica, 3rd Edition, Seattle, Eastland Press, 1986, 1993, 2004, P 562
[775] Zhang Bing Chen, *Convenient Reader of Materia Medica*, via Bensky, D, Clavey, S, Stöger, E & Gamble, A, Chinese Herbal Medicine Materia Medica, 3rd Edition, Seattle, Eastland Press, 1986, 1993, 2004, P 568
[776] Bensky, D, Clavey, S, Stöger, E & Gamble, A, Chinese Herbal Medicine Materia Medica, 3rd Edition, Seattle, Eastland Press, 1986, 1993, 2004, P 567
[777] Maciocia, G, The Channels of Acupuncture, Philadelphia, Elsevier, 2006, P 545
[778] Bensky, D, Clavey, S, Stöger, E & Gamble, A, Chinese Herbal Medicine Materia Medica, 3rd Edition, Seattle, Eastland Press, 1986, 1993, 2004, P 655
[779] Zhang Bing Chen, *Convenient Reader of Materia Medica*, via Bensky, D, Clavey, S, Stöger, E & Gamble, A, Chinese Herbal Medicine Materia Medica, 3rd Edition, Seattle, Eastland Press, 1986, 1993, 2004, P 607
[780] Bensky, D, Clavey, S, Stöger, E & Gamble, A, Chinese Herbal Medicine Materia Medica, 3rd Edition, Seattle, Eastland Press, 1986, 1993, 2004, P 653
[781] Bensky, D, Clavey, S, Stöger, E & Gamble, A, Chinese Herbal Medicine Materia Medica, 3rd Edition, Seattle, Eastland Press, 1986, 1993, 2004, P 612
[782] Bensky, D, Clavey, S, Stöger, E & Gamble, A, Chinese Herbal Medicine Materia Medica, 3rd Edition, Seattle, Eastland Press, 1986, 1993, 2004, P 664
[783] Bensky, D, Clavey, S, Stöger, E & Gamble, A, Chinese Herbal Medicine Materia Medica, 3rd Edition, Seattle, Eastland Press, 1986, 1993, 2004, P 664
[784] Brand, E & Wiseman, N, Concise Chinese Materia Medica, Taos, Paradigm Publications, 2008, P 293
[785] Bensky, D, Clavey, S, Stöger, E & Gamble, A, Chinese Herbal Medicine Materia Medica, 3rd Edition, Seattle, Eastland Press, 1986, 1993, 2004, P 605

[786] Bensky, D, Clavey, S, Stöger, E & Gamble, A, Chinese Herbal Medicine Materia Medica, 3rd Edition, Seattle, Eastland Press, 1986, 1993, 2004, P 605
[787] Brand, E & Wiseman, N, Concise Chinese Materia Medica, Taos, Paradigm Publications, 2008, P 284
[788] Bensky, D, Clavey, S, Stöger, E & Gamble, A, Chinese Herbal Medicine Materia Medica, 3rd Edition, Seattle, Eastland Press, 1986, 1993, 2004, P 650
[789] Bensky, D, Clavey, S, Stöger, E & Gamble, A, Chinese Herbal Medicine Materia Medica, 3rd Edition, Seattle, Eastland Press, 1986, 1993, 2004, P 650
[790] Chen, JK & TT, Chinese Medical Herbology and Pharmacology, City of Industry, Art of Medicine Press, 2001/2004, P 659
[791] Bensky, D, Clavey, S, Stöger, E & Gamble, A, Chinese Herbal Medicine Materia Medica, 3rd Edition, Seattle, Eastland Press, 1986, 1993, 2004, P 622
[792] Bensky, D, Clavey, S, Stöger, E & Gamble, A, Chinese Herbal Medicine Materia Medica, 3rd Edition, Seattle, Eastland Press, 1986, 1993, 2004, P 622
[793] Bensky, D, Clavey, S, Stöger, E & Gamble, A, Chinese Herbal Medicine Materia Medica, 3rd Edition, Seattle, Eastland Press, 1986, 1993, 2004, P 666
[794] Brand, E & Wiseman, N, Concise Chinese Materia Medica, Taos, Paradigm Publications, 2008, P 298, Bensky, D, Clavey, S, Stöger, E & Gamble, A, Chinese Herbal Medicine Materia Medica, 3rd Edition, Seattle, Eastland Press, 1986, 1993, 2004, P 633
[795] Tang Rong Chuan (Tang Zonghai), Ben Cao Wen Da, Personal Unpublished Translation, 2015, 1.5.18
[796] Chen, JK & TT, Chinese Medical Herbology and Pharmacology, City of Industry, Art of Medicine Press, 2001/2004, P 646
[797] Bensky, D, Clavey, S, Stöger, E & Gamble, A, Chinese Herbal Medicine Materia Medica, 3rd Edition, Seattle, Eastland Press, 1986, 1993, 2004, P 432
[798] Bensky, D, Clavey, S, Stöger, E & Gamble, A, Chinese Herbal Medicine Materia Medica, 3rd Edition, Seattle, Eastland Press, 1986, 1993, 2004, P 458
[799] Brand, E & Wiseman, N, Concise Chinese Materia Medica, Taos, Paradigm Publications, 2008, P 313
[800] Brand, E & Wiseman, N, Concise Chinese Materia Medica, Taos, Paradigm Publications, 2008, P 313
[801] Brand, E & Wiseman, N, Concise Chinese Materia Medica, Taos, Paradigm Publications, 2008, P 312
[802] Brand, E & Wiseman, N, Concise Chinese Materia Medica, Taos, Paradigm Publications, 2008, P 312, Bensky, D, Clavey, S, Stöger, E & Gamble, A, Chinese Herbal Medicine Materia Medica, 3rd Edition, Seattle, Eastland Press, 1986, 1993, 2004, P 421
[803] Bensky, D, Clavey, S, Stöger, E & Gamble, A, Chinese Herbal Medicine Materia Medica, 3rd Edition, Seattle, Eastland Press, 1986, 1993, 2004, P 655
[804] Brand, E & Wiseman, N, Concise Chinese Materia Medica, Taos, Paradigm Publications, 2008, P 311
[805] Chen, JK & TT, Chinese Medical Herbology and Pharmacology, City of Industry, Art of Medicine Press, 2001/2004, P 688
[806] Chen, JK & TT, Chinese Medical Herbology and Pharmacology, City of Industry, Art of Medicine Press, 2001/2004, P 688

[807] Brand, E & Wiseman, N, Concise Chinese Materia Medica, Taos, Paradigm Publications, 2008, P 311

[808] Bensky, D, Clavey, S, Stöger, E & Gamble, A, Chinese Herbal Medicine Materia Medica, 3rd Edition, Seattle, Eastland Press, 1986, 1993, 2004, P 458

[809] *Sichuan Chinese Materia Medica*, via Bensky, D, Clavey, S, Stöger, E & Gamble, A, Chinese Herbal Medicine Materia Medica, 3rd Edition, Seattle, Eastland Press, 1986, 1993, 2004, P 939

[810] *Sichuan Chinese Materia Medica*, via Bensky, D, Clavey, S, Stöger, E & Gamble, A, Chinese Herbal Medicine Materia Medica, 3rd Edition, Seattle, Eastland Press, 1986, 1993, 2004, P 939

[811] Bensky, D, Clavey, S, Stöger, E & Gamble, A, Chinese Herbal Medicine Materia Medica, 3rd Edition, Seattle, Eastland Press, 1986, 1993, 2004, P 543

[812] Brand, E & Wiseman, N, Concise Chinese Materia Medica, Taos, Paradigm Publications, 2008, P 350, Bensky, D, Clavey, S, Stöger, E & Gamble, A, Chinese Herbal Medicine Materia Medica, 3rd Edition, Seattle, Eastland Press, 1986, 1993, 2004, P 928

[813] Bensky, D, Clavey, S, Stöger, E & Gamble, A, Chinese Herbal Medicine Materia Medica, 3rd Edition, Seattle, Eastland Press, 1986, 1993, 2004, P 928

[814] Bensky, D, Clavey, S, Stöger, E & Gamble, A, Chinese Herbal Medicine Materia Medica, 3rd Edition, Seattle, Eastland Press, 1986, 1993, 2004, P 928

[815] Bensky, D, Clavey, S, Stöger, E & Gamble, A, Chinese Herbal Medicine Materia Medica, 3rd Edition, Seattle, Eastland Press, 1986, 1993, 2004, P 982

[816] Chen, JK & TT, Chinese Medical Herbology and Pharmacology, City of Industry, Art of Medicine Press, 2001/2004, P 794, Bensky, D, Clavey, S, Stöger, E & Gamble, A, Chinese Herbal Medicine Materia Medica, 3rd Edition, Seattle, Eastland Press, 1986, 1993, 2004, P 982

[817] Brand, E & Wiseman, N, Concise Chinese Materia Medica, Taos, Paradigm Publications, 2008, P 383

[818] Bensky, D, Clavey, S, Stöger, E & Gamble, A, Chinese Herbal Medicine Materia Medica, 3rd Edition, Seattle, Eastland Press, 1986, 1993, 2004, P 954

[819] Chen, JK & TT, Chinese Medical Herbology and Pharmacology, City of Industry, Art of Medicine Press, 2001/2004, P 825

[820] Chen, JK & TT, Chinese Medical Herbology and Pharmacology, City of Industry, Art of Medicine Press, 2001/2004, P 825

[821] Bensky, D, Clavey, S, Stöger, E & Gamble, A, Chinese Herbal Medicine Materia Medica, 3rd Edition, Seattle, Eastland Press, 1986, 1993, 2004, P 950

[822] *High Plateau Handbook of Treatment with Chinese Materia Medica*, via Bensky, D, Clavey, S, Stöger, E & Gamble, A, Chinese Herbal Medicine Materia Medica, 3rd Edition, Seattle, Eastland Press, 1986, 1993, 2004, P 742

[823] Bensky, D, Clavey, S, Stöger, E & Gamble, A, Chinese Herbal Medicine Materia Medica, 3rd Edition, Seattle, Eastland Press, 1986, 1993, 2004, P 742

[824] Maciocia, G, The Channels of Acupuncture, Philadelphia, Elsevier, 2006, P 545

[825] Bensky, D, Clavey, S, Stöger, E & Gamble, A, Chinese Herbal Medicine Materia Medica, 3rd Edition, Seattle, Eastland Press, 1986, 1993, 2004, P 718

[826] I think virtually anyone tasting Hong Jing Tian would immediately agree on its astringency.

[827] Brand, E & Wiseman, N, Concise Chinese Materia Medica, Taos, Paradigm Publications, 2008, P 411

[828] Brand, E & Wiseman, N, Concise Chinese Materia Medica, Taos, Paradigm Publications, 2008, P 411

[829] Chen, JK & TT, Chinese Medical Herbology and Pharmacology, City of Industry, Art of Medicine Press, 2001/2004, P 853

[830] Bensky, D, Clavey, S, Stöger, E & Gamble, A, Chinese Herbal Medicine Materia Medica, 3rd Edition, Seattle, Eastland Press, 1986, 1993, 2004, P 822

[831] Zhang, Shan Lei, *Rectification of the Meaning of Materia Medica,* via Bensky, D, Clavey, S, Stöger, E & Gamble, A, Chinese Herbal Medicine Materia Medica, 3rd Edition, Seattle, Eastland Press, 1986, 1993, 2004, P 823

[832] Brand, E & Wiseman, N, Concise Chinese Materia Medica, Taos, Paradigm Publications, 2008, P 398

[833] Brand, E & Wiseman, N, Concise Chinese Materia Medica, Taos, Paradigm Publications, 2008, P 395

[834] Brand, E & Wiseman, N, Concise Chinese Materia Medica, Taos, Paradigm Publications, 2008, P 395

[835] Brand, E & Wiseman, N, Concise Chinese Materia Medica, Taos, Paradigm Publications, 2008, P 409

[836] Tang Rong Chuan (Tang Zonghai), Ben Cao Wen Da, Personal Unpublished Translation, 2015, 1.3.3

[837] Maciocia, G, The Channels of Acupuncture, Philadelphia, Elsevier, 2006, P 545

[838] Me, on the basis of Tang Rong Chuan (Tang Zonghai), Ben Cao Wen Da, Personal Unpublished Translation, 2015, 1.2.1, etc., here contained. Although nowhere in the text does the author state that Huang Qi enters the San Jiao Jing-channel, he goes through such extensive and multiple descriptions of the structure and mechanisms of the San Jiao itself, plus his clear delineations of exactly how this herb physically enters and embodies the San Jiao, I would challenge anybody to prove that it *doesn't* enter the San Jiao Jing-channel. In addition, when we consider Huang Qi's central role in Bu Zhong Yi Qi Tang's use in treating qi deficiency with deficient heat symptoms, that is really all about the Shao Yang level of disease. I would put forth the question of why would one not use Huang Qi whenever its known set of qualities were needed to be applied to any aspect or dimension of the San Jiao Jing-channel?

[839] Tang Rong Chuan (Tang Zonghai), Ben Cao Wen Da, Personal Unpublished Translation, 2015, 2.2.5, and Bensky, D, Clavey, S, Stöger, E & Gamble, A, Chinese Herbal Medicine Materia Medica, 3rd Edition, Seattle, Eastland Press, 1986, 1993, 2004, P 727

[840] Huang Gong Xiu, *Seeking Accuracy in the Materia Medica,* via Bensky, D, Clavey, S, Stöger, E & Gamble, A, Chinese Herbal Medicine Materia Medica, 3rd Edition, Seattle, Eastland Press, 1986, 1993, 2004, P 727

[841] Brand, E & Wiseman, N, Concise Chinese Materia Medica, Taos, Paradigm Publications, 2008, P 407

[842] Tang Rong Chuan (Tang Zonghai), Ben Cao Wen Da, Personal Unpublished Translation, 2015, 2.2.5

[843] Bensky, D, Clavey, S, Stöger, E & Gamble, A, Chinese Herbal Medicine Materia Medica, 3rd Edition, Seattle, Eastland Press, 1986, 1993, 2004, P 739

[844] Bensky, D, Clavey, S, Stöger, E & Gamble, A, Chinese Herbal Medicine Materia Medica, 3rd Edition, Seattle, Eastland Press, 1986, 1993, 2004, P 787

[845] Brand, E & Wiseman, N, Concise Chinese Materia Medica, Taos, Paradigm Publications, 2008, P 425, Bensky, D, Clavey, S, Stöger, E & Gamble, A, Chinese Herbal Medicine Materia Medica, 3rd Edition, Seattle, Eastland Press, 1986, 1993, 2004, P 789
[846] Brand, E & Wiseman, N, Concise Chinese Materia Medica, Taos, Paradigm Publications, 2008, P 418
[847] Brand, E & Wiseman, N, Concise Chinese Materia Medica, Taos, Paradigm Publications, 2008, P 418
[848] Brand, E & Wiseman, N, Concise Chinese Materia Medica, Taos, Paradigm Publications, 2008, P 418
[849] Zhang Lu, *Encountering the Sources of the Classic of Materia Medica*, via Bensky, D, Clavey, S, Stöger, E & Gamble, A, Chinese Herbal Medicine Materia Medica, 3rd Edition, Seattle, Eastland Press, 1986, 1993, 2004, P 791
[850] Bensky, D, Clavey, S, Stöger, E & Gamble, A, Chinese Herbal Medicine Materia Medica, 3rd Edition, Seattle, Eastland Press, 1986, 1993, 2004, P 762
[851] Brand, E & Wiseman, N, Concise Chinese Materia Medica, Taos, Paradigm Publications, 2008, P 425
[852] Brand, E & Wiseman, N, Concise Chinese Materia Medica, Taos, Paradigm Publications, 2008, P 425
[853] Tang Rong Chuan (Tang Zonghai), Ben Cao Wen Da, Personal Unpublished Translation, 2015, 1.3.3
[854] Tang Rong Chuan (Tang Zonghai), Ben Cao Wen Da, Personal Unpublished Translation, 2015, 1.2.3
[855] Maciocia, G, The Channels of Acupuncture, Philadelphia, Elsevier, 2006, P 545
[856] Brand, E & Wiseman, N, Concise Chinese Materia Medica, Taos, Paradigm Publications, 2008, P 432
[857] Brand, E & Wiseman, N, Concise Chinese Materia Medica, Taos, Paradigm Publications, 2008, P 432, Bensky, D, Clavey, S, Stöger, E & Gamble, A, Chinese Herbal Medicine Materia Medica, 3rd Edition, Seattle, Eastland Press, 1986, 1993, 2004, P 754 says, 'slightly Cold.'
[858] Maciocia, G, The Channels of Acupuncture, Philadelphia, Elsevier, 2006, P 545
[859] Brand, E & Wiseman, N, Concise Chinese Materia Medica, Taos, Paradigm Publications, 2008, P 436, Bensky, D, Clavey, S, Stöger, E & Gamble, A, Chinese Herbal Medicine Materia Medica, 3rd Edition, Seattle, Eastland Press, 1986, 1993, 2004, P 825
[860] Chen, JK & TT, Chinese Medical Herbology and Pharmacology, City of Industry, Art of Medicine Press, 2001/2004, P 943
[861] Brand, E & Wiseman, N, Concise Chinese Materia Medica, Taos, Paradigm Publications, 2008, P 436, Bensky, D, Clavey, S, Stöger, E & Gamble, A, Chinese Herbal Medicine Materia Medica, 3rd Edition, Seattle, Eastland Press, 1986, 1993, 2004, P 825
[862] Bensky, D, Clavey, S, Stöger, E & Gamble, A, Chinese Herbal Medicine Materia Medica, 3rd Edition, Seattle, Eastland Press, 1986, 1993, 2004, P 822
[863] Zhang, Shan Lei, *Rectification of the Meaning of Materia Medica,* via Bensky, D, Clavey, S, Stöger, E & Gamble, A, Chinese Herbal Medicine Materia Medica, 3rd Edition, Seattle, Eastland Press, 1986, 1993, 2004, P 823
[864] Brand, E & Wiseman, N, Concise Chinese Materia Medica, Taos, Paradigm Publications, 2008, P 398

[865] Bensky, D, Clavey, S, Stöger, E & Gamble, A, Chinese Herbal Medicine Materia Medica, 3rd Edition, Seattle, Eastland Press, 1986, 1993, 2004, P 851
[866] Bensky, D, Clavey, S, Stöger, E & Gamble, A, Chinese Herbal Medicine Materia Medica, 3rd Edition, Seattle, Eastland Press, 1986, 1993, 2004, P 846
[867] Brand, E & Wiseman, N, Concise Chinese Materia Medica, Taos, Paradigm Publications, 2008, P 445
[868] Bensky, D, Clavey, S, Stöger, E & Gamble, A, Chinese Herbal Medicine Materia Medica, 3rd Edition, Seattle, Eastland Press, 1986, 1993, 2004, P 846
[869] *Materia Medica of Combinations*, via Bensky, D, Clavey, S, Stöger, E & Gamble, A, Chinese Herbal Medicine Materia Medica, 3rd Edition, Seattle, Eastland Press, 1986, 1993, 2004, P 844
[870] Bensky, D, Clavey, S, Stöger, E & Gamble, A, Chinese Herbal Medicine Materia Medica, 3rd Edition, Seattle, Eastland Press, 1986, 1993, 2004, P 864
[871] Chen, JK & TT, Chinese Medical Herbology and Pharmacology, City of Industry, Art of Medicine Press, 2001/2004, P 997, Brand, E & Wiseman, N, Concise Chinese Materia Medica, Taos, Paradigm Publications, 2008, P 463
[872] Bensky, D, Clavey, S, Stöger, E & Gamble, A, Chinese Herbal Medicine Materia Medica, 3rd Edition, Seattle, Eastland Press, 1986, 1993, 2004, P 877
[873] Bensky, D, Clavey, S, Stöger, E & Gamble, A, Chinese Herbal Medicine Materia Medica, 3rd Edition, Seattle, Eastland Press, 1986, 1993, 2004, P 193
[874] Zhang Bing Chen, *Convenient Reader of Materia Medica*, via Bensky, D, Clavey, S, Stöger, E & Gamble, A, Chinese Herbal Medicine Materia Medica, 3rd Edition, Seattle, Eastland Press, 1986, 1993, 2004, P 193
[875] Maciocia, G, The Channels of Acupuncture, Philadelphia, Elsevier, 2006, P 545
[876] Brand, E & Wiseman, N, Concise Chinese Materia Medica, Taos, Paradigm Publications, 2008, P 489
[877] Bensky, D, Clavey, S, Stöger, E & Gamble, A, Chinese Herbal Medicine Materia Medica, 3rd Edition, Seattle, Eastland Press, 1986, 1993, 2004, P 1014
[878] Li Shi Zhen, *Grand Materia Medica*, via Bensky, D, Clavey, S, Stöger, E & Gamble, A, Chinese Herbal Medicine Materia Medica, 3rd Edition, Seattle, Eastland Press, 1986, 1993, 2004, P 1022
[879] Chen, JK & TT, Chinese Medical Herbology and Pharmacology, City of Industry, Art of Medicine Press, 2001/2004, P 1045
[880] Li Shi Zhen, *Grand Materia Medica*, via Bensky, D, Clavey, S, Stöger, E & Gamble, A, Chinese Herbal Medicine Materia Medica, 3rd Edition, Seattle, Eastland Press, 1986, 1993, 2004, P 1022
[881] Li Shi Zhen, *Grand Materia Medica*, via Bensky, D, Clavey, S, Stöger, E & Gamble, A, Chinese Herbal Medicine Materia Medica, 3rd Edition, Seattle, Eastland Press, 1986, 1993, 2004, P 1022
[882] Bensky, D, Clavey, S, Stöger, E & Gamble, A, Chinese Herbal Medicine Materia Medica, 3rd Edition, Seattle, Eastland Press, 1986, 1993, 2004, P 655
[883] Bensky, D, Clavey, S, Stöger, E & Gamble, A, Chinese Herbal Medicine Materia Medica, 3rd Edition, Seattle, Eastland Press, 1986, 1993, 2004, P 1030
[884] Bensky, D, Clavey, S, Stöger, E & Gamble, A, Chinese Herbal Medicine Materia Medica, 3rd Edition, Seattle, Eastland Press, 1986, 1993, 2004, P 1026
[885] Brand, E & Wiseman, N, Concise Chinese Materia Medica, Taos, Paradigm Publications, 2008, P 491

[886] Bensky, D, Clavey, S, Stöger, E & Gamble, A, Chinese Herbal Medicine Materia Medica, 3rd Edition, Seattle, Eastland Press, 1986, 1993, 2004, P 1026
[887] Miao Xi Yong, *Commentary on the Divine Husbandman's Classic of Materia Medica*, via Bensky, D, Clavey, S, Stöger, E & Gamble, A, Chinese Herbal Medicine Materia Medica, 3rd Edition, Seattle, Eastland Press, 1986, 1993, 2004, P 1032
[888] Brand, E & Wiseman, N, Concise Chinese Materia Medica, Taos, Paradigm Publications, 2008, P 491
[889] Brand, E & Wiseman, N, Concise Chinese Materia Medica, Taos, Paradigm Publications, 2008, P 44
[890] Chen Shi Duo, via Bensky, D, Clavey, S, Stöger, E & Gamble, A, Chinese Herbal Medicine Materia Medica, 3rd Edition, Seattle, Eastland Press, 1986, 1993, 2004, P 37
[891] *Materia Medica of the Kai Bao Era*, via Bensky, D, Clavey, S, Stöger, E & Gamble, A, Chinese Herbal Medicine Materia Medica, 3rd Edition, Seattle, Eastland Press, 1986, 1993, 2004, P 46
[892] Chen, JK & TT, Chinese Medical Herbology and Pharmacology, City of Industry, Art of Medicine Press, 2001/2004, P 455
[893] Tang Rong Chuan (Tang Zonghai), Ben Cao Wen Da, Personal Unpublished Translation, 2015, 2.2.2
[894] Bensky, D, Clavey, S, Stöger, E & Gamble, A, Chinese Herbal Medicine Materia Medica, 3rd Edition, Seattle, Eastland Press, 1986, 1993, 2004, P 83
[895] Tang Rong Chuan (Tang Zonghai), Ben Cao Wen Da, Personal Unpublished Translation, 2015, 1.5.14
[896] Wang Ang, via Bensky, D, Clavey, S, Stöger, E & Gamble, A, Chinese Herbal Medicine Materia Medica, 3rd Edition, Seattle, Eastland Press, 1986, 1993, 2004, P 107
[897] Bensky, D, Clavey, S, Stöger, E & Gamble, A, Chinese Herbal Medicine Materia Medica, 3rd Edition, Seattle, Eastland Press, 1986, 1993, 2004, P 101
[898] Zhou Yan, *Records of Thoughtful Differentiation of Materia Medica*, via Bensky, D, Clavey, S, Stöger, E & Gamble, A, Chinese Herbal Medicine Materia Medica, 3rd Edition, Seattle, Eastland Press, 1986, 1993, 2004, P 96
[899] Bensky, D, Clavey, S, Stöger, E & Gamble, A, Chinese Herbal Medicine Materia Medica, 3rd Edition, Seattle, Eastland Press, 1986, 1993, 2004, P 105
[900] Chen, JK & TT, Chinese Medical Herbology and Pharmacology, City of Industry, Art of Medicine Press, 2001/2004, P 151
[901] Bensky, D, Clavey, S, Stöger, E & Gamble, A, Chinese Herbal Medicine Materia Medica, 3rd Edition, Seattle, Eastland Press, 1986, 1993, 2004, P 144
[902] Tang Rong Chuan (Tang Zonghai), Ben Cao Wen Da, Personal Unpublished Translation, 2015, 1.5.3
[903] Maciocia, G, The Channels of Acupuncture, Philadelphia, Elsevier, 2006, P 446
[904] Bensky, D, Clavey, S, Stöger, E & Gamble, A, Chinese Herbal Medicine Materia Medica, 3rd Edition, Seattle, Eastland Press, 1986, 1993, 2004, P 119
[905] *Grand Materia Medica*, via Bensky, D, Clavey, S, Stöger, E & Gamble, A, Chinese Herbal Medicine Materia Medica, 3rd Edition, Seattle, Eastland Press, 1986, 1993, 2004, P 127
[906] Brand, E & Wiseman, N, Concise Chinese Materia Medica, Taos, Paradigm Publications, 2008, P 98

[907] Wang, Hao Gu, *Harm and Benefit in the Materia Medica*, via Bensky, D, Clavey, S, Stöger, E & Gamble, A, Chinese Herbal Medicine Materia Medica, 3rd Edition, Seattle, Eastland Press, 1986, 1993, 2004, P 130
[908] Bensky, D, Clavey, S, Stöger, E & Gamble, A, Chinese Herbal Medicine Materia Medica, 3rd Edition, Seattle, Eastland Press, 1986, 1993, 2004, P 207
[909] Brand, E & Wiseman, N, Concise Chinese Materia Medica, Taos, Paradigm Publications, 2008, P 112
[910] Bensky, D, Clavey, S, Stöger, E & Gamble, A, Chinese Herbal Medicine Materia Medica, 3rd Edition, Seattle, Eastland Press, 1986, 1993, 2004, P 207
[911] Bensky, D, Clavey, S, Stöger, E & Gamble, A, Chinese Herbal Medicine Materia Medica, 3rd Edition, Seattle, Eastland Press, 1986, 1993, 2004, P 206
[912] Brand, E & Wiseman, N, Concise Chinese Materia Medica, Taos, Paradigm Publications, 2008, P 99
[913] Bensky, D, Clavey, S, Stöger, E & Gamble, A, Chinese Herbal Medicine Materia Medica, 3rd Edition, Seattle, Eastland Press, 1986, 1993, 2004, P 159
[914] Brand, E & Wiseman, N, Concise Chinese Materia Medica, Taos, Paradigm Publications, 2008, P 108
[915] Zhang Bing Cheng, *Convenient Reader of Materia Medica*, via Bensky, D, Clavey, S, Stöger, E & Gamble, A, Chinese Herbal Medicine Materia Medica, 3rd Edition, Seattle, Eastland Press, 1986, 1993, 2004, P 156
[916] Bensky, D, Clavey, S, Stöger, E & Gamble, A, Chinese Herbal Medicine Materia Medica, 3rd Edition, Seattle, Eastland Press, 1986, 1993, 2004, P 317
[917] Bensky, D, Clavey, S, Stöger, E & Gamble, A, Chinese Herbal Medicine Materia Medica, 3rd Edition, Seattle, Eastland Press, 1986, 1993, 2004, P317
[918] Bensky, D, Clavey, S, Stöger, E & Gamble, A, Chinese Herbal Medicine Materia Medica, 3rd Edition, Seattle, Eastland Press, 1986, 1993, 2004, P 317
[919] Bensky, D, Clavey, S, Stöger, E & Gamble, A, Chinese Herbal Medicine Materia Medica, 3rd Edition, Seattle, Eastland Press, 1986, 1993, 2004, P 317
[920] Bensky, D, Clavey, S, Stöger, E & Gamble, A, Chinese Herbal Medicine Materia Medica, 3rd Edition, Seattle, Eastland Press, 1986, 1993, 2004, P 153
[921] Bensky, D, Clavey, S, Stöger, E & Gamble, A, Chinese Herbal Medicine Materia Medica, 3rd Edition, Seattle, Eastland Press, 1986, 1993, 2004, P 153
[922] Bensky, D, Clavey, S, Stöger, E & Gamble, A, Chinese Herbal Medicine Materia Medica, 3rd Edition, Seattle, Eastland Press, 1986, 1993, 2004, P 215
[923] Bensky, D, Clavey, S, Stöger, E & Gamble, A, Chinese Herbal Medicine Materia Medica, 3rd Edition, Seattle, Eastland Press, 1986, 1993, 2004, P 215
[924] Bensky, D, Clavey, S, Stöger, E & Gamble, A, Chinese Herbal Medicine Materia Medica, 3rd Edition, Seattle, Eastland Press, 1986, 1993, 2004, P 215
[925] Brand, E & Wiseman, N, Concise Chinese Materia Medica, Taos, Paradigm Publications, 2008, P 102
[926] Zhang Bing Chen, *Convenient Reader of Materia Medica*, via Bensky, D, Clavey, S, Stöger, E & Gamble, A, Chinese Herbal Medicine Materia Medica, 3rd Edition, Seattle, Eastland Press, 1986, 1993, 2004, P 165

[927] Bensky, D, Clavey, S, Stöger, E & Gamble, A, Chinese Herbal Medicine Materia Medica, 3rd Edition, Seattle, Eastland Press, 1986, 1993, 2004, P 193
[928] Bensky, D, Clavey, S, Stöger, E & Gamble, A, Chinese Herbal Medicine Materia Medica, 3rd Edition, Seattle, Eastland Press, 1986, 1993, 2004, P 951
[929] Miao Xi Yong, *Commentary on the Divine Husbandman's Classic of Materia Medica*, via Bensky, D, Clavey, S, Stöger, E & Gamble, A, Chinese Herbal Medicine Materia Medica, 3rd Edition, Seattle, Eastland Press, 1986, 1993, 2004, P 961
[930] Tang Rong Chuan (Tang Zonghai), Ben Cao Wen Da, Personal Unpublished Translation, 2015, 1.3.4
[931] Brand, E & Wiseman, N, Concise Chinese Materia Medica, Taos, Paradigm Publications, 2008, P 132
[932] Tang Rong Chuan (Tang Zonghai), Ben Cao Wen Da, Personal Unpublished Translation, 2015, 1.5.3
[933] Bensky, D, Clavey, S, Stöger, E & Gamble, A, Chinese Herbal Medicine Materia Medica, 3rd Edition, Seattle, Eastland Press, 1986, 1993, 2004, P 239
[934] Tang Rong Chuan (Tang Zonghai), Ben Cao Wen Da, Personal Unpublished Translation, 2015, 1.5.2
[935] Maciocia, G, The Channels of Acupuncture, Philadelphia, Elsevier, 2006, P 446
[936] Ye Tian Shi, *Renewed Materia Medica*, via Bensky, D, Clavey, S, Stöger, E & Gamble, A, Chinese Herbal Medicine Materia Medica, 3rd Edition, Seattle, Eastland Press, 1986, 1993, 2004, P 351
[937] Ye Tian Shi, *Renewed Materia Medica*, via Bensky, D, Clavey, S, Stöger, E & Gamble, A, Chinese Herbal Medicine Materia Medica, 3rd Edition, Seattle, Eastland Press, 1986, 1993, 2004, P 351
[938] Bensky, D, Clavey, S, Stöger, E & Gamble, A, Chinese Herbal Medicine Materia Medica, 3rd Edition, Seattle, Eastland Press, 1986, 1993, 2004, P 360
[939] Bensky, D, Clavey, S, Stöger, E & Gamble, A, Chinese Herbal Medicine Materia Medica, 3rd Edition, Seattle, Eastland Press, 1986, 1993, 2004, P 267
[940] Brand, E & Wiseman, N, Concise Chinese Materia Medica, Taos, Paradigm Publications, 2008, P 198
[941] Bensky, D, Clavey, S, Stöger, E & Gamble, A, Chinese Herbal Medicine Materia Medica, 3rd Edition, Seattle, Eastland Press, 1986, 1993, 2004, P 317
[942] Bensky, D, Clavey, S, Stöger, E & Gamble, A, Chinese Herbal Medicine Materia Medica, 3rd Edition, Seattle, Eastland Press, 1986, 1993, 2004, P317
[943] Bensky, D, Clavey, S, Stöger, E & Gamble, A, Chinese Herbal Medicine Materia Medica, 3rd Edition, Seattle, Eastland Press, 1986, 1993, 2004, P 317
[944] Bensky, D, Clavey, S, Stöger, E & Gamble, A, Chinese Herbal Medicine Materia Medica, 3rd Edition, Seattle, Eastland Press, 1986, 1993, 2004, P 317
[945] Bensky, D, Clavey, S, Stöger, E & Gamble, A, Chinese Herbal Medicine Materia Medica, 3rd Edition, Seattle, Eastland Press, 1986, 1993, 2004, P 285
[946] Brand, E & Wiseman, N, Concise Chinese Materia Medica, Taos, Paradigm Publications, 2008, P 194
[947] Chen, JK & TT, Chinese Medical Herbology and Pharmacology, City of Industry, Art of Medicine Press, 2001/2004, P 455
[948] Tang Rong Chuan (Tang Zonghai), Ben Cao Wen Da, Personal Unpublished Translation, 2015, 2.2.2

[949] Bensky, D, Clavey, S, Stöger, E & Gamble, A, Chinese Herbal Medicine Materia Medica, 3rd Edition, Seattle, Eastland Press, 1986, 1993, 2004, P 83
[950] Bensky, D, Clavey, S, Stöger, E & Gamble, A, Chinese Herbal Medicine Materia Medica, 3rd Edition, Seattle, Eastland Press, 1986, 1993, 2004, P 680
[951] Tang Rong Chuan (Tang Zonghai), Ben Cao Wen Da, Personal Unpublished Translation, 2015, 1.2.4
[952] Tang Rong Chuan (Tang Zonghai), Ben Cao Wen Da, Personal Unpublished Translation, 2015, 1.2.4
[953] Chen, JK & TT, Chinese Medical Herbology and Pharmacology, City of Industry, Art of Medicine Press, 2001/2004, P 441
[954] Brand, E & Wiseman, N, Concise Chinese Materia Medica, Taos, Paradigm Publications, 2008, P 208
[955] Zhang, Shan Lei, *Rectification of the Meaning of Materia Medica,* via Bensky, D, Clavey, S, Stöger, E & Gamble, A, Chinese Herbal Medicine Materia Medica, 3rd Edition, Seattle, Eastland Press, 1986, 1993, 2004, P 675
[956] Tang Rong Chuan (Tang Zonghai), Ben Cao Wen Da, Personal Unpublished Translation, 2015, 2.2.2
[957] Maciocia, G, The Channels of Acupuncture, Philadelphia, Elsevier, 2006, P 446
[958] Brand, E & Wiseman, N, Concise Chinese Materia Medica, Taos, Paradigm Publications, 2008, P 269
[959] Bensky, D, Clavey, S, Stöger, E & Gamble, A, Chinese Herbal Medicine Materia Medica, 3rd Edition, Seattle, Eastland Press, 1986, 1993, 2004, P 588
[960] Bensky, D, Clavey, S, Stöger, E & Gamble, A, Chinese Herbal Medicine Materia Medica, 3rd Edition, Seattle, Eastland Press, 1986, 1993, 2004, P 588
[961] Bensky, D, Clavey, S, Stöger, E & Gamble, A, Chinese Herbal Medicine Materia Medica, 3rd Edition, Seattle, Eastland Press, 1986, 1993, 2004, P 563
[962] Bensky, D, Clavey, S, Stöger, E & Gamble, A, Chinese Herbal Medicine Materia Medica, 3rd Edition, Seattle, Eastland Press, 1986, 1993, 2004, P 562
[963] Bensky, D, Clavey, S, Stöger, E & Gamble, A, Chinese Herbal Medicine Materia Medica, 3rd Edition, Seattle, Eastland Press, 1986, 1993, 2004, P 652
[964] Chen, JK & TT, Chinese Medical Herbology and Pharmacology, City of Industry, Art of Medicine Press, 2001/2004, P 593
[965] Brand, E & Wiseman, N, Concise Chinese Materia Medica, Taos, Paradigm Publications, 2008, P 266
[966] Bensky, D, Clavey, S, Stöger, E & Gamble, A, Chinese Herbal Medicine Materia Medica, 3rd Edition, Seattle, Eastland Press, 1986, 1993, 2004, P 562
[967] Zhang Bing Chen, *Convenient Reader of Materia Medica*, via Bensky, D, Clavey, S, Stöger, E & Gamble, A, Chinese Herbal Medicine Materia Medica, 3rd Edition, Seattle, Eastland Press, 1986, 1993, 2004, P 568
[968] Bensky, D, Clavey, S, Stöger, E & Gamble, A, Chinese Herbal Medicine Materia Medica, 3rd Edition, Seattle, Eastland Press, 1986, 1993, 2004, P 567
[969] Brand, E & Wiseman, N, Concise Chinese Materia Medica, Taos, Paradigm Publications, 2008, P 260

[970] Zhang Bing Chen, *Convenient Reader of Materia Medica*, via Bensky, D, Clavey, S, Stöger, E & Gamble, A, Chinese Herbal Medicine Materia Medica, 3rd Edition, Seattle, Eastland Press, 1986, 1993, 2004, P 569
[971] Zhang Bing Chen, *Convenient Reader of Materia Medica*, via Bensky, D, Clavey, S, Stöger, E & Gamble, A, Chinese Herbal Medicine Materia Medica, 3rd Edition, Seattle, Eastland Press, 1986, 1993, 2004, P 569
[972] Bensky, D, Clavey, S, Stöger, E & Gamble, A, Chinese Herbal Medicine Materia Medica, 3rd Edition, Seattle, Eastland Press, 1986, 1993, 2004, P 564
[973] Brand, E & Wiseman, N, Concise Chinese Materia Medica, Taos, Paradigm Publications, 2008, P 288, Bensky, D, Clavey, S, Stöger, E & Gamble, A, Chinese Herbal Medicine Materia Medica, 3rd Edition, Seattle, Eastland Press, 1986, 1993, 2004, P 624
[974] Bensky, D, Clavey, S, Stöger, E & Gamble, A, Chinese Herbal Medicine Materia Medica, 3rd Edition, Seattle, Eastland Press, 1986, 1993, 2004, P 610
[975] Zhang Bing Chen, *Convenient Reader of Materia Medica*, via Bensky, D, Clavey, S, Stöger, E & Gamble, A, Chinese Herbal Medicine Materia Medica, 3rd Edition, Seattle, Eastland Press, 1986, 1993, 2004, P 607
[976] Bensky, D, Clavey, S, Stöger, E & Gamble, A, Chinese Herbal Medicine Materia Medica, 3rd Edition, Seattle, Eastland Press, 1986, 1993, 2004, P 653
[977] Bensky, D, Clavey, S, Stöger, E & Gamble, A, Chinese Herbal Medicine Materia Medica, 3rd Edition, Seattle, Eastland Press, 1986, 1993, 2004, P 664
[978] Bensky, D, Clavey, S, Stöger, E & Gamble, A, Chinese Herbal Medicine Materia Medica, 3rd Edition, Seattle, Eastland Press, 1986, 1993, 2004, P 664
[979] Brand, E & Wiseman, N, Concise Chinese Materia Medica, Taos, Paradigm Publications, 2008, P 293
[980] Bensky, D, Clavey, S, Stöger, E & Gamble, A, Chinese Herbal Medicine Materia Medica, 3rd Edition, Seattle, Eastland Press, 1986, 1993, 2004, P 605
[981] Bensky, D, Clavey, S, Stöger, E & Gamble, A, Chinese Herbal Medicine Materia Medica, 3rd Edition, Seattle, Eastland Press, 1986, 1993, 2004, P 605
[982] Brand, E & Wiseman, N, Concise Chinese Materia Medica, Taos, Paradigm Publications, 2008, P 284
[983] Bensky, D, Clavey, S, Stöger, E & Gamble, A, Chinese Herbal Medicine Materia Medica, 3rd Edition, Seattle, Eastland Press, 1986, 1993, 2004, P 650
[984] Bensky, D, Clavey, S, Stöger, E & Gamble, A, Chinese Herbal Medicine Materia Medica, 3rd Edition, Seattle, Eastland Press, 1986, 1993, 2004, P 650
[985] Chen, JK & TT, Chinese Medical Herbology and Pharmacology, City of Industry, Art of Medicine Press, 2001/2004, P 659
[986] Brand, E & Wiseman, N, Concise Chinese Materia Medica, Taos, Paradigm Publications, 2008, P 289, Bensky, D, Clavey, S, Stöger, E & Gamble, A, Chinese Herbal Medicine Materia Medica, 3rd Edition, Seattle, Eastland Press, 1986, 1993, 2004, P 614
[987] *Grand Materia Medica*, via Bensky, D, Clavey, S, Stöger, E & Gamble, A, Chinese Herbal Medicine Materia Medica, 3rd Edition, Seattle, Eastland Press, 1986, 1993, 2004, P 127
[988] Brand, E & Wiseman, N, Concise Chinese Materia Medica, Taos, Paradigm Publications, 2008, P 286

[989] Wang, Hao Gu, *Harm and Benefit in the Materia Medica*, via Bensky, D, Clavey, S, Stöger, E & Gamble, A, Chinese Herbal Medicine Materia Medica, 3rd Edition, Seattle, Eastland Press, 1986, 1993, 2004, P 603
[990] Chen, JK & TT, Chinese Medical Herbology and Pharmacology, City of Industry, Art of Medicine Press, 2001/2004, P 636 , Bensky, D, Clavey, S, Stöger, E & Gamble, A, Chinese Herbal Medicine Materia Medica, 3rd Edition, Seattle, Eastland Press, 1986, 1993, 2004, P 602
[991] Tang Rong Chuan (Tang Zonghai), Ben Cao Wen Da, Personal Unpublished Translation, 2015, 1.2.3
[992] Zhang, Shan Lei, *Rectification of the Meaning of Materia Medica,* via Bensky, D, Clavey, S, Stöger, E & Gamble, A, Chinese Herbal Medicine Materia Medica, 3rd Edition, Seattle, Eastland Press, 1986, 1993, 2004, P 628
[993] Zhang, Shan Lei, *Rectification of the Meaning of Materia Medica,* via Bensky, D, Clavey, S, Stöger, E & Gamble, A, Chinese Herbal Medicine Materia Medica, 3rd Edition, Seattle, Eastland Press, 1986, 1993, 2004, P 628
[994] Brand, E & Wiseman, N, Concise Chinese Materia Medica, Taos, Paradigm Publications, 2008, P 288
[995] Chen, JK & TT, Chinese Medical Herbology and Pharmacology, City of Industry, Art of Medicine Press, 2001/2004, P 642
[996] Brand, E & Wiseman, N, Concise Chinese Materia Medica, Taos, Paradigm Publications, 2008, P 296
[997] Chen, JK & TT, Chinese Medical Herbology and Pharmacology, City of Industry, Art of Medicine Press, 2001/2004, P 1058
[998] Brand, E & Wiseman, N, Concise Chinese Materia Medica, Taos, Paradigm Publications, 2008, P 322
[999] Brand, E & Wiseman, N, Concise Chinese Materia Medica, Taos, Paradigm Publications, 2008, P 322
[1000] Brand, E & Wiseman, N, Concise Chinese Materia Medica, Taos, Paradigm Publications, 2008, P 318
[1001] Brand, E & Wiseman, N, Concise Chinese Materia Medica, Taos, Paradigm Publications, 2008, P 321
[1002] Brand, E & Wiseman, N, Concise Chinese Materia Medica, Taos, Paradigm Publications, 2008, P 330
[1003] Chen Shi Duo, *New Edition of Materia Medica*, via Bensky, D, Clavey, S, Stöger, E & Gamble, A, Chinese Herbal Medicine Materia Medica, 3rd Edition, Seattle, Eastland Press, 1986, 1993, 2004, P 443
[1004] Chen, JK & TT, Chinese Medical Herbology and Pharmacology, City of Industry, Art of Medicine Press, 2001/2004, P 729
[1005] Chen Shi Duo, *New Edition of Materia Medica*, via Bensky, D, Clavey, S, Stöger, E & Gamble, A, Chinese Herbal Medicine Materia Medica, 3rd Edition, Seattle, Eastland Press, 1986, 1993, 2004, P 443
[1006] *Sichuan Chinese Materia Medica*, via Bensky, D, Clavey, S, Stöger, E & Gamble, A, Chinese Herbal Medicine Materia Medica, 3rd Edition, Seattle, Eastland Press, 1986, 1993, 2004, P 939
[1007] *Sichuan Chinese Materia Medica*, via Bensky, D, Clavey, S, Stöger, E & Gamble, A, Chinese Herbal Medicine Materia Medica, 3rd Edition, Seattle, Eastland Press, 1986, 1993, 2004, P 939

[1008] Bensky, D, Clavey, S, Stöger, E & Gamble, A, Chinese Herbal Medicine Materia Medica, 3rd Edition, Seattle, Eastland Press, 1986, 1993, 2004, P 543

[1009] Brand, E & Wiseman, N, Concise Chinese Materia Medica, Taos, Paradigm Publications, 2008, P 352

[1010] Li Shi Zhen, *Grand Materia Medica*, via Bensky, D, Clavey, S, Stöger, E & Gamble, A, Chinese Herbal Medicine Materia Medica, 3rd Edition, Seattle, Eastland Press, 1986, 1993, 2004, P 931

[1011] Zhang, Jie Bin, *Rectification of the Meaning of Materia Medica*, via Bensky, D, Clavey, S, Stöger, E & Gamble, A, Chinese Herbal Medicine Materia Medica, 3rd Edition, Seattle, Eastland Press, 1986, 1993, 2004, P 931

[1012] Zhang, Jie Bin, *Rectification of the Meaning of Materia Medica*, via Bensky, D, Clavey, S, Stöger, E & Gamble, A, Chinese Herbal Medicine Materia Medica, 3rd Edition, Seattle, Eastland Press, 1986, 1993, 2004, P 931

[1013] Brand, E & Wiseman, N, Concise Chinese Materia Medica, Taos, Paradigm Publications, 2008, P 350, Bensky, D, Clavey, S, Stöger, E & Gamble, A, Chinese Herbal Medicine Materia Medica, 3rd Edition, Seattle, Eastland Press, 1986, 1993, 2004, P 928

[1014] Bensky, D, Clavey, S, Stöger, E & Gamble, A, Chinese Herbal Medicine Materia Medica, 3rd Edition, Seattle, Eastland Press, 1986, 1993, 2004, P 928

[1015] Bensky, D, Clavey, S, Stöger, E & Gamble, A, Chinese Herbal Medicine Materia Medica, 3rd Edition, Seattle, Eastland Press, 1986, 1993, 2004, P 928

[1016] Brand, E & Wiseman, N, Concise Chinese Materia Medica, Taos, Paradigm Publications, 2008, P 355

[1017] Brand, E & Wiseman, N, Concise Chinese Materia Medica, Taos, Paradigm Publications, 2008, P 355

[1018] This is my call, but I think that virtually anyone smelling magnolia flower would agree that it is very aromatic.

[1019] Bensky, D, Clavey, S, Stöger, E & Gamble, A, Chinese Herbal Medicine Materia Medica, 3rd Edition, Seattle, Eastland Press, 1986, 1993, 2004, P 912

[1020] Wang, Hao Gu, *Harm and Benefit in the Materia Medica*, via Bensky, D, Clavey, S, Stöger, E & Gamble, A, Chinese Herbal Medicine Materia Medica, 3rd Edition, Seattle, Eastland Press, 1986, 1993, 2004, P 924

[1021] Chen, JK & TT, Chinese Medical Herbology and Pharmacology, City of Industry, Art of Medicine Press, 2001/2004, P 760, and Bensky, D, Clavey, S, Stöger, E & Gamble, A, Chinese Herbal Medicine Materia Medica, 3rd Edition, Seattle, Eastland Press, 1986, 1993, 2004, P 923

[1022] Chen, JK & TT, Chinese Medical Herbology and Pharmacology, City of Industry, Art of Medicine Press, 2001/2004, P 346, and *Thoroughly Revised Materia Medica*, via Bensky, D, Clavey, S, Stöger, E & Gamble, A, Chinese Herbal Medicine Materia Medica, 3rd Edition, Seattle, Eastland Press, 1986, 1993, 2004, P 916

[1023] Zhang Xi Chun, *Essays on Medicine Esteeming the Chinese and Respecting the Western*, via Bensky, D, Clavey, S, Stöger, E & Gamble, A, Chinese Herbal Medicine Materia Medica, 3rd Edition, Seattle, Eastland Press, 1986, 1993, 2004, P 911

[1024] Brand, E & Wiseman, N, Concise Chinese Materia Medica, Taos, Paradigm Publications, 2008, P 348

[1025] Bensky, D, Clavey, S, Stöger, E & Gamble, A, Chinese Herbal Medicine Materia Medica, 3rd Edition, Seattle, Eastland Press, 1986, 1993, 2004, P 910

[1026] Bensky, D, Clavey, S, Stöger, E & Gamble, A, Chinese Herbal Medicine Materia Medica, 3rd Edition, Seattle, Eastland Press, 1986, 1993, 2004, P 910
[1027] Brand, E & Wiseman, N, Concise Chinese Materia Medica, Taos, Paradigm Publications, 2008, P 347, Bensky, D, Clavey, S, Stöger, E & Gamble, A, Chinese Herbal Medicine Materia Medica, 3rd Edition, Seattle, Eastland Press, 1986, 1993, 2004, P 910
[1028] Maciocia, G, The Channels of Acupuncture, Philadelphia, Elsevier, 2006, P 545
[1029] Zhang Bing Chen, *Convenient Reader of Materia Medica*, via Bensky, D, Clavey, S, Stöger, E & Gamble, A, Chinese Herbal Medicine Materia Medica, 3rd Edition, Seattle, Eastland Press, 1986, 1993, 2004, P 919
[1030] Brand, E & Wiseman, N, Concise Chinese Materia Medica, Taos, Paradigm Publications, 2008, P 365
[1031] Bensky, D, Clavey, S, Stöger, E & Gamble, A, Chinese Herbal Medicine Materia Medica, 3rd Edition, Seattle, Eastland Press, 1986, 1993, 2004, P 920
[1032] Bensky, D, Clavey, S, Stöger, E & Gamble, A, Chinese Herbal Medicine Materia Medica, 3rd Edition, Seattle, Eastland Press, 1986, 1993, 2004, P 921
[1033] Yao Lan, *Materia Medica Arranged by Channel*, via Bensky, D, Clavey, S, Stöger, E & Gamble, A, Chinese Herbal Medicine Materia Medica, 3rd Edition, Seattle, Eastland Press, 1986, 1993, 2004, P 922
[1034] Bensky, D, Clavey, S, Stöger, E & Gamble, A, Chinese Herbal Medicine Materia Medica, 3rd Edition, Seattle, Eastland Press, 1986, 1993, 2004, P 991
[1035] Brand, E & Wiseman, N, Concise Chinese Materia Medica, Taos, Paradigm Publications, 2008, P 369, Bensky, D, Clavey, S, Stöger, E & Gamble, A, Chinese Herbal Medicine Materia Medica, 3rd Edition, Seattle, Eastland Press, 1986, 1993, 2004, P 970
[1036] Bensky, D, Clavey, S, Stöger, E & Gamble, A, Chinese Herbal Medicine Materia Medica, 3rd Edition, Seattle, Eastland Press, 1986, 1993, 2004, P 987
[1037] Zhang Bing Chen, *Convenient Reader of Materia Medica*, via Bensky, D, Clavey, S, Stöger, E & Gamble, A, Chinese Herbal Medicine Materia Medica, 3rd Edition, Seattle, Eastland Press, 1986, 1993, 2004, P 919
[1038] Brand, E & Wiseman, N, Concise Chinese Materia Medica, Taos, Paradigm Publications, 2008, P 365
[1039] Bensky, D, Clavey, S, Stöger, E & Gamble, A, Chinese Herbal Medicine Materia Medica, 3rd Edition, Seattle, Eastland Press, 1986, 1993, 2004, P 920
[1040] Bensky, D, Clavey, S, Stöger, E & Gamble, A, Chinese Herbal Medicine Materia Medica, 3rd Edition, Seattle, Eastland Press, 1986, 1993, 2004, P 921
[1041] Yao Lan, *Materia Medica Arranged by Channel*, via Bensky, D, Clavey, S, Stöger, E & Gamble, A, Chinese Herbal Medicine Materia Medica, 3rd Edition, Seattle, Eastland Press, 1986, 1993, 2004, P 922
[1042] Brand, E & Wiseman, N, Concise Chinese Materia Medica, Taos, Paradigm Publications, 2008, P 383
[1043] Bensky, D, Clavey, S, Stöger, E & Gamble, A, Chinese Herbal Medicine Materia Medica, 3rd Edition, Seattle, Eastland Press, 1986, 1993, 2004, P 954
[1044] Chen, JK & TT, Chinese Medical Herbology and Pharmacology, City of Industry, Art of Medicine Press, 2001/2004, P 825

[1045] Chen, JK & TT, Chinese Medical Herbology and Pharmacology, City of Industry, Art of Medicine Press, 2001/2004, P 825
[1046] Brand, E & Wiseman, N, Concise Chinese Materia Medica, Taos, Paradigm Publications, 2008, P 385, Bensky, D, Clavey, S, Stöger, E & Gamble, A, Chinese Herbal Medicine Materia Medica, 3rd Edition, Seattle, Eastland Press, 1986, 1993, 2004, P 956
[1047] Bensky, D, Clavey, S, Stöger, E & Gamble, A, Chinese Herbal Medicine Materia Medica, 3rd Edition, Seattle, Eastland Press, 1986, 1993, 2004, P 950
[1048] Bensky, D, Clavey, S, Stöger, E & Gamble, A, Chinese Herbal Medicine Materia Medica, 3rd Edition, Seattle, Eastland Press, 1986, 1993, 2004, P 951
[1049] Miao Xi Yong, *Commentary on the Divine Husbandman's Classic of Materia Medica*, via Bensky, D, Clavey, S, Stöger, E & Gamble, A, Chinese Herbal Medicine Materia Medica, 3rd Edition, Seattle, Eastland Press, 1986, 1993, 2004, P 961
[1050] Maciocia, G, The Channels of Acupuncture, Philadelphia, Elsevier, 2006, P 545
[1051] Brand, E & Wiseman, N, Concise Chinese Materia Medica, Taos, Paradigm Publications, 2008, P 411
[1052] Brand, E & Wiseman, N, Concise Chinese Materia Medica, Taos, Paradigm Publications, 2008, P 411
[1053] Chen, JK & TT, Chinese Medical Herbology and Pharmacology, City of Industry, Art of Medicine Press, 2001/2004, P 853
[1054] Bensky, D, Clavey, S, Stöger, E & Gamble, A, Chinese Herbal Medicine Materia Medica, 3rd Edition, Seattle, Eastland Press, 1986, 1993, 2004, P 822
[1055] Zhang, Shan Lei, *Rectification of the Meaning of Materia Medica,* via Bensky, D, Clavey, S, Stöger, E & Gamble, A, Chinese Herbal Medicine Materia Medica, 3rd Edition, Seattle, Eastland Press, 1986, 1993, 2004, P 823
[1056] Brand, E & Wiseman, N, Concise Chinese Materia Medica, Taos, Paradigm Publications, 2008, P 398
[1057] Brand, E & Wiseman, N, Concise Chinese Materia Medica, Taos, Paradigm Publications, 2008, P 395
[1058] Brand, E & Wiseman, N, Concise Chinese Materia Medica, Taos, Paradigm Publications, 2008, P 395
[1059] Brand, E & Wiseman, N, Concise Chinese Materia Medica, Taos, Paradigm Publications, 2008, P 409
[1060] Chen, JK & TT, Chinese Medical Herbology and Pharmacology, City of Industry, Art of Medicine Press, 2001/2004, P 883
[1061] Brand, E & Wiseman, N, Concise Chinese Materia Medica, Taos, Paradigm Publications, 2008, P 432
[1062] Chen, JK & TT, Chinese Medical Herbology and Pharmacology, City of Industry, Art of Medicine Press, 2001/2004, P 928
[1063] Tang Rong Chuan (Tang Zonghai), Ben Cao Wen Da, Personal Unpublished Translation, 2015, 1.3.3
[1064] Tang Rong Chuan (Tang Zonghai), Ben Cao Wen Da, Personal Unpublished Translation, 2015, 1.2.3
[1065] Maciocia, G, The Channels of Acupuncture, Philadelphia, Elsevier, 2006, P 545

[1066] Chen, JK & TT, Chinese Medical Herbology and Pharmacology, City of Industry, Art of Medicine Press, 2001/2004, P 959, Bensky, D, Clavey, S, Stöger, E & Gamble, A, Chinese Herbal Medicine Materia Medica, 3rd Edition, Seattle, Eastland Press, 1986, 1993, 2004, P 763
[1067] Bensky, D, Clavey, S, Stöger, E & Gamble, A, Chinese Herbal Medicine Materia Medica, 3rd Edition, Seattle, Eastland Press, 1986, 1993, 2004, P 744
[1068] Brand, E & Wiseman, N, Concise Chinese Materia Medica, Taos, Paradigm Publications, 2008, P 436, Bensky, D, Clavey, S, Stöger, E & Gamble, A, Chinese Herbal Medicine Materia Medica, 3rd Edition, Seattle, Eastland Press, 1986, 1993, 2004, P 825
[1069] Chen, JK & TT, Chinese Medical Herbology and Pharmacology, City of Industry, Art of Medicine Press, 2001/2004, P 943
[1070] Brand, E & Wiseman, N, Concise Chinese Materia Medica, Taos, Paradigm Publications, 2008, P 436, Bensky, D, Clavey, S, Stöger, E & Gamble, A, Chinese Herbal Medicine Materia Medica, 3rd Edition, Seattle, Eastland Press, 1986, 1993, 2004, P 825
[1071] Bensky, D, Clavey, S, Stöger, E & Gamble, A, Chinese Herbal Medicine Materia Medica, 3rd Edition, Seattle, Eastland Press, 1986, 1993, 2004, P 822
[1072] Zhang, Shan Lei, *Rectification of the Meaning of Materia Medica,* via Bensky, D, Clavey, S, Stöger, E & Gamble, A, Chinese Herbal Medicine Materia Medica, 3rd Edition, Seattle, Eastland Press, 1986, 1993, 2004, P 823
[1073] Brand, E & Wiseman, N, Concise Chinese Materia Medica, Taos, Paradigm Publications, 2008, P 398
[1074] Bensky, D, Clavey, S, Stöger, E & Gamble, A, Chinese Herbal Medicine Materia Medica, 3rd Edition, Seattle, Eastland Press, 1986, 1993, 2004, P 835
[1075] Zhang, Shan Lei, *Rectification of the Meaning of Materia Medica,* via Bensky, D, Clavey, S, Stöger, E & Gamble, A, Chinese Herbal Medicine Materia Medica, 3rd Edition, Seattle, Eastland Press, 1986, 1993, 2004, P 836
[1076] Zhang, Shan Lei, *Rectification of the Meaning of Materia Medica,* via Bensky, D, Clavey, S, Stöger, E & Gamble, A, Chinese Herbal Medicine Materia Medica, 3rd Edition, Seattle, Eastland Press, 1986, 1993, 2004, P 836
[1077] Brand, E & Wiseman, N, Concise Chinese Materia Medica, Taos, Paradigm Publications, 2008, P 440, Bensky, D, Clavey, S, Stöger, E & Gamble, A, Chinese Herbal Medicine Materia Medica, 3rd Edition, Seattle, Eastland Press, 1986, 1993, 2004, P 835
[1078] Chen, JK & TT, Chinese Medical Herbology and Pharmacology, City of Industry, Art of Medicine Press, 2001/2004, P 959, Bensky, D, Clavey, S, Stöger, E & Gamble, A, Chinese Herbal Medicine Materia Medica, 3rd Edition, Seattle, Eastland Press, 1986, 1993, 2004, P 763
[1079] Ye Tian Shi, *Case Records as a Guide to Clinical Practice*, via Bensky, D, Clavey, S, Stöger, E & Gamble, A, Chinese Herbal Medicine Materia Medica, 3rd Edition, Seattle, Eastland Press, 1986, 1993, 2004, P 844
[1080] Brand, E & Wiseman, N, Concise Chinese Materia Medica, Taos, Paradigm Publications, 2008, P 457, Bensky, D, Clavey, S, Stöger, E & Gamble, A, Chinese Herbal Medicine Materia Medica, 3rd Edition, Seattle, Eastland Press, 1986, 1993, 2004, P 860
[1081] Li Shi Zhen, *Grand Materia Medica*, via Bensky, D, Clavey, S, Stöger, E & Gamble, A, Chinese Herbal Medicine Materia Medica, 3rd Edition, Seattle, Eastland Press, 1986, 1993, 2004, P 861
[1082] Li Shi Zhen, *Grand Materia Medica*, via Bensky, D, Clavey, S, Stöger, E & Gamble, A, Chinese Herbal Medicine Materia Medica, 3rd Edition, Seattle, Eastland Press, 1986, 1993, 2004, P 861

[1083] Li Shi Zhen, *Grand Materia Medica*, via Bensky, D, Clavey, S, Stöger, E & Gamble, A, Chinese Herbal Medicine Materia Medica, 3rd Edition, Seattle, Eastland Press, 1986, 1993, 2004, P 861
[1084] Maciocia, G, The Channels of Acupuncture, Philadelphia, Elsevier, 2006, P 545
[1085] Bensky, D, Clavey, S, Stöger, E & Gamble, A, Chinese Herbal Medicine Materia Medica, 3rd Edition, Seattle, Eastland Press, 1986, 1993, 2004, P 193
[1086] Zhang Bing Chen, *Convenient Reader of Materia Medica*, via Bensky, D, Clavey, S, Stöger, E & Gamble, A, Chinese Herbal Medicine Materia Medica, 3rd Edition, Seattle, Eastland Press, 1986, 1993, 2004, P 193
[1087] Bensky, D, Clavey, S, Stöger, E & Gamble, A, Chinese Herbal Medicine Materia Medica, 3rd Edition, Seattle, Eastland Press, 1986, 1993, 2004, P 896
[1088] Li Shi Zhen, *Grand Materia Medica*, via Bensky, D, Clavey, S, Stöger, E & Gamble, A, Chinese Herbal Medicine Materia Medica, 3rd Edition, Seattle, Eastland Press, 1986, 1993, 2004, P 896
[1089] Li Shi Zhen, *Grand Materia Medica*, via Bensky, D, Clavey, S, Stöger, E & Gamble, A, Chinese Herbal Medicine Materia Medica, 3rd Edition, Seattle, Eastland Press, 1986, 1993, 2004, P 898
[1090] Li Shi Zhen, *Grand Materia Medica*, via Bensky, D, Clavey, S, Stöger, E & Gamble, A, Chinese Herbal Medicine Materia Medica, 3rd Edition, Seattle, Eastland Press, 1986, 1993, 2004, P 898
[1091] Bensky, D, Clavey, S, Stöger, E & Gamble, A, Chinese Herbal Medicine Materia Medica, 3rd Edition, Seattle, Eastland Press, 1986, 1993, 2004, P 105
[1092] Bensky, D, Clavey, S, Stöger, E & Gamble, A, Chinese Herbal Medicine Materia Medica, 3rd Edition, Seattle, Eastland Press, 1986, 1993, 2004, P 883
[1093] Bensky, D, Clavey, S, Stöger, E & Gamble, A, Chinese Herbal Medicine Materia Medica, 3rd Edition, Seattle, Eastland Press, 1986, 1993, 2004, P 1017
[1094] Chen, JK & TT, Chinese Medical Herbology and Pharmacology, City of Industry, Art of Medicine Press, 2001/2004, P 1039
[1095] Brand, E & Wiseman, N, Concise Chinese Materia Medica, Taos, Paradigm Publications, 2008, P 484
[1096] Brand, E & Wiseman, N, Concise Chinese Materia Medica, Taos, Paradigm Publications, 2008, P 484
[1097] Brand, E & Wiseman, N, Concise Chinese Materia Medica, Taos, Paradigm Publications, 2008, P 484
[1098] Brand, E & Wiseman, N, Concise Chinese Materia Medica, Taos, Paradigm Publications, 2008, P 490, Bensky, D, Clavey, S, Stöger, E & Gamble, A, Chinese Herbal Medicine Materia Medica, 3rd Edition, Seattle, Eastland Press, 1986, 1993, 2004, P 1038
[1099] Bensky, D, Clavey, S, Stöger, E & Gamble, A, Chinese Herbal Medicine Materia Medica, 3rd Edition, Seattle, Eastland Press, 1986, 1993, 2004, P 1026
[1100] Brand, E & Wiseman, N, Concise Chinese Materia Medica, Taos, Paradigm Publications, 2008, P 491
[1101] Bensky, D, Clavey, S, Stöger, E & Gamble, A, Chinese Herbal Medicine Materia Medica, 3rd Edition, Seattle, Eastland Press, 1986, 1993, 2004, P 1026
[1102] Brand, E & Wiseman, N, Concise Chinese Materia Medica, Taos, Paradigm Publications, 2008, P 296
[1103] Chen, JK & TT, Chinese Medical Herbology and Pharmacology, City of Industry, Art of Medicine Press, 2001/2004, P 1058

[1104] Tang Rong Chuan (Tang Zonghai), Ben Cao Wen Da, Personal Unpublished Translation, 2015, 2.1.6

[1105] Tang Rong Chuan (Tang Zonghai), Ben Cao Wen Da, Personal Unpublished Translation, 2015, 2.1.3

[1106] Bensky, D, Clavey, S, Stöger, E & Gamble, A, Chinese Herbal Medicine Materia Medica, 3rd Edition, Seattle, Eastland Press, 1986, 1993, 2004, P 20/21

[1107] Maciocia, G, The Channels of Acupuncture, Philadelphia, Elsevier, 2006, P 446

[1108] Tang Rong Chuan (Tang Zonghai), Ben Cao Wen Da, Personal Unpublished Translation, 2015, 2.1.3

[1109] Tang Rong Chuan (Tang Zonghai), Ben Cao Wen Da, Personal Unpublished Translation, 2015, 1.5.10

[1110] Tang Rong Chuan (Tang Zonghai), Ben Cao Wen Da, Personal Unpublished Translation, 2015, 1.4.6

[1111] Tang Rong Chuan (Tang Zonghai), Ben Cao Wen Da, Personal Unpublished Translation, 2015, 1.5.9

[1112] Tang Rong Chuan (Tang Zonghai), Ben Cao Wen Da, Personal Unpublished Translation, 2015, 1.5.9

[1113] Tang Rong Chuan (Tang Zonghai), Ben Cao Wen Da, Personal Unpublished Translation, 2015, 1.4.6

[1114] Chen, JK & TT, Chinese Medical Herbology and Pharmacology, City of Industry, Art of Medicine Press, 2001/2004, P 151

[1115] Bensky, D, Clavey, S, Stöger, E & Gamble, A, Chinese Herbal Medicine Materia Medica, 3rd Edition, Seattle, Eastland Press, 1986, 1993, 2004, P 144

[1116] Bensky, D, Clavey, S, Stöger, E & Gamble, A, Chinese Herbal Medicine Materia Medica, 3rd Edition, Seattle, Eastland Press, 1986, 1993, 2004, P 317

[1117] Bensky, D, Clavey, S, Stöger, E & Gamble, A, Chinese Herbal Medicine Materia Medica, 3rd Edition, Seattle, Eastland Press, 1986, 1993, 2004, P317

[1118] Bensky, D, Clavey, S, Stöger, E & Gamble, A, Chinese Herbal Medicine Materia Medica, 3rd Edition, Seattle, Eastland Press, 1986, 1993, 2004, P 317

[1119] Bensky, D, Clavey, S, Stöger, E & Gamble, A, Chinese Herbal Medicine Materia Medica, 3rd Edition, Seattle, Eastland Press, 1986, 1993, 2004, P 317

[1120] Bensky, D, Clavey, S, Stöger, E & Gamble, A, Chinese Herbal Medicine Materia Medica, 3rd Edition, Seattle, Eastland Press, 1986, 1993, 2004, P 183

[1121] Chen, JK & TT, Chinese Medical Herbology and Pharmacology, City of Industry, Art of Medicine Press, 2001/2004, P 290

[1122] Bensky, D, Clavey, S, Stöger, E & Gamble, A, Chinese Herbal Medicine Materia Medica, 3rd Edition, Seattle, Eastland Press, 1986, 1993, 2004, P 249

[1123] Brand, E & Wiseman, N, Concise Chinese Materia Medica, Taos, Paradigm Publications, 2008, P 188

[1124] Bensky, D, Clavey, S, Stöger, E & Gamble, A, Chinese Herbal Medicine Materia Medica, 3rd Edition, Seattle, Eastland Press, 1986, 1993, 2004, P 407

[1125] Bensky, D, Clavey, S, Stöger, E & Gamble, A, Chinese Herbal Medicine Materia Medica, 3rd Edition, Seattle, Eastland Press, 1986, 1993, 2004, P 407

[1126] Brand, E & Wiseman, N, Concise Chinese Materia Medica, Taos, Paradigm Publications, 2008, P 198
[1127] Bensky, D, Clavey, S, Stöger, E & Gamble, A, Chinese Herbal Medicine Materia Medica, 3rd Edition, Seattle, Eastland Press, 1986, 1993, 2004, P 317
[1128] Bensky, D, Clavey, S, Stöger, E & Gamble, A, Chinese Herbal Medicine Materia Medica, 3rd Edition, Seattle, Eastland Press, 1986, 1993, 2004, P317
[1129] Bensky, D, Clavey, S, Stöger, E & Gamble, A, Chinese Herbal Medicine Materia Medica, 3rd Edition, Seattle, Eastland Press, 1986, 1993, 2004, P 317
[1130] Bensky, D, Clavey, S, Stöger, E & Gamble, A, Chinese Herbal Medicine Materia Medica, 3rd Edition, Seattle, Eastland Press, 1986, 1993, 2004, P 317
[1131] Bensky, D, Clavey, S, Stöger, E & Gamble, A, Chinese Herbal Medicine Materia Medica, 3rd Edition, Seattle, Eastland Press, 1986, 1993, 2004, P 285
[1132] Brand, E & Wiseman, N, Concise Chinese Materia Medica, Taos, Paradigm Publications, 2008, P 194
[1133] Bensky, D, Clavey, S, Stöger, E & Gamble, A, Chinese Herbal Medicine Materia Medica, 3rd Edition, Seattle, Eastland Press, 1986, 1993, 2004, P 297
[1134] Bensky, D, Clavey, S, Stöger, E & Gamble, A, Chinese Herbal Medicine Materia Medica, 3rd Edition, Seattle, Eastland Press, 1986, 1993, 2004, P 278
[1135] Brand, E & Wiseman, N, Concise Chinese Materia Medica, Taos, Paradigm Publications, 2008, P 191
[1136] Zhang Bing Chen, *Convenient Reader of Materia Medica*, via Bensky, D, Clavey, S, Stöger, E & Gamble, A, Chinese Herbal Medicine Materia Medica, 3rd Edition, Seattle, Eastland Press, 1986, 1993, 2004, P 299
[1137] Zhang Bing Chen, *Convenient Reader of Materia Medica*, via Bensky, D, Clavey, S, Stöger, E & Gamble, A, Chinese Herbal Medicine Materia Medica, 3rd Edition, Seattle, Eastland Press, 1986, 1993, 2004, P 299
[1138] Brand, E & Wiseman, N, Concise Chinese Materia Medica, Taos, Paradigm Publications, 2008, P 196
[1139] Zhang Xi Chun, *Essays on Medicine Esteeming the Chinese and Respecting the Western*, via Bensky, D, Clavey, S, Stöger, E & Gamble, A, Chinese Herbal Medicine Materia Medica, 3rd Edition, Seattle, Eastland Press, 1986, 1993, 2004, P 545
[1140] Bensky, D, Clavey, S, Stöger, E & Gamble, A, Chinese Herbal Medicine Materia Medica, 3rd Edition, Seattle, Eastland Press, 1986, 1993, 2004, P 579
[1141] Brand, E & Wiseman, N, Concise Chinese Materia Medica, Taos, Paradigm Publications, 2008, P 260
[1142] Zhang Bing Chen, *Convenient Reader of Materia Medica*, via Bensky, D, Clavey, S, Stöger, E & Gamble, A, Chinese Herbal Medicine Materia Medica, 3rd Edition, Seattle, Eastland Press, 1986, 1993, 2004, P 569
[1143] Zhang Bing Chen, *Convenient Reader of Materia Medica*, via Bensky, D, Clavey, S, Stöger, E & Gamble, A, Chinese Herbal Medicine Materia Medica, 3rd Edition, Seattle, Eastland Press, 1986, 1993, 2004, P 569
[1144] Bensky, D, Clavey, S, Stöger, E & Gamble, A, Chinese Herbal Medicine Materia Medica, 3rd Edition, Seattle, Eastland Press, 1986, 1993, 2004, P 407

[1145] Bensky, D, Clavey, S, Stöger, E & Gamble, A, Chinese Herbal Medicine Materia Medica, 3rd Edition, Seattle, Eastland Press, 1986, 1993, 2004, P 407
[1146] *High Plateau Handbook of Treatment with Chinese Materia Medica*, via Bensky, D, Clavey, S, Stöger, E & Gamble, A, Chinese Herbal Medicine Materia Medica, 3rd Edition, Seattle, Eastland Press, 1986, 1993, 2004, P 742
[1147] Brand, E & Wiseman, N, Concise Chinese Materia Medica, Taos, Paradigm Publications, 2008, P 492
[1148] Brand, E & Wiseman, N, Concise Chinese Materia Medica, Taos, Paradigm Publications, 2008, P 492
[1149] Brand, E & Wiseman, N, Concise Chinese Materia Medica, Taos, Paradigm Publications, 2008, P 492
[1150] Bensky, D, Clavey, S, Stöger, E & Gamble, A, Chinese Herbal Medicine Materia Medica, 3rd Edition, Seattle, Eastland Press, 1986, 1993, 2004, P 4
[1151] Tang Rong Chuan (Tang Zonghai), Ben Cao Wen Da, Personal Unpublished Translation, 2015, 1.4.6
[1152] Maciocia, G, The Channels of Acupuncture, Philadelphia, Elsevier, 2006, P 585
[1153] Maciocia, G, The Channels of Acupuncture, Philadelphia, Elsevier, 2006, P 446
[1154] Maciocia, G, The Channels of Acupuncture, Philadelphia, Elsevier, 2006, P 585
[1155] Tang Rong Chuan (Tang Zonghai), Ben Cao Wen Da, Personal Unpublished Translation, 2015, 2.1.6
[1156] Tang Rong Chuan (Tang Zonghai), Ben Cao Wen Da, Personal Unpublished Translation, 2015, 2.1.3
[1157] Bensky, D, Clavey, S, Stöger, E & Gamble, A, Chinese Herbal Medicine Materia Medica, 3rd Edition, Seattle, Eastland Press, 1986, 1993, 2004, P 20/21
[1158] Maciocia, G, The Channels of Acupuncture, Philadelphia, Elsevier, 2006, P 446
[1159] Tang Rong Chuan (Tang Zonghai), Ben Cao Wen Da, Personal Unpublished Translation, 2015, 2.1.3
[1160] Chen, JK & TT, Chinese Medical Herbology and Pharmacology, City of Industry, Art of Medicine Press, 2001/2004, P 55, and Bensky, D, Clavey, S, Stöger, E & Gamble, A, Chinese Herbal Medicine Materia Medica, 3rd Edition, Seattle, Eastland Press, 1986, 1993, 2004, P 22
[1161] Zhou Yan, *Thoughtful Differention of Materia Medica*, via Bensky, D, Clavey, S, Stöger, E & Gamble, A, Chinese Herbal Medicine Materia Medica, 3rd Edition, Seattle, Eastland Press, 1986, 1993, 2004, P 62
[1162] Brand, E & Wiseman, N, Concise Chinese Materia Medica, Taos, Paradigm Publications, 2008, P 58
[1163] Chen, JK & TT, Chinese Medical Herbology and Pharmacology, City of Industry, Art of Medicine Press, 2001/2004, P 77
[1164] Tang Rong Chuan (Tang Zonghai), Ben Cao Wen Da, Personal Unpublished Translation, 2015, 2.1.6
[1165] Tang Rong Chuan (Tang Zonghai), Ben Cao Wen Da, Personal Unpublished Translation, 2015, 2.1.6
[1166] Tang Rong Chuan (Tang Zonghai), Ben Cao Wen Da, Personal Unpublished Translation, 2015, 1.5.10

[1167] Tang Rong Chuan (Tang Zonghai), Ben Cao Wen Da, Personal Unpublished Translation, 2015, 1.4.6
[1168] Tang Rong Chuan (Tang Zonghai), Ben Cao Wen Da, Personal Unpublished Translation, 2015, 1.5.9
[1169] Tang Rong Chuan (Tang Zonghai), Ben Cao Wen Da, Personal Unpublished Translation, 2015, 1.5.9
[1170] Tang Rong Chuan (Tang Zonghai), Ben Cao Wen Da, Personal Unpublished Translation, 2015, 1.4.6
[1171] Bensky, D, Clavey, S, Stöger, E & Gamble, A, Chinese Herbal Medicine Materia Medica, 3rd Edition, Seattle, Eastland Press, 1986, 1993, 2004, P 101
[1172] Chen, JK & TT, Chinese Medical Herbology and Pharmacology, City of Industry, Art of Medicine Press, 2001/2004, P 151
[1173] Bensky, D, Clavey, S, Stöger, E & Gamble, A, Chinese Herbal Medicine Materia Medica, 3rd Edition, Seattle, Eastland Press, 1986, 1993, 2004, P 144
[1174] Tang Rong Chuan (Tang Zonghai), Ben Cao Wen Da, Personal Unpublished Translation, 2015, 1.3.4
[1175] Brand, E & Wiseman, N, Concise Chinese Materia Medica, Taos, Paradigm Publications, 2008, P 90
[1176] *Encountering the Sources of the Classic of Materia Medica*, via Bensky, D, Clavey, S, Stöger, E & Gamble, A, Chinese Herbal Medicine Materia Medica, 3rd Edition, Seattle, Eastland Press, 1986, 1993, 2004, P172
[1177] *Encountering the Sources of the Classic of Materia Medica*, via Bensky, D, Clavey, S, Stöger, E & Gamble, A, Chinese Herbal Medicine Materia Medica, 3rd Edition, Seattle, Eastland Press, 1986, 1993, 2004, P172
[1178] Bensky, D, Clavey, S, Stöger, E & Gamble, A, Chinese Herbal Medicine Materia Medica, 3rd Edition, Seattle, Eastland Press, 1986, 1993, 2004, P 171
[1179] Brand, E & Wiseman, N, Concise Chinese Materia Medica, Taos, Paradigm Publications, 2008, P 143, Bensky, D, Clavey, S, Stöger, E & Gamble, A, Chinese Herbal Medicine Materia Medica, 3rd Edition, Seattle, Eastland Press, 1986, 1993, 2004, P 261
[1180] Bensky, D, Clavey, S, Stöger, E & Gamble, A, Chinese Herbal Medicine Materia Medica, 3rd Edition, Seattle, Eastland Press, 1986, 1993, 2004, P 261
[1181] Bensky, D, Clavey, S, Stöger, E & Gamble, A, Chinese Herbal Medicine Materia Medica, 3rd Edition, Seattle, Eastland Press, 1986, 1993, 2004, P 313
[1182] Bensky, D, Clavey, S, Stöger, E & Gamble, A, Chinese Herbal Medicine Materia Medica, 3rd Edition, Seattle, Eastland Press, 1986, 1993, 2004, P 313
[1183] Chen, JK & TT, Chinese Medical Herbology and Pharmacology, City of Industry, Art of Medicine Press, 2001/2004, P 308
[1184] Brand, E & Wiseman, N, Concise Chinese Materia Medica, Taos, Paradigm Publications, 2008, P 158
[1185] Maciocia, G, The Channels of Acupuncture, Philadelphia, Elsevier, 2006, P 585
[1186] '…circulates the Còu Lǐ-interstices and the Sān Jiāo.' Tang Rong Chuan (Tang Zonghai), Ben Cao Wen Da, Personal Unpublished Translation, 2015, 2.2.5
[1187] Maciocia, G, The Channels of Acupuncture, Philadelphia, Elsevier, 2006, P 585

[1188] Bensky, D, Clavey, S, Stöger, E & Gamble, A, Chinese Herbal Medicine Materia Medica, 3rd Edition, Seattle, Eastland Press, 1986, 1993, 2004, P 327

[1189] Tang Rong Chuan (Tang Zonghai), Ben Cao Wen Da, Personal Unpublished Translation, 2015, 2.1.6

[1190] Chen, JK & TT, Chinese Medical Herbology and Pharmacology, City of Industry, Art of Medicine Press, 2001/2004, P 304, Bensky, D, Clavey, S, Stöger, E & Gamble, A, Chinese Herbal Medicine Materia Medica, 3rd Edition, Seattle, Eastland Press, 1986, 1993, 2004, P 323, Tang Rong Chuan (Tang Zonghai), Ben Cao Wen Da, Personal Unpublished Translation, 2015, 1.3.7

[1191] Maciocia, G, The Channels of Acupuncture, Philadelphia, Elsevier, 2006, P 446

[1192] Bensky, D, Clavey, S, Stöger, E & Gamble, A, Chinese Herbal Medicine Materia Medica, 3rd Edition, Seattle, Eastland Press, 1986, 1993, 2004, P 285

[1193] Brand, E & Wiseman, N, Concise Chinese Materia Medica, Taos, Paradigm Publications, 2008, P 194

[1194] Bensky, D, Clavey, S, Stöger, E & Gamble, A, Chinese Herbal Medicine Materia Medica, 3rd Edition, Seattle, Eastland Press, 1986, 1993, 2004, P 278

[1195] Brand, E & Wiseman, N, Concise Chinese Materia Medica, Taos, Paradigm Publications, 2008, P 191

[1196] Brand, E & Wiseman, N, Concise Chinese Materia Medica, Taos, Paradigm Publications, 2008, P 197

[1197] Zhang Bing Chen, *Convenient Reader of Materia Medica*, via Bensky, D, Clavey, S, Stöger, E & Gamble, A, Chinese Herbal Medicine Materia Medica, 3rd Edition, Seattle, Eastland Press, 1986, 1993, 2004, P 299

[1198] Zhang Bing Chen, *Convenient Reader of Materia Medica*, via Bensky, D, Clavey, S, Stöger, E & Gamble, A, Chinese Herbal Medicine Materia Medica, 3rd Edition, Seattle, Eastland Press, 1986, 1993, 2004, P 299

[1199] Brand, E & Wiseman, N, Concise Chinese Materia Medica, Taos, Paradigm Publications, 2008, P 196

[1200] Brand, E & Wiseman, N, Concise Chinese Materia Medica, Taos, Paradigm Publications, 2008, P 195

[1201] Chen, JK & TT, Chinese Medical Herbology and Pharmacology, City of Industry, Art of Medicine Press, 2001/2004, P 400

[1202] Bensky, D, Clavey, S, Stöger, E & Gamble, A, Chinese Herbal Medicine Materia Medica, 3rd Edition, Seattle, Eastland Press, 1986, 1993, 2004, P 294

[1203] Tang Rong Chuan (Tang Zonghai), Ben Cao Wen Da, Personal Unpublished Translation, 2015, 1.4.4

[1204] Brand, E & Wiseman, N, Concise Chinese Materia Medica, Taos, Paradigm Publications, 2008, P 189

[1205] Bensky, D, Clavey, S, Stöger, E & Gamble, A, Chinese Herbal Medicine Materia Medica, 3rd Edition, Seattle, Eastland Press, 1986, 1993, 2004, P 304

[1206] Brand, E & Wiseman, N, Concise Chinese Materia Medica, Taos, Paradigm Publications, 2008, P 200

[1207] Bensky, D, Clavey, S, Stöger, E & Gamble, A, Chinese Herbal Medicine Materia Medica, 3rd Edition, Seattle, Eastland Press, 1986, 1993, 2004, P 700

[1208] Li Shi Zhen, via Bensky, D, Clavey, S, Stöger, E & Gamble, A, Chinese Herbal Medicine Materia Medica, 3rd Edition, Seattle, Eastland Press, 1986, 1993, 2004, P 534

[1209] Zhang Xi Chun, *Essays on Medicine Esteeming the Chinese and Respecting the Western*, via Bensky, D, Clavey, S, Stöger, E & Gamble, A, Chinese Herbal Medicine Materia Medica, 3rd Edition, Seattle, Eastland Press, 1986, 1993, 2004, P 545

[1210] Miao Xi Yong, *Commentary on the Divine Husbandman's Classic of Materia Medica*, via Bensky, D, Clavey, S, Stöger, E & Gamble, A, Chinese Herbal Medicine Materia Medica, 3rd Edition, Seattle, Eastland Press, 1986, 1993, 2004, P 512

[1211] Miao Xi Yong, *Commentary on the Divine Husbandman's Classic of Materia Medica*, via Bensky, D, Clavey, S, Stöger, E & Gamble, A, Chinese Herbal Medicine Materia Medica, 3rd Edition, Seattle, Eastland Press, 1986, 1993, 2004, P 512

[1212] Bensky, D, Clavey, S, Stöger, E & Gamble, A, Chinese Herbal Medicine Materia Medica, 3rd Edition, Seattle, Eastland Press, 1986, 1993, 2004, P 579

[1213] Brand, E & Wiseman, N, Concise Chinese Materia Medica, Taos, Paradigm Publications, 2008, P 260

[1214] Zhang Bing Chen, *Convenient Reader of Materia Medica*, via Bensky, D, Clavey, S, Stöger, E & Gamble, A, Chinese Herbal Medicine Materia Medica, 3rd Edition, Seattle, Eastland Press, 1986, 1993, 2004, P 569

[1215] Zhang Bing Chen, *Convenient Reader of Materia Medica*, via Bensky, D, Clavey, S, Stöger, E & Gamble, A, Chinese Herbal Medicine Materia Medica, 3rd Edition, Seattle, Eastland Press, 1986, 1993, 2004, P 569

[1216] Brand, E & Wiseman, N, Concise Chinese Materia Medica, Taos, Paradigm Publications, 2008, P 293

[1217] Brand, E & Wiseman, N, Concise Chinese Materia Medica, Taos, Paradigm Publications, 2008, P 293

[1218] Brand, E & Wiseman, N, Concise Chinese Materia Medica, Taos, Paradigm Publications, 2008, P 289, Bensky, D, Clavey, S, Stöger, E & Gamble, A, Chinese Herbal Medicine Materia Medica, 3rd Edition, Seattle, Eastland Press, 1986, 1993, 2004, P 614

[1219] Bensky, D, Clavey, S, Stöger, E & Gamble, A, Chinese Herbal Medicine Materia Medica, 3rd Edition, Seattle, Eastland Press, 1986, 1993, 2004, P 656

[1220] Brand, E & Wiseman, N, Concise Chinese Materia Medica, Taos, Paradigm Publications, 2008, P 332

[1221] Wang, Hao Gu, *Harm and Benefit in the Materia Medica*, via Bensky, D, Clavey, S, Stöger, E & Gamble, A, Chinese Herbal Medicine Materia Medica, 3rd Edition, Seattle, Eastland Press, 1986, 1993, 2004, P 924

[1222] Chen, JK & TT, Chinese Medical Herbology and Pharmacology, City of Industry, Art of Medicine Press, 2001/2004, P 760, and Bensky, D, Clavey, S, Stöger, E & Gamble, A, Chinese Herbal Medicine Materia Medica, 3rd Edition, Seattle, Eastland Press, 1986, 1993, 2004, P 923

[1223] Bensky, D, Clavey, S, Stöger, E & Gamble, A, Chinese Herbal Medicine Materia Medica, 3rd Edition, Seattle, Eastland Press, 1986, 1993, 2004, P 982

[1224] Chen, JK & TT, Chinese Medical Herbology and Pharmacology, City of Industry, Art of Medicine Press, 2001/2004, P 794, Bensky, D, Clavey, S, Stöger, E & Gamble, A, Chinese Herbal Medicine Materia Medica, 3rd Edition, Seattle, Eastland Press, 1986, 1993, 2004, P 982

[1225] Miao Xi Yong, *Commentary on the Divine Husbandman's Classic of Materia Medica*, via Bensky, D, Clavey, S, Stöger, E & Gamble, A, Chinese Herbal Medicine Materia Medica, 3rd Edition, Seattle, Eastland Press, 1986, 1993, 2004, P 888

[1226] Chen, JK & TT, Chinese Medical Herbology and Pharmacology, City of Industry, Art of Medicine Press, 2001/2004, P 455

[1227] Tang Rong Chuan (Tang Zonghai), Ben Cao Wen Da, Personal Unpublished Translation, 2015, 2.2.2

[1228] Bensky, D, Clavey, S, Stöger, E & Gamble, A, Chinese Herbal Medicine Materia Medica, 3rd Edition, Seattle, Eastland Press, 1986, 1993, 2004, P 83

[1229] Tang Rong Chuan (Tang Zonghai), Ben Cao Wen Da, Personal Unpublished Translation, 2015, 2.1.6

[1230] Tang Rong Chuan (Tang Zonghai), Ben Cao Wen Da, Personal Unpublished Translation, 2015, 2.1.3

[1231] Bensky, D, Clavey, S, Stöger, E & Gamble, A, Chinese Herbal Medicine Materia Medica, 3rd Edition, Seattle, Eastland Press, 1986, 1993, 2004, P 20/21

[1232] Maciocia, G, The Channels of Acupuncture, Philadelphia, Elsevier, 2006, P 446

[1233] Tang Rong Chuan (Tang Zonghai), Ben Cao Wen Da, Personal Unpublished Translation, 2015, 2.1.3

[1234] Brand, E & Wiseman, N, Concise Chinese Materia Medica, Taos, Paradigm Publications, 2008, P 84, and Huang Gong Xiu, *Seeking Accuracy in the Materia Medica*, via Bensky, D, Clavey, S, Stöger, E & Gamble, A, Chinese Herbal Medicine Materia Medica, 3rd Edition, Seattle, Eastland Press, 1986, 1993, 2004, P 112

[1235] Brand, E & Wiseman, N, Concise Chinese Materia Medica, Taos, Paradigm Publications, 2008, P 84

[1236] *Grand Materia Medica*, via Bensky, D, Clavey, S, Stöger, E & Gamble, A, Chinese Herbal Medicine Materia Medica, 3rd Edition, Seattle, Eastland Press, 1986, 1993, 2004, P 104

[1237] Bensky, D, Clavey, S, Stöger, E & Gamble, A, Chinese Herbal Medicine Materia Medica, 3rd Edition, Seattle, Eastland Press, 1986, 1993, 2004, P 904

[1238] Bensky, D, Clavey, S, Stöger, E & Gamble, A, Chinese Herbal Medicine Materia Medica, 3rd Edition, Seattle, Eastland Press, 1986, 1993, 2004, P 905

[1239] *Grand Materia Medica*, via Bensky, D, Clavey, S, Stöger, E & Gamble, A, Chinese Herbal Medicine Materia Medica, 3rd Edition, Seattle, Eastland Press, 1986, 1993, 2004, P 127

[1240] Brand, E & Wiseman, N, Concise Chinese Materia Medica, Taos, Paradigm Publications, 2008, P 107

[1241] Bensky, D, Clavey, S, Stöger, E & Gamble, A, Chinese Herbal Medicine Materia Medica, 3rd Edition, Seattle, Eastland Press, 1986, 1993, 2004, P 205

[1242] *Convenient Reader of Materia Medica*, Bensky, D, Clavey, S, Stöger, E & Gamble, A, Chinese Herbal Medicine Materia Medica, 3rd Edition, Seattle, Eastland Press, 1986, 1993, 2004, P 214

[1243] *Convenient Reader of Materia Medica*, Bensky, D, Clavey, S, Stöger, E & Gamble, A, Chinese Herbal Medicine Materia Medica, 3rd Edition, Seattle, Eastland Press, 1986, 1993, 2004, P 214

[1244] Zhang Bing Chen, *Convenient Reader of Materia Medica*, via Bensky, D, Clavey, S, Stöger, E & Gamble, A, Chinese Herbal Medicine Materia Medica, 3rd Edition, Seattle, Eastland Press, 1986, 1993, 2004, P 214

[1245] Brand, E & Wiseman, N, Concise Chinese Materia Medica, Taos, Paradigm Publications, 2008, P 120, Bensky, D, Clavey, S, Stöger, E & Gamble, A, Chinese Herbal Medicine Materia Medica, 3rd Edition, Seattle, Eastland Press, 1986, 1993, 2004, P 224
[1246] Bensky, D, Clavey, S, Stöger, E & Gamble, A, Chinese Herbal Medicine Materia Medica, 3rd Edition, Seattle, Eastland Press, 1986, 1993, 2004, P 224
[1247] Chen, JK & TT, Chinese Medical Herbology and Pharmacology, City of Industry, Art of Medicine Press, 2001/2004, P 247
[1248] Tang Rong Chuan (Tang Zonghai), Ben Cao Wen Da, Personal Unpublished Translation, 2015, 2.3.5
[1249] Brand, E & Wiseman, N, Concise Chinese Materia Medica, Taos, Paradigm Publications, 2008, P 121, Bensky, D, Clavey, S, Stöger, E & Gamble, A, Chinese Herbal Medicine Materia Medica, 3rd Edition, Seattle, Eastland Press, 1986, 1993, 2004, P 222
[1250] Chen, JK & TT, Chinese Medical Herbology and Pharmacology, City of Industry, Art of Medicine Press, 2001/2004, P 244
[1251] Brand, E & Wiseman, N, Concise Chinese Materia Medica, Taos, Paradigm Publications, 2008, P 119
[1252] Brand, E & Wiseman, N, Concise Chinese Materia Medica, Taos, Paradigm Publications, 2008, P 143, Bensky, D, Clavey, S, Stöger, E & Gamble, A, Chinese Herbal Medicine Materia Medica, 3rd Edition, Seattle, Eastland Press, 1986, 1993, 2004, P 261
[1253] Bensky, D, Clavey, S, Stöger, E & Gamble, A, Chinese Herbal Medicine Materia Medica, 3rd Edition, Seattle, Eastland Press, 1986, 1993, 2004, P 261
[1254] Chen, JK & TT, Chinese Medical Herbology and Pharmacology, City of Industry, Art of Medicine Press, 2001/2004, P 287
[1255] Brand, E & Wiseman, N, Concise Chinese Materia Medica, Taos, Paradigm Publications, 2008, P 139
[1256] *Seeking Accuracy in the Materia Medica*, via Bensky, D, Clavey, S, Stöger, E & Gamble, A, Chinese Herbal Medicine Materia Medica, 3rd Edition, Seattle, Eastland Press, 1986, 1993, 2004, P 254
[1257] *Seeking Accuracy in the Materia Medica*, via Bensky, D, Clavey, S, Stöger, E & Gamble, A, Chinese Herbal Medicine Materia Medica, 3rd Edition, Seattle, Eastland Press, 1986, 1993, 2004, P 254
[1258] Chen, JK & TT, Chinese Medical Herbology and Pharmacology, City of Industry, Art of Medicine Press, 2001/2004, P 290
[1259] Bensky, D, Clavey, S, Stöger, E & Gamble, A, Chinese Herbal Medicine Materia Medica, 3rd Edition, Seattle, Eastland Press, 1986, 1993, 2004, P 249
[1260] Bensky, D, Clavey, S, Stöger, E & Gamble, A, Chinese Herbal Medicine Materia Medica, 3rd Edition, Seattle, Eastland Press, 1986, 1993, 2004, P 313
[1261] Bensky, D, Clavey, S, Stöger, E & Gamble, A, Chinese Herbal Medicine Materia Medica, 3rd Edition, Seattle, Eastland Press, 1986, 1993, 2004, P 313
[1262] Chen, JK & TT, Chinese Medical Herbology and Pharmacology, City of Industry, Art of Medicine Press, 2001/2004, P 308
[1263] Brand, E & Wiseman, N, Concise Chinese Materia Medica, Taos, Paradigm Publications, 2008, P 158
[1264] Maciocia, G, The Channels of Acupuncture, Philadelphia, Elsevier, 2006, P 585

1265 '...circulates the Còu Lǐ-interstices and the Sān Jiāo.' Tang Rong Chuan (Tang Zonghai), Ben Cao Wen Da, Personal Unpublished Translation, 2015, 2.2.5

1266 Bensky, D, Clavey, S, Stöger, E & Gamble, A, Chinese Herbal Medicine Materia Medica, 3rd Edition, Seattle, Eastland Press, 1986, 1993, 2004, P 342

1267 Bensky, D, Clavey, S, Stöger, E & Gamble, A, Chinese Herbal Medicine Materia Medica, 3rd Edition, Seattle, Eastland Press, 1986, 1993, 2004, P 342

1268 Bensky, D, Clavey, S, Stöger, E & Gamble, A, Chinese Herbal Medicine Materia Medica, 3rd Edition, Seattle, Eastland Press, 1986, 1993, 2004, P 329

1269 Bensky, D, Clavey, S, Stöger, E & Gamble, A, Chinese Herbal Medicine Materia Medica, 3rd Edition, Seattle, Eastland Press, 1986, 1993, 2004, P 329

1270 Brand, E & Wiseman, N, Concise Chinese Materia Medica, Taos, Paradigm Publications, 2008, P 155

1271 Brand, E & Wiseman, N, Concise Chinese Materia Medica, Taos, Paradigm Publications, 2008, P 155

1272 Ye Tian Shi, *Renewed Materia Medica*, via Bensky, D, Clavey, S, Stöger, E & Gamble, A, Chinese Herbal Medicine Materia Medica, 3rd Edition, Seattle, Eastland Press, 1986, 1993, 2004, P 351

1273 Ye Tian Shi, *Renewed Materia Medica*, via Bensky, D, Clavey, S, Stöger, E & Gamble, A, Chinese Herbal Medicine Materia Medica, 3rd Edition, Seattle, Eastland Press, 1986, 1993, 2004, P 351

1274 Tang Rong Chuan (Tang Zonghai), Ben Cao Wen Da, Personal Unpublished Translation, 2015, 2.1.6

1275 Chen, JK & TT, Chinese Medical Herbology and Pharmacology, City of Industry, Art of Medicine Press, 2001/2004, P 304, Bensky, D, Clavey, S, Stöger, E & Gamble, A, Chinese Herbal Medicine Materia Medica, 3rd Edition, Seattle, Eastland Press, 1986, 1993, 2004, P 323, Tang Rong Chuan (Tang Zonghai), Ben Cao Wen Da, Personal Unpublished Translation, 2015, 1.3.7

1276 Maciocia, G, The Channels of Acupuncture, Philadelphia, Elsevier, 2006, P 446

1277 Brand, E & Wiseman, N, Concise Chinese Materia Medica, Taos, Paradigm Publications, 2008, P 160

1278 Li Zhong Zhi, *Penetrating the Mysteries of the Materia Medica*, via Bensky, D, Clavey, S, Stöger, E & Gamble, A, Chinese Herbal Medicine Materia Medica, 3rd Edition, Seattle, Eastland Press, 1986, 1993, 2004, P 358

1279 Brand, E & Wiseman, N, Concise Chinese Materia Medica, Taos, Paradigm Publications, 2008, P 156

1280 Brand, E & Wiseman, N, Concise Chinese Materia Medica, Taos, Paradigm Publications, 2008, P 156

1281 Zhang, Jie Bin, *Rectification of the Meaning of Materia Medica*, via Bensky, D, Clavey, S, Stöger, E & Gamble, A, Chinese Herbal Medicine Materia Medica, 3rd Edition, Seattle, Eastland Press, 1986, 1993, 2004, P 352

1282 Bensky, D, Clavey, S, Stöger, E & Gamble, A, Chinese Herbal Medicine Materia Medica, 3rd Edition, Seattle, Eastland Press, 1986, 1993, 2004, P 353

1283 Brand, E & Wiseman, N, Concise Chinese Materia Medica, Taos, Paradigm Publications, 2008, P 163

1284 Tang Rong Chuan (Tang Zonghai), Ben Cao Wen Da, Personal Unpublished Translation, 2015, 2.1.6

[1285] Bensky, D, Clavey, S, Stöger, E & Gamble, A, Chinese Herbal Medicine Materia Medica, 3rd Edition, Seattle, Eastland Press, 1986, 1993, 2004, P 337
[1286] Zhang, Jie Bin, *Rectification of the Meaning of Materia Medica*, via Bensky, D, Clavey, S, Stöger, E & Gamble, A, Chinese Herbal Medicine Materia Medica, 3rd Edition, Seattle, Eastland Press, 1986, 1993, 2004, P 352
[1287] Bensky, D, Clavey, S, Stöger, E & Gamble, A, Chinese Herbal Medicine Materia Medica, 3rd Edition, Seattle, Eastland Press, 1986, 1993, 2004, P 353
[1288] Brand, E & Wiseman, N, Concise Chinese Materia Medica, Taos, Paradigm Publications, 2008, P186
[1289] Bensky, D, Clavey, S, Stöger, E & Gamble, A, Chinese Herbal Medicine Materia Medica, 3rd Edition, Seattle, Eastland Press, 1986, 1993, 2004, P 267
[1290] Bensky, D, Clavey, S, Stöger, E & Gamble, A, Chinese Herbal Medicine Materia Medica, 3rd Edition, Seattle, Eastland Press, 1986, 1993, 2004, P 278
[1291] Brand, E & Wiseman, N, Concise Chinese Materia Medica, Taos, Paradigm Publications, 2008, P 191
[1292] Chen, JK & TT, Chinese Medical Herbology and Pharmacology, City of Industry, Art of Medicine Press, 2001/2004, P 400
[1293] Bensky, D, Clavey, S, Stöger, E & Gamble, A, Chinese Herbal Medicine Materia Medica, 3rd Edition, Seattle, Eastland Press, 1986, 1993, 2004, P 294
[1294] Tang Rong Chuan (Tang Zonghai), Ben Cao Wen Da, Personal Unpublished Translation, 2015, 1.4.4
[1295] Brand, E & Wiseman, N, Concise Chinese Materia Medica, Taos, Paradigm Publications, 2008, P 189
[1296] Bensky, D, Clavey, S, Stöger, E & Gamble, A, Chinese Herbal Medicine Materia Medica, 3rd Edition, Seattle, Eastland Press, 1986, 1993, 2004, P 304
[1297] Brand, E & Wiseman, N, Concise Chinese Materia Medica, Taos, Paradigm Publications, 2008, P 200
[1298] Chen, JK & TT, Chinese Medical Herbology and Pharmacology, City of Industry, Art of Medicine Press, 2001/2004, P 455
[1299] Tang Rong Chuan (Tang Zonghai), Ben Cao Wen Da, Personal Unpublished Translation, 2015, 2.2.2
[1300] Bensky, D, Clavey, S, Stöger, E & Gamble, A, Chinese Herbal Medicine Materia Medica, 3rd Edition, Seattle, Eastland Press, 1986, 1993, 2004, P 83
[1301] Bensky, D, Clavey, S, Stöger, E & Gamble, A, Chinese Herbal Medicine Materia Medica, 3rd Edition, Seattle, Eastland Press, 1986, 1993, 2004, P 700
[1302] Tang Rong Chuan (Tang Zonghai), Ben Cao Wen Da, Personal Unpublished Translation, 2015, 1.5.13
[1303] Brand, E & Wiseman, N, Concise Chinese Materia Medica, Taos, Paradigm Publications, 2008, P 212
[1304] Bensky, D, Clavey, S, Stöger, E & Gamble, A, Chinese Herbal Medicine Materia Medica, 3rd Edition, Seattle, Eastland Press, 1986, 1993, 2004, P 680
[1305] Tang Rong Chuan (Tang Zonghai), Ben Cao Wen Da, Personal Unpublished Translation, 2015, 1.2.4

[1306] Tang Rong Chuan (Tang Zonghai), Ben Cao Wen Da, Personal Unpublished Translation, 2015, 1.2.4

[1307] Chen, JK & TT, Chinese Medical Herbology and Pharmacology, City of Industry, Art of Medicine Press, 2001/2004, P 441

[1308] Brand, E & Wiseman, N, Concise Chinese Materia Medica, Taos, Paradigm Publications, 2008, P 208

[1309] Zhang, Shan Lei, *Rectification of the Meaning of Materia Medica,* via Bensky, D, Clavey, S, Stöger, E & Gamble, A, Chinese Herbal Medicine Materia Medica, 3rd Edition, Seattle, Eastland Press, 1986, 1993, 2004, P 675

[1310] Tang Rong Chuan (Tang Zonghai), Ben Cao Wen Da, Personal Unpublished Translation, 2015, 2.2.2

[1311] Li Shi Zhen, via Bensky, D, Clavey, S, Stöger, E & Gamble, A, Chinese Herbal Medicine Materia Medica, 3rd Edition, Seattle, Eastland Press, 1986, 1993, 2004, P 534

[1312] Bensky, D, Clavey, S, Stöger, E & Gamble, A, Chinese Herbal Medicine Materia Medica, 3rd Edition, Seattle, Eastland Press, 1986, 1993, 2004, P 543

[1313] Bensky, D, Clavey, S, Stöger, E & Gamble, A, Chinese Herbal Medicine Materia Medica, 3rd Edition, Seattle, Eastland Press, 1986, 1993, 2004, P 544

[1314] Miao Xi Yong, *Commentary on the Divine Husbandman's Classic of Materia Medica*, via Bensky, D, Clavey, S, Stöger, E & Gamble, A, Chinese Herbal Medicine Materia Medica, 3rd Edition, Seattle, Eastland Press, 1986, 1993, 2004, P 512

[1315] Miao Xi Yong, *Commentary on the Divine Husbandman's Classic of Materia Medica*, via Bensky, D, Clavey, S, Stöger, E & Gamble, A, Chinese Herbal Medicine Materia Medica, 3rd Edition, Seattle, Eastland Press, 1986, 1993, 2004, P 512

[1316] Brand, E & Wiseman, N, Concise Chinese Materia Medica, Taos, Paradigm Publications, 2008, P 269

[1317] Bensky, D, Clavey, S, Stöger, E & Gamble, A, Chinese Herbal Medicine Materia Medica, 3rd Edition, Seattle, Eastland Press, 1986, 1993, 2004, P 588

[1318] Bensky, D, Clavey, S, Stöger, E & Gamble, A, Chinese Herbal Medicine Materia Medica, 3rd Edition, Seattle, Eastland Press, 1986, 1993, 2004, P 588

[1319] Maciocia, G, The Channels of Acupuncture, Philadelphia, Elsevier, 2006, P 545

[1320] *Convenient Reader of Materia Medica*, Bensky, D, Clavey, S, Stöger, E & Gamble, A, Chinese Herbal Medicine Materia Medica, 3rd Edition, Seattle, Eastland Press, 1986, 1993, 2004, P 214

[1321] *Convenient Reader of Materia Medica*, Bensky, D, Clavey, S, Stöger, E & Gamble, A, Chinese Herbal Medicine Materia Medica, 3rd Edition, Seattle, Eastland Press, 1986, 1993, 2004, P 214

[1322] Zhang Bing Chen, *Convenient Reader of Materia Medica*, via Bensky, D, Clavey, S, Stöger, E & Gamble, A, Chinese Herbal Medicine Materia Medica, 3rd Edition, Seattle, Eastland Press, 1986, 1993, 2004, P 214

[1323] *Grand Materia Medica*, via Bensky, D, Clavey, S, Stöger, E & Gamble, A, Chinese Herbal Medicine Materia Medica, 3rd Edition, Seattle, Eastland Press, 1986, 1993, 2004, P 127

[1324] Brand, E & Wiseman, N, Concise Chinese Materia Medica, Taos, Paradigm Publications, 2008, P 291

[1325] Chen, JK & TT, Chinese Medical Herbology and Pharmacology, City of Industry, Art of Medicine Press, 2001/2004, P 715

[1326] Chen, JK & TT, Chinese Medical Herbology and Pharmacology, City of Industry, Art of Medicine Press, 2001/2004, P 715
[1327] Bensky, D, Clavey, S, Stöger, E & Gamble, A, Chinese Herbal Medicine Materia Medica, 3rd Edition, Seattle, Eastland Press, 1986, 1993, 2004, P 404
[1328] Brand, E & Wiseman, N, Concise Chinese Materia Medica, Taos, Paradigm Publications, 2008, P 326
[1329] Bensky, D, Clavey, S, Stöger, E & Gamble, A, Chinese Herbal Medicine Materia Medica, 3rd Edition, Seattle, Eastland Press, 1986, 1993, 2004, P 813
[1330] Brand, E & Wiseman, N, Concise Chinese Materia Medica, Taos, Paradigm Publications, 2008, P 333, Bensky, D, Clavey, S, Stöger, E & Gamble, A, Chinese Herbal Medicine Materia Medica, 3rd Edition, Seattle, Eastland Press, 1986, 1993, 2004, P 894
[1331] Brand, E & Wiseman, N, Concise Chinese Materia Medica, Taos, Paradigm Publications, 2008, P 352
[1332] Li Shi Zhen, *Grand Materia Medica*, via Bensky, D, Clavey, S, Stöger, E & Gamble, A, Chinese Herbal Medicine Materia Medica, 3rd Edition, Seattle, Eastland Press, 1986, 1993, 2004, P 931
[1333] Zhang, Jie Bin, *Rectification of the Meaning of Materia Medica*, via Bensky, D, Clavey, S, Stöger, E & Gamble, A, Chinese Herbal Medicine Materia Medica, 3rd Edition, Seattle, Eastland Press, 1986, 1993, 2004, P 931
[1334] Zhang, Jie Bin, *Rectification of the Meaning of Materia Medica*, via Bensky, D, Clavey, S, Stöger, E & Gamble, A, Chinese Herbal Medicine Materia Medica, 3rd Edition, Seattle, Eastland Press, 1986, 1993, 2004, P 931
[1335] Chen, JK & TT, Chinese Medical Herbology and Pharmacology, City of Industry, Art of Medicine Press, 2001/2004, P 346, and *Thoroughly Revised Materia Medica*, via Bensky, D, Clavey, S, Stöger, E & Gamble, A, Chinese Herbal Medicine Materia Medica, 3rd Edition, Seattle, Eastland Press, 1986, 1993, 2004, P 916
[1336] Zhang Xi Chun, *Essays on Medicine Esteeming the Chinese and Respecting the Western*, via Bensky, D, Clavey, S, Stöger, E & Gamble, A, Chinese Herbal Medicine Materia Medica, 3rd Edition, Seattle, Eastland Press, 1986, 1993, 2004, P 911
[1337] Brand, E & Wiseman, N, Concise Chinese Materia Medica, Taos, Paradigm Publications, 2008, P 348
[1338] Bensky, D, Clavey, S, Stöger, E & Gamble, A, Chinese Herbal Medicine Materia Medica, 3rd Edition, Seattle, Eastland Press, 1986, 1993, 2004, P 910
[1339] Bensky, D, Clavey, S, Stöger, E & Gamble, A, Chinese Herbal Medicine Materia Medica, 3rd Edition, Seattle, Eastland Press, 1986, 1993, 2004, P 910
[1340] Brand, E & Wiseman, N, Concise Chinese Materia Medica, Taos, Paradigm Publications, 2008, P 347, Bensky, D, Clavey, S, Stöger, E & Gamble, A, Chinese Herbal Medicine Materia Medica, 3rd Edition, Seattle, Eastland Press, 1986, 1993, 2004, P 910
[1341] Maciocia, G, The Channels of Acupuncture, Philadelphia, Elsevier, 2006, P 545
[1342] Brand, E & Wiseman, N, Concise Chinese Materia Medica, Taos, Paradigm Publications, 2008, P 365, and Wang, An, *Essentials of the Materia Medica*, via Bensky, D, Clavey, S, Stöger, E & Gamble, A, Chinese Herbal Medicine Materia Medica, 3rd Edition, Seattle, Eastland Press, 1986, 1993, 2004, P 914
[1343] Bensky, D, Clavey, S, Stöger, E & Gamble, A, Chinese Herbal Medicine Materia Medica, 3rd Edition, Seattle, Eastland Press, 1986, 1993, 2004, P 982

1344 Chen, JK & TT, Chinese Medical Herbology and Pharmacology, City of Industry, Art of Medicine Press, 2001/2004, P 794, Bensky, D, Clavey, S, Stöger, E & Gamble, A, Chinese Herbal Medicine Materia Medica, 3rd Edition, Seattle, Eastland Press, 1986, 1993, 2004, P 982

1345 Brand, E & Wiseman, N, Concise Chinese Materia Medica, Taos, Paradigm Publications, 2008, P 84, and Huang Gong Xiu, *Seeking Accuracy in the Materia Medica*, via Bensky, D, Clavey, S, Stöger, E & Gamble, A, Chinese Herbal Medicine Materia Medica, 3rd Edition, Seattle, Eastland Press, 1986, 1993, 2004, P 112

1346 Brand, E & Wiseman, N, Concise Chinese Materia Medica, Taos, Paradigm Publications, 2008, P 84

1347 Brand, E & Wiseman, N, Concise Chinese Materia Medica, Taos, Paradigm Publications, 2008, P 365, and Wang, An, *Essentials of the Materia Medica*, via Bensky, D, Clavey, S, Stöger, E & Gamble, A, Chinese Herbal Medicine Materia Medica, 3rd Edition, Seattle, Eastland Press, 1986, 1993, 2004, P 914

1348 Bensky, D, Clavey, S, Stöger, E & Gamble, A, Chinese Herbal Medicine Materia Medica, 3rd Edition, Seattle, Eastland Press, 1986, 1993, 2004, P 980

1349 Bensky, D, Clavey, S, Stöger, E & Gamble, A, Chinese Herbal Medicine Materia Medica, 3rd Edition, Seattle, Eastland Press, 1986, 1993, 2004, P 822

1350 Zhang, Shan Lei, *Rectification of the Meaning of Materia Medica,* via Bensky, D, Clavey, S, Stöger, E & Gamble, A, Chinese Herbal Medicine Materia Medica, 3rd Edition, Seattle, Eastland Press, 1986, 1993, 2004, P 823

1351 Brand, E & Wiseman, N, Concise Chinese Materia Medica, Taos, Paradigm Publications, 2008, P 398

1352 Brand, E & Wiseman, N, Concise Chinese Materia Medica, Taos, Paradigm Publications, 2008, P 395

1353 Brand, E & Wiseman, N, Concise Chinese Materia Medica, Taos, Paradigm Publications, 2008, P 395

1354 Brand, E & Wiseman, N, Concise Chinese Materia Medica, Taos, Paradigm Publications, 2008, P 409

1355 Tang Rong Chuan (Tang Zonghai), Ben Cao Wen Da, Personal Unpublished Translation, 2015, 1.3.3

1356 Maciocia, G, The Channels of Acupuncture, Philadelphia, Elsevier, 2006, P 545

1357 Brand, E & Wiseman, N, Concise Chinese Materia Medica, Taos, Paradigm Publications, 2008, P 415

1358 Bensky, D, Clavey, S, Stöger, E & Gamble, A, Chinese Herbal Medicine Materia Medica, 3rd Edition, Seattle, Eastland Press, 1986, 1993, 2004, P 813

1359 Li Shi Zhen, *Grand Materia Medica*, via Bensky, D, Clavey, S, Stöger, E & Gamble, A, Chinese Herbal Medicine Materia Medica, 3rd Edition, Seattle, Eastland Press, 1986, 1993, 2004, P 779

1360 Li Shi Zhen says that Yin Yang Huo is an herb of the Arm and Leg Yang Ming, San Jiao and Ming Men, Li Shi Zhen, *Grand Materia Medica*, via Bensky, D, Clavey, S, Stöger, E & Gamble, A, Chinese Herbal Medicine Materia Medica, 3rd Edition, Seattle, Eastland Press, 1986, 1993, 2004, P 779

1361 Bensky, D, Clavey, S, Stöger, E & Gamble, A, Chinese Herbal Medicine Materia Medica, 3rd Edition, Seattle, Eastland Press, 1986, 1993, 2004, P 787

[1362] Brand, E & Wiseman, N, Concise Chinese Materia Medica, Taos, Paradigm Publications, 2008, P 425, Bensky, D, Clavey, S, Stöger, E & Gamble, A, Chinese Herbal Medicine Materia Medica, 3rd Edition, Seattle, Eastland Press, 1986, 1993, 2004, P 789
[1363] Brand, E & Wiseman, N, Concise Chinese Materia Medica, Taos, Paradigm Publications, 2008, P 418
[1364] Brand, E & Wiseman, N, Concise Chinese Materia Medica, Taos, Paradigm Publications, 2008, P 418
[1365] Brand, E & Wiseman, N, Concise Chinese Materia Medica, Taos, Paradigm Publications, 2008, P 418
[1366] Zhang Lu, *Encountering the Sources of the Classic of Materia Medica*, via Bensky, D, Clavey, S, Stöger, E & Gamble, A, Chinese Herbal Medicine Materia Medica, 3rd Edition, Seattle, Eastland Press, 1986, 1993, 2004, P 791
[1367] Bensky, D, Clavey, S, Stöger, E & Gamble, A, Chinese Herbal Medicine Materia Medica, 3rd Edition, Seattle, Eastland Press, 1986, 1993, 2004, P 762
[1368] Brand, E & Wiseman, N, Concise Chinese Materia Medica, Taos, Paradigm Publications, 2008, P 425
[1369] Brand, E & Wiseman, N, Concise Chinese Materia Medica, Taos, Paradigm Publications, 2008, P 425
[1370] Chen, JK & TT, Chinese Medical Herbology and Pharmacology, City of Industry, Art of Medicine Press, 2001/2004, P 883
[1371] Zhou Yan/Zhou Bo Du, *Records of Thoughtful Differentiation of Materia Medica*, via Bensky, D, Clavey, S, Stöger, E & Gamble, A, Chinese Herbal Medicine Materia Medica, 3rd Edition, Seattle, Eastland Press, 1986, 1993, 2004, P 809
[1372] Brand, E & Wiseman, N, Concise Chinese Materia Medica, Taos, Paradigm Publications, 2008, P 427
[1373] Zhang, Shan Lei, *Rectification of the Meaning of Materia Medica,* via Bensky, D, Clavey, S, Stöger, E & Gamble, A, Chinese Herbal Medicine Materia Medica, 3rd Edition, Seattle, Eastland Press, 1986, 1993, 2004, P 783
[1374] Chen, JK & TT, Chinese Medical Herbology and Pharmacology, City of Industry, Art of Medicine Press, 2001/2004, P 908
[1375] Chen, JK & TT, Chinese Medical Herbology and Pharmacology, City of Industry, Art of Medicine Press, 2001/2004, P 907, Brand, E & Wiseman, N, Concise Chinese Materia Medica, Taos, Paradigm Publications, 2008, P 423
[1376] *The Divine Husbandman's Classic of the Materia Medica*, via Bensky, D, Clavey, S, Stöger, E & Gamble, A, Chinese Herbal Medicine Materia Medica, 3rd Edition, Seattle, Eastland Press, 1986, 1993, 2004, P 796
[1377] Wang, An, *Essentials of the Materia Medica*, via Bensky, D, Clavey, S, Stöger, E & Gamble, A, Chinese Herbal Medicine Materia Medica, 3rd Edition, Seattle, Eastland Press, 1986, 1993, 2004, P 792, and Jeffrey Yuen San Francisco 6-26-2017
[1378] Brand, E & Wiseman, N, Concise Chinese Materia Medica, Taos, Paradigm Publications, 2008, P 427, Bensky, D, Clavey, S, Stöger, E & Gamble, A, Chinese Herbal Medicine Materia Medica, 3rd Edition, Seattle, Eastland Press, 1986, 1993, 2004, P 805
[1379] Tang Rong Chuan (Tang Zonghai), Ben Cao Wen Da, Personal Unpublished Translation, 2015, 1.3.6

[1380] Brand, E & Wiseman, N, Concise Chinese Materia Medica, Taos, Paradigm Publications, 2008, P 417

[1381] Zhang Lu, *Encountering the Sources of the Classic of Materia Medica*, via Bensky, D, Clavey, S, Stöger, E & Gamble, A, Chinese Herbal Medicine Materia Medica, 3rd Edition, Seattle, Eastland Press, 1986, 1993, 2004, P 781

[1382] Ye Tian Shi, *Case Records as a Guide to Clinical Practice*, via Bensky, D, Clavey, S, Stöger, E & Gamble, A, Chinese Herbal Medicine Materia Medica, 3rd Edition, Seattle, Eastland Press, 1986, 1993, 2004, P 767

[1383] Maciocia, G, The Channels of Acupuncture, Philadelphia, Elsevier, 2006, P 545

[1384] Chen, JK & TT, Chinese Medical Herbology and Pharmacology, City of Industry, Art of Medicine Press, 2001/2004, P 959, Bensky, D, Clavey, S, Stöger, E & Gamble, A, Chinese Herbal Medicine Materia Medica, 3rd Edition, Seattle, Eastland Press, 1986, 1993, 2004, P 763

[1385] Bensky, D, Clavey, S, Stöger, E & Gamble, A, Chinese Herbal Medicine Materia Medica, 3rd Edition, Seattle, Eastland Press, 1986, 1993, 2004, P 744

[1386] Brand, E & Wiseman, N, Concise Chinese Materia Medica, Taos, Paradigm Publications, 2008, P 437

[1387] Bensky, D, Clavey, S, Stöger, E & Gamble, A, Chinese Herbal Medicine Materia Medica, 3rd Edition, Seattle, Eastland Press, 1986, 1993, 2004, P 822

[1388] Zhang, Shan Lei, *Rectification of the Meaning of Materia Medica,* via Bensky, D, Clavey, S, Stöger, E & Gamble, A, Chinese Herbal Medicine Materia Medica, 3rd Edition, Seattle, Eastland Press, 1986, 1993, 2004, P 823

[1389] Brand, E & Wiseman, N, Concise Chinese Materia Medica, Taos, Paradigm Publications, 2008, P 398

[1390] Brand, E & Wiseman, N, Concise Chinese Materia Medica, Taos, Paradigm Publications, 2008, P 447

[1391] Brand, E & Wiseman, N, Concise Chinese Materia Medica, Taos, Paradigm Publications, 2008, P 446, Bensky, D, Clavey, S, Stöger, E & Gamble, A, Chinese Herbal Medicine Materia Medica, 3rd Edition, Seattle, Eastland Press, 1986, 1993, 2004, P 841

[1392] Bensky, D, Clavey, S, Stöger, E & Gamble, A, Chinese Herbal Medicine Materia Medica, 3rd Edition, Seattle, Eastland Press, 1986, 1993, 2004, P 830

[1393] Bensky, D, Clavey, S, Stöger, E & Gamble, A, Chinese Herbal Medicine Materia Medica, 3rd Edition, Seattle, Eastland Press, 1986, 1993, 2004, P 830

[1394] Bensky, D, Clavey, S, Stöger, E & Gamble, A, Chinese Herbal Medicine Materia Medica, 3rd Edition, Seattle, Eastland Press, 1986, 1993, 2004, P 851

[1395] Bensky, D, Clavey, S, Stöger, E & Gamble, A, Chinese Herbal Medicine Materia Medica, 3rd Edition, Seattle, Eastland Press, 1986, 1993, 2004, P 846

[1396] Brand, E & Wiseman, N, Concise Chinese Materia Medica, Taos, Paradigm Publications, 2008, P 445

[1397] Bensky, D, Clavey, S, Stöger, E & Gamble, A, Chinese Herbal Medicine Materia Medica, 3rd Edition, Seattle, Eastland Press, 1986, 1993, 2004, P 846

[1398] *Materia Medica of Combinations*, via Bensky, D, Clavey, S, Stöger, E & Gamble, A, Chinese Herbal Medicine Materia Medica, 3rd Edition, Seattle, Eastland Press, 1986, 1993, 2004, P 844

1399 Chen, JK & TT, Chinese Medical Herbology and Pharmacology, City of Industry, Art of Medicine Press, 2001/2004, P 959, Bensky, D, Clavey, S, Stöger, E & Gamble, A, Chinese Herbal Medicine Materia Medica, 3rd Edition, Seattle, Eastland Press, 1986, 1993, 2004, P 763

1400 Ye Tian Shi, *Case Records as a Guide to Clinical Practice*, via Bensky, D, Clavey, S, Stöger, E & Gamble, A, Chinese Herbal Medicine Materia Medica, 3rd Edition, Seattle, Eastland Press, 1986, 1993, 2004, P 844

1401 Bensky, D, Clavey, S, Stöger, E & Gamble, A, Chinese Herbal Medicine Materia Medica, 3rd Edition, Seattle, Eastland Press, 1986, 1993, 2004, P 839

1402 Bensky, D, Clavey, S, Stöger, E & Gamble, A, Chinese Herbal Medicine Materia Medica, 3rd Edition, Seattle, Eastland Press, 1986, 1993, 2004, P 838

1403 Bensky, D, Clavey, S, Stöger, E & Gamble, A, Chinese Herbal Medicine Materia Medica, 3rd Edition, Seattle, Eastland Press, 1986, 1993, 2004, P 893

1404 Brand, E & Wiseman, N, Concise Chinese Materia Medica, Taos, Paradigm Publications, 2008, P 457, Bensky, D, Clavey, S, Stöger, E & Gamble, A, Chinese Herbal Medicine Materia Medica, 3rd Edition, Seattle, Eastland Press, 1986, 1993, 2004, P 860

1405 Li Shi Zhen, *Grand Materia Medica*, via Bensky, D, Clavey, S, Stöger, E & Gamble, A, Chinese Herbal Medicine Materia Medica, 3rd Edition, Seattle, Eastland Press, 1986, 1993, 2004, P 861

1406 Li Shi Zhen, *Grand Materia Medica*, via Bensky, D, Clavey, S, Stöger, E & Gamble, A, Chinese Herbal Medicine Materia Medica, 3rd Edition, Seattle, Eastland Press, 1986, 1993, 2004, P 861

1407 Li Shi Zhen, *Grand Materia Medica*, via Bensky, D, Clavey, S, Stöger, E & Gamble, A, Chinese Herbal Medicine Materia Medica, 3rd Edition, Seattle, Eastland Press, 1986, 1993, 2004, P 861

1408 Maciocia, G, The Channels of Acupuncture, Philadelphia, Elsevier, 2006, P 545

1409 Brand, E & Wiseman, N, Concise Chinese Materia Medica, Taos, Paradigm Publications, 2008, P 333, Bensky, D, Clavey, S, Stöger, E & Gamble, A, Chinese Herbal Medicine Materia Medica, 3rd Edition, Seattle, Eastland Press, 1986, 1993, 2004, P 894

1410 Ye Gui, *Renewed Materia Medica*, via Bensky, D, Clavey, S, Stöger, E & Gamble, A, Chinese Herbal Medicine Materia Medica, 3rd Edition, Seattle, Eastland Press, 1986, 1993, 2004, P 900

1411 Ye Gui, *Renewed Materia Medica*, via Bensky, D, Clavey, S, Stöger, E & Gamble, A, Chinese Herbal Medicine Materia Medica, 3rd Edition, Seattle, Eastland Press, 1986, 1993, 2004, P 900

1412 Miao Xi Yong, *Commentary on the Divine Husbandman's Classic of Materia Medica*, via Bensky, D, Clavey, S, Stöger, E & Gamble, A, Chinese Herbal Medicine Materia Medica, 3rd Edition, Seattle, Eastland Press, 1986, 1993, 2004, P 888

1413 Bensky, D, Clavey, S, Stöger, E & Gamble, A, Chinese Herbal Medicine Materia Medica, 3rd Edition, Seattle, Eastland Press, 1986, 1993, 2004, P 904

1414 Bensky, D, Clavey, S, Stöger, E & Gamble, A, Chinese Herbal Medicine Materia Medica, 3rd Edition, Seattle, Eastland Press, 1986, 1993, 2004, P 905

1415 Bensky, D, Clavey, S, Stöger, E & Gamble, A, Chinese Herbal Medicine Materia Medica, 3rd Edition, Seattle, Eastland Press, 1986, 1993, 2004, P 900

1416 Maciocia, G, The Channels of Acupuncture, Philadelphia, Elsevier, 2006, P 545

1417 Bensky, D, Clavey, S, Stöger, E & Gamble, A, Chinese Herbal Medicine Materia Medica, 3rd Edition, Seattle, Eastland Press, 1986, 1993, 2004, P 883

1418 Miao Xi Yong, *Commentary on the Divine Husbandman's Classic of Materia Medica*, via Bensky, D, Clavey, S, Stöger, E & Gamble, A, Chinese Herbal Medicine Materia Medica, 3rd Edition, Seattle, Eastland Press, 1986, 1993, 2004, P 859

[1419] Bensky, D, Clavey, S, Stöger, E & Gamble, A, Chinese Herbal Medicine Materia Medica, 3rd Edition, Seattle, Eastland Press, 1986, 1993, 2004, P 889

[1420] Maciocia, G, The Channels of Acupuncture, Philadelphia, Elsevier, 2006, P 545

[1421][1421] Bensky, D, Clavey, S, Stöger, E & Gamble, A, Chinese Herbal Medicine Materia Medica, 3rd Edition, Seattle, Eastland Press, 1986, 1993, 2004, P 903

[1422] Maciocia, G, The Channels of Acupuncture, Philadelphia, Elsevier, 2006, P 545

[1423] Chen, JK & TT, Chinese Medical Herbology and Pharmacology, City of Industry, Art of Medicine Press, 2001/2004, P 1039

[1424] Brand, E & Wiseman, N, Concise Chinese Materia Medica, Taos, Paradigm Publications, 2008, P 484

[1425] Brand, E & Wiseman, N, Concise Chinese Materia Medica, Taos, Paradigm Publications, 2008, P 484

[1426] Brand, E & Wiseman, N, Concise Chinese Materia Medica, Taos, Paradigm Publications, 2008, P 484

[1427] Brand, E & Wiseman, N, Concise Chinese Materia Medica, Taos, Paradigm Publications, 2008, P 492

[1428] Brand, E & Wiseman, N, Concise Chinese Materia Medica, Taos, Paradigm Publications, 2008, P 492

[1429] Brand, E & Wiseman, N, Concise Chinese Materia Medica, Taos, Paradigm Publications, 2008, P 492

[1430] Brand, E & Wiseman, N, Concise Chinese Materia Medica, Taos, Paradigm Publications, 2008, P 485

[1431] Bensky, D, Clavey, S, Stöger, E & Gamble, A, Chinese Herbal Medicine Materia Medica, 3rd Edition, Seattle, Eastland Press, 1986, 1993, 2004, P 1025

[1432] Bensky, D, Clavey, S, Stöger, E & Gamble, A, Chinese Herbal Medicine Materia Medica, 3rd Edition, Seattle, Eastland Press, 1986, 1993, 2004, P 1025

[1433] Miao Xi Yong, *Commentary on the Divine Husbandman's Classic of Materia Medica*, via Bensky, D, Clavey, S, Stöger, E & Gamble, A, Chinese Herbal Medicine Materia Medica, 3rd Edition, Seattle, Eastland Press, 1986, 1993, 2004, P 1032

[1434] Chen, JK & TT, Chinese Medical Herbology and Pharmacology, City of Industry, Art of Medicine Press, 2001/2004, P 84

[1435] *Divine Husbandman's Classic of the Materia Medica*, via Bensky, D, Clavey, S, Stöger, E & Gamble, A, Chinese Herbal Medicine Materia Medica, 3rd Edition, Seattle, Eastland Press, 1986, 1993, 2004, P 75

[1436] Brand, E & Wiseman, N, Concise Chinese Materia Medica, Taos, Paradigm Publications, 2008, P 61

[1437] Bensky, D, Clavey, S, Stöger, E & Gamble, A, Chinese Herbal Medicine Materia Medica, 3rd Edition, Seattle, Eastland Press, 1986, 1993, 2004, P 74

[1438] Bensky, D, Clavey, S, Stöger, E & Gamble, A, Chinese Herbal Medicine Materia Medica, 3rd Edition, Seattle, Eastland Press, 1986, 1993, 2004, P 74

[1439] Bensky, D, Clavey, S, Stöger, E & Gamble, A, Chinese Herbal Medicine Materia Medica, 3rd Edition, Seattle, Eastland Press, 1986, 1993, 2004, P 105

[1440] *Grand Materia Medica*, via Bensky, D, Clavey, S, Stöger, E & Gamble, A, Chinese Herbal Medicine Materia Medica, 3rd Edition, Seattle, Eastland Press, 1986, 1993, 2004, P 127

[1441] Brand, E & Wiseman, N, Concise Chinese Materia Medica, Taos, Paradigm Publications, 2008, P 102

[1442] Zhang Bing Chen, *Convenient Reader of Materia Medica*, via Bensky, D, Clavey, S, Stöger, E & Gamble, A, Chinese Herbal Medicine Materia Medica, 3rd Edition, Seattle, Eastland Press, 1986, 1993, 2004, P 165

[1443] Chen, JK & TT, Chinese Medical Herbology and Pharmacology, City of Industry, Art of Medicine Press, 2001/2004, P 587, Bensky, D, Clavey, S, Stöger, E & Gamble, A, Chinese Herbal Medicine Materia Medica, 3rd Edition, Seattle, Eastland Press, 1986, 1993, 2004, P 559

[1444] Brand, E & Wiseman, N, Concise Chinese Materia Medica, Taos, Paradigm Publications, 2008, P 264

[1445] Zhang Bing Chen, *Convenient Reader of Materia Medica*, via Bensky, D, Clavey, S, Stöger, E & Gamble, A, Chinese Herbal Medicine Materia Medica, 3rd Edition, Seattle, Eastland Press, 1986, 1993, 2004, P 560

[1446] Zhang Bing Chen, *Convenient Reader of Materia Medica*, via Bensky, D, Clavey, S, Stöger, E & Gamble, A, Chinese Herbal Medicine Materia Medica, 3rd Edition, Seattle, Eastland Press, 1986, 1993, 2004, P 560. In this section Bensky, D, Clavey, S, Stöger, E & Gamble, A, Chinese Herbal Medicine Materia Medica, 3rd Edition, Seattle, Eastland Press, 1986, 1993, 2004, P, et al. quote Zhang as saying that san qi enters the Yang Ming and Jue Yin channels. For some reason they only include the large intestine in their assessment, but not the pericardium. I include it here as it is at least as reasonable a conclusion, and I have used clinically san qi as a pericardium herb for many years with excellent effects.

[1447] Bensky, D, Clavey, S, Stöger, E & Gamble, A, Chinese Herbal Medicine Materia Medica, 3rd Edition, Seattle, Eastland Press, 1986, 1993, 2004, P 563

[1448] Bensky, D, Clavey, S, Stöger, E & Gamble, A, Chinese Herbal Medicine Materia Medica, 3rd Edition, Seattle, Eastland Press, 1986, 1993, 2004, P 562

[1449] Bensky, D, Clavey, S, Stöger, E & Gamble, A, Chinese Herbal Medicine Materia Medica, 3rd Edition, Seattle, Eastland Press, 1986, 1993, 2004, P 652

[1450] Chen, JK & TT, Chinese Medical Herbology and Pharmacology, City of Industry, Art of Medicine Press, 2001/2004, P 593

[1451] Brand, E & Wiseman, N, Concise Chinese Materia Medica, Taos, Paradigm Publications, 2008, P 266

[1452] Bensky, D, Clavey, S, Stöger, E & Gamble, A, Chinese Herbal Medicine Materia Medica, 3rd Edition, Seattle, Eastland Press, 1986, 1993, 2004, P 562

[1453] *Grand Materia Medica*, via Bensky, D, Clavey, S, Stöger, E & Gamble, A, Chinese Herbal Medicine Materia Medica, 3rd Edition, Seattle, Eastland Press, 1986, 1993, 2004, P 127

[1454] Brand, E & Wiseman, N, Concise Chinese Materia Medica, Taos, Paradigm Publications, 2008, P 286

[1455] Wang, Hao Gu, *Harm and Benefit in the Materia Medica*, via Bensky, D, Clavey, S, Stöger, E & Gamble, A, Chinese Herbal Medicine Materia Medica, 3rd Edition, Seattle, Eastland Press, 1986, 1993, 2004, P 603

[1456] Chen, JK & TT, Chinese Medical Herbology and Pharmacology, City of Industry, Art of Medicine Press, 2001/2004, P 636 , Bensky, D, Clavey, S, Stöger, E & Gamble, A, Chinese Herbal Medicine Materia Medica, 3rd Edition, Seattle, Eastland Press, 1986, 1993, 2004, P 602

[1457] Tang Rong Chuan (Tang Zonghai), Ben Cao Wen Da, Personal Unpublished Translation, 2015, 1.2.3
[1458] Bensky, D, Clavey, S, Stöger, E & Gamble, A, Chinese Herbal Medicine Materia Medica, 3rd Edition, Seattle, Eastland Press, 1986, 1993, 2004, P 601
[1459] Chen, JK & TT, Chinese Medical Herbology and Pharmacology, City of Industry, Art of Medicine Press, 2001/2004, P 614
[1460] Zhang, Shan Lei, *Rectification of the Meaning of Materia Medica,* via Bensky, D, Clavey, S, Stöger, E & Gamble, A, Chinese Herbal Medicine Materia Medica, 3rd Edition, Seattle, Eastland Press, 1986, 1993, 2004, P 663
[1461] Bensky, D, Clavey, S, Stöger, E & Gamble, A, Chinese Herbal Medicine Materia Medica, 3rd Edition, Seattle, Eastland Press, 1986, 1993, 2004, P 991
[1462] Brand, E & Wiseman, N, Concise Chinese Materia Medica, Taos, Paradigm Publications, 2008, P 369, Bensky, D, Clavey, S, Stöger, E & Gamble, A, Chinese Herbal Medicine Materia Medica, 3rd Edition, Seattle, Eastland Press, 1986, 1993, 2004, P 970
[1463] Bensky, D, Clavey, S, Stöger, E & Gamble, A, Chinese Herbal Medicine Materia Medica, 3rd Edition, Seattle, Eastland Press, 1986, 1993, 2004, P 987
[1464] Chen, JK & TT, Chinese Medical Herbology and Pharmacology, City of Industry, Art of Medicine Press, 2001/2004, P 883
[1465] Bensky, D, Clavey, S, Stöger, E & Gamble, A, Chinese Herbal Medicine Materia Medica, 3rd Edition, Seattle, Eastland Press, 1986, 1993, 2004, P 105
[1466] Brand, E & Wiseman, N, Concise Chinese Materia Medica, Taos, Paradigm Publications, 2008, P 485
[1467] Bensky, D, Clavey, S, Stöger, E & Gamble, A, Chinese Herbal Medicine Materia Medica, 3rd Edition, Seattle, Eastland Press, 1986, 1993, 2004, P 1025
[1468] Bensky, D, Clavey, S, Stöger, E & Gamble, A, Chinese Herbal Medicine Materia Medica, 3rd Edition, Seattle, Eastland Press, 1986, 1993, 2004, P 1025
[1469] Tang Rong Chuan (Tang Zonghai), Ben Cao Wen Da, Personal Unpublished Translation, 2015, 2.2.2
[1470] Tang Rong Chuan (Tang Zonghai), Ben Cao Wen Da, Personal Unpublished Translation, 2015, 2.2.2
[1471] Maciocia, G, The Channels of Acupuncture, Philadelphia, Elsevier, 2006, P 446
[1472] Zhou Yan, *Thoughtful Differention of Materia Medica*, via Bensky, D, Clavey, S, Stöger, E & Gamble, A, Chinese Herbal Medicine Materia Medica, 3rd Edition, Seattle, Eastland Press, 1986, 1993, 2004, P 62
[1473] Brand, E & Wiseman, N, Concise Chinese Materia Medica, Taos, Paradigm Publications, 2008, P 58
[1474] Chen, JK & TT, Chinese Medical Herbology and Pharmacology, City of Industry, Art of Medicine Press, 2001/2004, P 77
[1475] Tang Rong Chuan (Tang Zonghai), Ben Cao Wen Da, Personal Unpublished Translation, 2015, 2.1.6
[1476] Tang Rong Chuan (Tang Zonghai), Ben Cao Wen Da, Personal Unpublished Translation, 2015, 2.1.6
[1477] Chen, JK & TT, Chinese Medical Herbology and Pharmacology, City of Industry, Art of Medicine Press, 2001/2004, P 84

[1478] *Divine Husbandman's Classic of the Materia Medica*, via Bensky, D, Clavey, S, Stöger, E & Gamble, A, Chinese Herbal Medicine Materia Medica, 3rd Edition, Seattle, Eastland Press, 1986, 1993, 2004, P 75

[1479] Brand, E & Wiseman, N, Concise Chinese Materia Medica, Taos, Paradigm Publications, 2008, P 61

[1480] Bensky, D, Clavey, S, Stöger, E & Gamble, A, Chinese Herbal Medicine Materia Medica, 3rd Edition, Seattle, Eastland Press, 1986, 1993, 2004, P 74

[1481] Bensky, D, Clavey, S, Stöger, E & Gamble, A, Chinese Herbal Medicine Materia Medica, 3rd Edition, Seattle, Eastland Press, 1986, 1993, 2004, P 74

[1482] Zhou Yan, *Records of Thoughtful Differentiation of Materia Medica*, via Bensky, D, Clavey, S, Stöger, E & Gamble, A, Chinese Herbal Medicine Materia Medica, 3rd Edition, Seattle, Eastland Press, 1986, 1993, 2004, P 96

[1483] Tang Rong Chuan (Tang Zonghai), Ben Cao Wen Da, Personal Unpublished Translation, 2015, 2.3.5

[1484] Bensky, D, Clavey, S, Stöger, E & Gamble, A, Chinese Herbal Medicine Materia Medica, 3rd Edition, Seattle, Eastland Press, 1986, 1993, 2004, P 313

[1485] Bensky, D, Clavey, S, Stöger, E & Gamble, A, Chinese Herbal Medicine Materia Medica, 3rd Edition, Seattle, Eastland Press, 1986, 1993, 2004, P 313

[1486] Chen, JK & TT, Chinese Medical Herbology and Pharmacology, City of Industry, Art of Medicine Press, 2001/2004, P 308

[1487] Brand, E & Wiseman, N, Concise Chinese Materia Medica, Taos, Paradigm Publications, 2008, P 158

[1488] Maciocia, G, The Channels of Acupuncture, Philadelphia, Elsevier, 2006, P 585

[1489] '…circulates the Còu Lǐ-interstices and the Sān Jiāo.' Tang Rong Chuan (Tang Zonghai), Ben Cao Wen Da, Personal Unpublished Translation, 2015, 2.2.5

[1490] Zhang, Shan Lei, *Rectification of the Meaning of Materia Medica,* via Bensky, D, Clavey, S, Stöger, E & Gamble, A, Chinese Herbal Medicine Materia Medica, 3rd Edition, Seattle, Eastland Press, 1986, 1993, 2004, P 482

[1491] Zhang, Shan Lei, *Rectification of the Meaning of Materia Medica,* via Bensky, D, Clavey, S, Stöger, E & Gamble, A, Chinese Herbal Medicine Materia Medica, 3rd Edition, Seattle, Eastland Press, 1986, 1993, 2004, P 482

[1492] Huang Gong Xiu, *Seeking Accuracy in the Materia Medica*, and, *Harm and Benefit in the Materia Medica*, both via Bensky, D, Clavey, S, Stöger, E & Gamble, A, Chinese Herbal Medicine Materia Medica, 3rd Edition, Seattle, Eastland Press, 1986, 1993, 2004, P 482

[1493] Bensky, D, Clavey, S, Stöger, E & Gamble, A, Chinese Herbal Medicine Materia Medica, 3rd Edition, Seattle, Eastland Press, 1986, 1993, 2004, P 530

[1494] Brand, E & Wiseman, N, Concise Chinese Materia Medica, Taos, Paradigm Publications, 2008, P 228, Bensky, D, Clavey, S, Stöger, E & Gamble, A, Chinese Herbal Medicine Materia Medica, 3rd Edition, Seattle, Eastland Press, 1986, 1993, 2004, P 530

[1495] Zhang, Jie Bin, *Rectification of the Meaning of Materia Medica*, via Bensky, D, Clavey, S, Stöger, E & Gamble, A, Chinese Herbal Medicine Materia Medica, 3rd Edition, Seattle, Eastland Press, 1986, 1993, 2004, P 515

[1496] Zhang, Jie Bin, *Rectification of the Meaning of Materia Medica*, via Bensky, D, Clavey, S, Stöger, E & Gamble, A, Chinese Herbal Medicine Materia Medica, 3rd Edition, Seattle, Eastland Press, 1986, 1993, 2004, P 515

[1497] Zhang, Shan Lei, *Rectification of the Meaning of Materia Medica,* via Bensky, D, Clavey, S, Stöger, E & Gamble, A, Chinese Herbal Medicine Materia Medica, 3rd Edition, Seattle, Eastland Press, 1986, 1993, 2004, P 528

[1498] Brand, E & Wiseman, N, Concise Chinese Materia Medica, Taos, Paradigm Publications, 2008, P 229

[1499] Bensky, D, Clavey, S, Stöger, E & Gamble, A, Chinese Herbal Medicine Materia Medica, 3rd Edition, Seattle, Eastland Press, 1986, 1993, 2004, P 527

[1500] Tang Rong Chuan (Tang Zonghai), Ben Cao Wen Da, Personal Unpublished Translation, 2015, 1.2.3

[1501] Bensky, D, Clavey, S, Stöger, E & Gamble, A, Chinese Herbal Medicine Materia Medica, 3rd Edition, Seattle, Eastland Press, 1986, 1993, 2004, P 601

[1502] Chen, JK & TT, Chinese Medical Herbology and Pharmacology, City of Industry, Art of Medicine Press, 2001/2004, P 614

[1503] Me, on the basis of Tang Rong Chuan (Tang Zonghai), Ben Cao Wen Da, Personal Unpublished Translation, 2015, 1.2.1, etc., here contained. Although nowhere in the text does the author state that Huang Qi enters the San Jiao Jing-channel, he goes through such extensive and multiple descriptions of the structure and mechanisms of the San Jiao itself, plus his clear delineations of exactly how this herb physically enters and embodies the San Jiao, I would challenge anybody to prove that it *doesn't* enter the San Jiao Jing-channel. In addition, when we consider Huang Qi's central role in Bu Zhong Yi Qi Tang's use in treating qi deficiency with deficient heat symptoms, that is really all about the Shao Yang level of disease. I would put forth the question of why would one not use Huang Qi whenever its known set of qualities were needed to be applied to any aspect or dimension of the San Jiao Jing-channel?

[1504] Li Shi Zhen, *Grand Materia Medica*, via Bensky, D, Clavey, S, Stöger, E & Gamble, A, Chinese Herbal Medicine Materia Medica, 3rd Edition, Seattle, Eastland Press, 1986, 1993, 2004, P 779

[1505] Li Shi Zhen says that Yin Yang Huo is an herb of the Arm and Leg Yang Ming, San Jiao and Ming Men, Li Shi Zhen, *Grand Materia Medica*, via Bensky, D, Clavey, S, Stöger, E & Gamble, A, Chinese Herbal Medicine Materia Medica, 3rd Edition, Seattle, Eastland Press, 1986, 1993, 2004, P 779

[1506] Brand, E & Wiseman, N, Concise Chinese Materia Medica, Taos, Paradigm Publications, 2008, P 418

[1507] Brand, E & Wiseman, N, Concise Chinese Materia Medica, Taos, Paradigm Publications, 2008, P 418

[1508] Brand, E & Wiseman, N, Concise Chinese Materia Medica, Taos, Paradigm Publications, 2008, P 418

[1509] Zhang Lu, *Encountering the Sources of the Classic of Materia Medica*, via Bensky, D, Clavey, S, Stöger, E & Gamble, A, Chinese Herbal Medicine Materia Medica, 3rd Edition, Seattle, Eastland Press, 1986, 1993, 2004, P 791

[1510] Tang Rong Chuan (Tang Zonghai), Ben Cao Wen Da, Personal Unpublished Translation, 2015, 2.2.2

[1511] Tang Rong Chuan (Tang Zonghai), Ben Cao Wen Da, Personal Unpublished Translation, 2015, 2.2.2

[1512] Maciocia, G, The Channels of Acupuncture, Philadelphia, Elsevier, 2006, P 446
[1513] Zhou Yan, *Thoughtful Differention of Materia Medica*, via Bensky, D, Clavey, S, Stöger, E & Gamble, A, Chinese Herbal Medicine Materia Medica, 3rd Edition, Seattle, Eastland Press, 1986, 1993, 2004, P 62
[1514] Brand, E & Wiseman, N, Concise Chinese Materia Medica, Taos, Paradigm Publications, 2008, P 58
[1515] Chen, JK & TT, Chinese Medical Herbology and Pharmacology, City of Industry, Art of Medicine Press, 2001/2004, P 77
[1516] Tang Rong Chuan (Tang Zonghai), Ben Cao Wen Da, Personal Unpublished Translation, 2015, 2.1.6
[1517] Tang Rong Chuan (Tang Zonghai), Ben Cao Wen Da, Personal Unpublished Translation, 2015, 2.1.6
[1518] Chen, JK & TT, Chinese Medical Herbology and Pharmacology, City of Industry, Art of Medicine Press, 2001/2004, P 79, and Bensky, D, Clavey, S, Stöger, E & Gamble, A, Chinese Herbal Medicine Materia Medica, 3rd Edition, Seattle, Eastland Press, 1986, 1993, 2004, P 69
[1519] Chen, JK & TT, Chinese Medical Herbology and Pharmacology, City of Industry, Art of Medicine Press, 2001/2004, P 84
[1520] *Divine Husbandman's Classic of the Materia Medica*, via Bensky, D, Clavey, S, Stöger, E & Gamble, A, Chinese Herbal Medicine Materia Medica, 3rd Edition, Seattle, Eastland Press, 1986, 1993, 2004, P 75
[1521] Brand, E & Wiseman, N, Concise Chinese Materia Medica, Taos, Paradigm Publications, 2008, P 61
[1522] Bensky, D, Clavey, S, Stöger, E & Gamble, A, Chinese Herbal Medicine Materia Medica, 3rd Edition, Seattle, Eastland Press, 1986, 1993, 2004, P 74
[1523] Bensky, D, Clavey, S, Stöger, E & Gamble, A, Chinese Herbal Medicine Materia Medica, 3rd Edition, Seattle, Eastland Press, 1986, 1993, 2004, P 74
[1524] Tang Rong Chuan (Tang Zonghai), Ben Cao Wen Da, Personal Unpublished Translation, 2015, 1.3.4 Although this text indicates that Huang Qin enters the San Jiao, the author is also quite specific in distinguishing between the organs and their Jing-channels. Here he does not indicate the Jing-channel, so I do not indicate otherwise.
[1525] Brand, E & Wiseman, N, Concise Chinese Materia Medica, Taos, Paradigm Publications, 2008, P 114
[1526] Brand, E & Wiseman, N, Concise Chinese Materia Medica, Taos, Paradigm Publications, 2008, P114, Bensky, D, Clavey, S, Stöger, E & Gamble, A, Chinese Herbal Medicine Materia Medica, 3rd Edition, Seattle, Eastland Press, 1986, 1993, 2004, P 147
[1527] Bensky, D, Clavey, S, Stöger, E & Gamble, A, Chinese Herbal Medicine Materia Medica, 3rd Edition, Seattle, Eastland Press, 1986, 1993, 2004, P 147
[1528] Tang Rong Chuan (Tang Zonghai), Ben Cao Wen Da, Personal Unpublished Translation, 2015, 1.3.4
[1529] Brand, E & Wiseman, N, Concise Chinese Materia Medica, Taos, Paradigm Publications, 2008, P 90
[1530] Bensky, D, Clavey, S, Stöger, E & Gamble, A, Chinese Herbal Medicine Materia Medica, 3rd Edition, Seattle, Eastland Press, 1986, 1993, 2004, P 153

[1531] Bensky, D, Clavey, S, Stöger, E & Gamble, A, Chinese Herbal Medicine Materia Medica, 3rd Edition, Seattle, Eastland Press, 1986, 1993, 2004, P 153
[1532] Brand, E & Wiseman, N, Concise Chinese Materia Medica, Taos, Paradigm Publications, 2008, P 114
[1533] Brand, E & Wiseman, N, Concise Chinese Materia Medica, Taos, Paradigm Publications, 2008, P114, Bensky, D, Clavey, S, Stöger, E & Gamble, A, Chinese Herbal Medicine Materia Medica, 3rd Edition, Seattle, Eastland Press, 1986, 1993, 2004, P 147
[1534] Bensky, D, Clavey, S, Stöger, E & Gamble, A, Chinese Herbal Medicine Materia Medica, 3rd Edition, Seattle, Eastland Press, 1986, 1993, 2004, P 147
[1535] Bensky, D, Clavey, S, Stöger, E & Gamble, A, Chinese Herbal Medicine Materia Medica, 3rd Edition, Seattle, Eastland Press, 1986, 1993, 2004, P 951
[1536] Miao Xi Yong, *Commentary on the Divine Husbandman's Classic of Materia Medica*, via Bensky, D, Clavey, S, Stöger, E & Gamble, A, Chinese Herbal Medicine Materia Medica, 3rd Edition, Seattle, Eastland Press, 1986, 1993, 2004, P 961
[1537] *Nanning City Medicines*, via Bensky, D, Clavey, S, Stöger, E & Gamble, A, Chinese Herbal Medicine Materia Medica, 3rd Edition, Seattle, Eastland Press, 1986, 1993, 2004, P 203
[1538] Chen, JK & TT, Chinese Medical Herbology and Pharmacology, City of Industry, Art of Medicine Press, 2001/2004, P 244
[1539] Brand, E & Wiseman, N, Concise Chinese Materia Medica, Taos, Paradigm Publications, 2008, P 119
[1540] Chen, JK & TT, Chinese Medical Herbology and Pharmacology, City of Industry, Art of Medicine Press, 2001/2004, P 287
[1541] Brand, E & Wiseman, N, Concise Chinese Materia Medica, Taos, Paradigm Publications, 2008, P 139
[1542] *Seeking Accuracy in the Materia Medica*, via Bensky, D, Clavey, S, Stöger, E & Gamble, A, Chinese Herbal Medicine Materia Medica, 3rd Edition, Seattle, Eastland Press, 1986, 1993, 2004, P 254
[1543] *Seeking Accuracy in the Materia Medica*, via Bensky, D, Clavey, S, Stöger, E & Gamble, A, Chinese Herbal Medicine Materia Medica, 3rd Edition, Seattle, Eastland Press, 1986, 1993, 2004, P 254
[1544] Bensky, D, Clavey, S, Stöger, E & Gamble, A, Chinese Herbal Medicine Materia Medica, 3rd Edition, Seattle, Eastland Press, 1986, 1993, 2004, P 355
[1545] Bensky, D, Clavey, S, Stöger, E & Gamble, A, Chinese Herbal Medicine Materia Medica, 3rd Edition, Seattle, Eastland Press, 1986, 1993, 2004, P 354
[1546] Bensky, D, Clavey, S, Stöger, E & Gamble, A, Chinese Herbal Medicine Materia Medica, 3rd Edition, Seattle, Eastland Press, 1986, 1993, 2004, P 354
[1547] Brand, E & Wiseman, N, Concise Chinese Materia Medica, Taos, Paradigm Publications, 2008, P 200
[1548] Brand, E & Wiseman, N, Concise Chinese Materia Medica, Taos, Paradigm Publications, 2008, P 189
[1549] Bensky, D, Clavey, S, Stöger, E & Gamble, A, Chinese Herbal Medicine Materia Medica, 3rd Edition, Seattle, Eastland Press, 1986, 1993, 2004, P 304
[1550] Brand, E & Wiseman, N, Concise Chinese Materia Medica, Taos, Paradigm Publications, 2008, P 200

[1551] Bensky, D, Clavey, S, Stöger, E & Gamble, A, Chinese Herbal Medicine Materia Medica, 3rd Edition, Seattle, Eastland Press, 1986, 1993, 2004, P 530
[1552] Brand, E & Wiseman, N, Concise Chinese Materia Medica, Taos, Paradigm Publications, 2008, P 228, Bensky, D, Clavey, S, Stöger, E & Gamble, A, Chinese Herbal Medicine Materia Medica, 3rd Edition, Seattle, Eastland Press, 1986, 1993, 2004, P 530
[1553] Zhang, Jie Bin, *Rectification of the Meaning of Materia Medica*, via Bensky, D, Clavey, S, Stöger, E & Gamble, A, Chinese Herbal Medicine Materia Medica, 3rd Edition, Seattle, Eastland Press, 1986, 1993, 2004, P 515
[1554] Zhang, Jie Bin, *Rectification of the Meaning of Materia Medica*, via Bensky, D, Clavey, S, Stöger, E & Gamble, A, Chinese Herbal Medicine Materia Medica, 3rd Edition, Seattle, Eastland Press, 1986, 1993, 2004, P 515
[1555] Zhang, Shan Lei, *Rectification of the Meaning of Materia Medica,* via Bensky, D, Clavey, S, Stöger, E & Gamble, A, Chinese Herbal Medicine Materia Medica, 3rd Edition, Seattle, Eastland Press, 1986, 1993, 2004, P 528
[1556] Brand, E & Wiseman, N, Concise Chinese Materia Medica, Taos, Paradigm Publications, 2008, P 229
[1557] Bensky, D, Clavey, S, Stöger, E & Gamble, A, Chinese Herbal Medicine Materia Medica, 3rd Edition, Seattle, Eastland Press, 1986, 1993, 2004, P 527
[1558] Huang Gong Xiu, *Seeking Accuracy in the Materia Medica*, via Bensky, D, Clavey, S, Stöger, E & Gamble, A, Chinese Herbal Medicine Materia Medica, 3rd Edition, Seattle, Eastland Press, 1986, 1993, 2004, P 576
[1559] Bensky, D, Clavey, S, Stöger, E & Gamble, A, Chinese Herbal Medicine Materia Medica, 3rd Edition, Seattle, Eastland Press, 1986, 1993, 2004, P 610
[1560] Tang Rong Chuan (Tang Zonghai), Ben Cao Wen Da, Personal Unpublished Translation, 2015, 1.2.3
[1561] Bensky, D, Clavey, S, Stöger, E & Gamble, A, Chinese Herbal Medicine Materia Medica, 3rd Edition, Seattle, Eastland Press, 1986, 1993, 2004, P 601
[1562] Chen, JK & TT, Chinese Medical Herbology and Pharmacology, City of Industry, Art of Medicine Press, 2001/2004, P 614
[1563] Brand, E & Wiseman, N, Concise Chinese Materia Medica, Taos, Paradigm Publications, 2008, P 321
[1564] Brand, E & Wiseman, N, Concise Chinese Materia Medica, Taos, Paradigm Publications, 2008, P 321
[1565] Brand, E & Wiseman, N, Concise Chinese Materia Medica, Taos, Paradigm Publications, 2008, P 311
[1566] Chen, JK & TT, Chinese Medical Herbology and Pharmacology, City of Industry, Art of Medicine Press, 2001/2004, P 688
[1567] Chen, JK & TT, Chinese Medical Herbology and Pharmacology, City of Industry, Art of Medicine Press, 2001/2004, P 688
[1568] Brand, E & Wiseman, N, Concise Chinese Materia Medica, Taos, Paradigm Publications, 2008, P 311
[1569] Brand, E & Wiseman, N, Concise Chinese Materia Medica, Taos, Paradigm Publications, 2008, P 316

[1570] Bensky, D, Clavey, S, Stöger, E & Gamble, A, Chinese Herbal Medicine Materia Medica, 3rd Edition, Seattle, Eastland Press, 1986, 1993, 2004, P 377
[1571] Bensky, D, Clavey, S, Stöger, E & Gamble, A, Chinese Herbal Medicine Materia Medica, 3rd Edition, Seattle, Eastland Press, 1986, 1993, 2004, P 377
[1572] Brand, E & Wiseman, N, Concise Chinese Materia Medica, Taos, Paradigm Publications, 2008, P 321
[1573] Brand, E & Wiseman, N, Concise Chinese Materia Medica, Taos, Paradigm Publications, 2008, P 350, Bensky, D, Clavey, S, Stöger, E & Gamble, A, Chinese Herbal Medicine Materia Medica, 3rd Edition, Seattle, Eastland Press, 1986, 1993, 2004, P 928
[1574] Bensky, D, Clavey, S, Stöger, E & Gamble, A, Chinese Herbal Medicine Materia Medica, 3rd Edition, Seattle, Eastland Press, 1986, 1993, 2004, P 928
[1575] Bensky, D, Clavey, S, Stöger, E & Gamble, A, Chinese Herbal Medicine Materia Medica, 3rd Edition, Seattle, Eastland Press, 1986, 1993, 2004, P 928
[1576] Bensky, D, Clavey, S, Stöger, E & Gamble, A, Chinese Herbal Medicine Materia Medica, 3rd Edition, Seattle, Eastland Press, 1986, 1993, 2004, P 951
[1577] Miao Xi Yong, *Commentary on the Divine Husbandman's Classic of Materia Medica*, via Bensky, D, Clavey, S, Stöger, E & Gamble, A, Chinese Herbal Medicine Materia Medica, 3rd Edition, Seattle, Eastland Press, 1986, 1993, 2004, P 961
[1578] Tang Rong Chuan (Tang Zonghai), Ben Cao Wen Da, Personal Unpublished Translation, 2015, 2.2.2
[1579] Tang Rong Chuan (Tang Zonghai), Ben Cao Wen Da, Personal Unpublished Translation, 2015, 2.2.2
[1580] Maciocia, G, The Channels of Acupuncture, Philadelphia, 2006, P 446
[1581] Chen, JK & TT, Chinese Medical Herbology and Pharmacology, City of Industry, Art of Medicine Press, 2001/2004, P 57
[1582] Bensky, D, Clavey, S, Stöger, E & Gamble, A, Chinese Herbal Medicine Materia Medica, 3rd Edition, Seattle, Eastland Press, 1986, 1993, 2004, P 44
[1583] Bensky, D, Clavey, S, Stöger, E & Gamble, A, Chinese Herbal Medicine Materia Medica, 3rd Edition, Seattle, Eastland Press, 1986, 1993, 2004, P 39
[1584] Chen, JK & TT, Chinese Medical Herbology and Pharmacology, City of Industry, Art of Medicine Press, 2001/2004, P 62, Tang Rong Chuan (Tang Zonghai), Ben Cao Wen Da, Personal Unpublished Translation, 2015, 2.1.6
[1585] Maciocia, G, The Channels of Acupuncture, Philadelphia, 2006, P 446
[1586] Maciocia, G, The Channels of Acupuncture, Philadelphia, 2006, P 446
[1587] Maciocia, G, The Channels of Acupuncture, Philadelphia, 2006, P 585
[1588] Tang Rong Chuan (Tang Zonghai), Ben Cao Wen Da, Personal Unpublished Translation, 2015, 2.1.6
[1589] Tang Rong Chuan (Tang Zonghai), Ben Cao Wen Da, Personal Unpublished Translation, 2015, 2.1.3
[1590] Bensky, D, Clavey, S, Stöger, E & Gamble, A, Chinese Herbal Medicine Materia Medica, 3rd Edition, Seattle, Eastland Press, 1986, 1993, 2004, P 20/21
[1591] Maciocia, G, The Channels of Acupuncture, Philadelphia, 2006, P 446
[1592] Tang Rong Chuan (Tang Zonghai), Ben Cao Wen Da, Personal Unpublished Translation, 2015, 2.1.3

[1593] Brand, E & Wiseman, N, Concise Chinese Materia Medica, Taos, Paradigm Publications, 2008, P 56

[1594] Li Shi Zhen, *Grand Materia Medica*, via Bensky, D, Clavey, S, Stöger, E & Gamble, A, Chinese Herbal Medicine Materia Medica, 3rd Edition, Seattle, Eastland Press, 1986, 1993, 2004, P 56

[1595] Li Shi Zhen, *Grand Materia Medica*, via Bensky, D, Clavey, S, Stöger, E & Gamble, A, Chinese Herbal Medicine Materia Medica, 3rd Edition, Seattle, Eastland Press, 1986, 1993, 2004, P 56

[1596] Zhou Yan, *Thoughtful Differention of Materia Medica*, via Bensky, D, Clavey, S, Stöger, E & Gamble, A, Chinese Herbal Medicine Materia Medica, 3rd Edition, Seattle, Eastland Press, 1986, 1993, 2004, P 62

[1597] Brand, E & Wiseman, N, Concise Chinese Materia Medica, Taos, Paradigm Publications, 2008, P 58

[1598] Chen, JK & TT, Chinese Medical Herbology and Pharmacology, City of Industry, Art of Medicine Press, 2001/2004, P 77

[1599] Tang Rong Chuan (Tang Zonghai), Ben Cao Wen Da, Personal Unpublished Translation, 2015, 2.1.6

[1600] Tang Rong Chuan (Tang Zonghai), Ben Cao Wen Da, Personal Unpublished Translation, 2015, 2.1.6

[1601] Chen, JK & TT, Chinese Medical Herbology and Pharmacology, City of Industry, Art of Medicine Press, 2001/2004, P 79, and Bensky, D, Clavey, S, Stöger, E & Gamble, A, Chinese Herbal Medicine Materia Medica, 3rd Edition, Seattle, Eastland Press, 1986, 1993, 2004, P 69

[1602] Brand, E & Wiseman, N, Concise Chinese Materia Medica, Taos, Paradigm Publications, 2008, P 56, Chen, JK & TT, Chinese Medical Herbology and Pharmacology, City of Industry, Art of Medicine Press, 2001/2004, P 75

[1603] Bensky, D, Clavey, S, Stöger, E & Gamble, A, Chinese Herbal Medicine Materia Medica, 3rd Edition, Seattle, Eastland Press, 1986, 1993, 2004, P 58

[1604] Bensky, D, Clavey, S, Stöger, E & Gamble, A, Chinese Herbal Medicine Materia Medica, 3rd Edition, Seattle, Eastland Press, 1986, 1993, 2004, P 58

[1605] Bensky, D, Clavey, S, Stöger, E & Gamble, A, Chinese Herbal Medicine Materia Medica, 3rd Edition, Seattle, Eastland Press, 1986, 1993, 2004, P 166

[1606] Zhang Xi Chun, *Essays on Medicine Esteeming the Chinese and Respecting the Western*, via Bensky, D, Clavey, S, Stöger, E & Gamble, A, Chinese Herbal Medicine Materia Medica, 3rd Edition, Seattle, Eastland Press, 1986, 1993, 2004, P 53

[1607] Bensky, D, Clavey, S, Stöger, E & Gamble, A, Chinese Herbal Medicine Materia Medica, 3rd Edition, Seattle, Eastland Press, 1986, 1993, 2004, P 52

[1608] Chen, JK & TT, Chinese Medical Herbology and Pharmacology, City of Industry, Art of Medicine Press, 2001/2004, P 84

[1609] *Divine Husbandman's Classic of the Materia Medica*, via Bensky, D, Clavey, S, Stöger, E & Gamble, A, Chinese Herbal Medicine Materia Medica, 3rd Edition, Seattle, Eastland Press, 1986, 1993, 2004, P 75

[1610] Brand, E & Wiseman, N, Concise Chinese Materia Medica, Taos, Paradigm Publications, 2008, P 61

[1611] Bensky, D, Clavey, S, Stöger, E & Gamble, A, Chinese Herbal Medicine Materia Medica, 3rd Edition, Seattle, Eastland Press, 1986, 1993, 2004, P 74

[1612] Bensky, D, Clavey, S, Stöger, E & Gamble, A, Chinese Herbal Medicine Materia Medica, 3rd Edition, Seattle, Eastland Press, 1986, 1993, 2004, P 74
[1613] Zhou Yan, *Records of Thoughtful Differentiation of Materia Medica*, via Bensky, D, Clavey, S, Stöger, E & Gamble, A, Chinese Herbal Medicine Materia Medica, 3rd Edition, Seattle, Eastland Press, 1986, 1993, 2004, P 96
[1614] Brand, E & Wiseman, N, Concise Chinese Materia Medica, Taos, Paradigm Publications, 2008, P 84, and Huang Gong Xiu, *Seeking Accuracy in the Materia Medica*, via Bensky, D, Clavey, S, Stöger, E & Gamble, A, Chinese Herbal Medicine Materia Medica, 3rd Edition, Seattle, Eastland Press, 1986, 1993, 2004, P 112
[1615] Brand, E & Wiseman, N, Concise Chinese Materia Medica, Taos, Paradigm Publications, 2008, P 84
[1616] Brand, E & Wiseman, N, Concise Chinese Materia Medica, Taos, Paradigm Publications, 2008, P 85
[1617] Brand, E & Wiseman, N, Concise Chinese Materia Medica, Taos, Paradigm Publications, 2008, P 85
[1618] Zhang Shan Lei, via Bensky, D, Clavey, S, Stöger, E & Gamble, A, Chinese Herbal Medicine Materia Medica, 3rd Edition, Seattle, Eastland Press, 1986, 1993, 2004, P 116
[1619] Bensky, D, Clavey, S, Stöger, E & Gamble, A, Chinese Herbal Medicine Materia Medica, 3rd Edition, Seattle, Eastland Press, 1986, 1993, 2004, P 113
[1620] Bensky, D, Clavey, S, Stöger, E & Gamble, A, Chinese Herbal Medicine Materia Medica, 3rd Edition, Seattle, Eastland Press, 1986, 1993, 2004, P 114
[1621] Bensky, D, Clavey, S, Stöger, E & Gamble, A, Chinese Herbal Medicine Materia Medica, 3rd Edition, Seattle, Eastland Press, 1986, 1993, 2004, P 115
[1622] Chen, JK & TT, Chinese Medical Herbology and Pharmacology, City of Industry, Art of Medicine Press, 2001/2004, P 151
[1623] Bensky, D, Clavey, S, Stöger, E & Gamble, A, Chinese Herbal Medicine Materia Medica, 3rd Edition, Seattle, Eastland Press, 1986, 1993, 2004, P 144
[1624] Tang Rong Chuan (Tang Zonghai), Ben Cao Wen Da, Personal Unpublished Translation, 2015, 1.5.3
[1625] Maciocia, G, The Channels of Acupuncture, Philadelphia, 2006, P 446
[1626] Brand, E & Wiseman, N, Concise Chinese Materia Medica, Taos, Paradigm Publications, 2008, P 114
[1627] Brand, E & Wiseman, N, Concise Chinese Materia Medica, Taos, Paradigm Publications, 2008, P114, Bensky, D, Clavey, S, Stöger, E & Gamble, A, Chinese Herbal Medicine Materia Medica, 3rd Edition, Seattle, Eastland Press, 1986, 1993, 2004, P 147
[1628] Bensky, D, Clavey, S, Stöger, E & Gamble, A, Chinese Herbal Medicine Materia Medica, 3rd Edition, Seattle, Eastland Press, 1986, 1993, 2004, P 147
[1629] Tang Rong Chuan (Tang Zonghai), Ben Cao Wen Da, Personal Unpublished Translation, 2015, 1.3.4
[1630] Brand, E & Wiseman, N, Concise Chinese Materia Medica, Taos, Paradigm Publications, 2008, P 90
[1631] Bensky, D, Clavey, S, Stöger, E & Gamble, A, Chinese Herbal Medicine Materia Medica, 3rd Edition, Seattle, Eastland Press, 1986, 1993, 2004, P 904

[1632] Bensky, D, Clavey, S, Stöger, E & Gamble, A, Chinese Herbal Medicine Materia Medica, 3rd Edition, Seattle, Eastland Press, 1986, 1993, 2004, P 905
[1633] Bensky, D, Clavey, S, Stöger, E & Gamble, A, Chinese Herbal Medicine Materia Medica, 3rd Edition, Seattle, Eastland Press, 1986, 1993, 2004, P 119
[1634] Bensky, D, Clavey, S, Stöger, E & Gamble, A, Chinese Herbal Medicine Materia Medica, 3rd Edition, Seattle, Eastland Press, 1986, 1993, 2004, P 622
[1635] Bensky, D, Clavey, S, Stöger, E & Gamble, A, Chinese Herbal Medicine Materia Medica, 3rd Edition, Seattle, Eastland Press, 1986, 1993, 2004, P 622
[1636] *Grand Materia Medica*, via Bensky, D, Clavey, S, Stöger, E & Gamble, A, Chinese Herbal Medicine Materia Medica, 3rd Edition, Seattle, Eastland Press, 1986, 1993, 2004, P 127
[1637] Brand, E & Wiseman, N, Concise Chinese Materia Medica, Taos, Paradigm Publications, 2008, P 98
[1638] Wang, Hao Gu, *Harm and Benefit in the Materia Medica*, via Bensky, D, Clavey, S, Stöger, E & Gamble, A, Chinese Herbal Medicine Materia Medica, 3rd Edition, Seattle, Eastland Press, 1986, 1993, 2004, P 130
[1639] Brand, E & Wiseman, N, Concise Chinese Materia Medica, Taos, Paradigm Publications, 2008, P 107
[1640] Bensky, D, Clavey, S, Stöger, E & Gamble, A, Chinese Herbal Medicine Materia Medica, 3rd Edition, Seattle, Eastland Press, 1986, 1993, 2004, P 205
[1641] Brand, E & Wiseman, N, Concise Chinese Materia Medica, Taos, Paradigm Publications, 2008, P 108
[1642] Zhang Bing Cheng, *Convenient Reader of Materia Medica*, via Bensky, D, Clavey, S, Stöger, E & Gamble, A, Chinese Herbal Medicine Materia Medica, 3rd Edition, Seattle, Eastland Press, 1986, 1993, 2004, P 156
[1643] Bensky, D, Clavey, S, Stöger, E & Gamble, A, Chinese Herbal Medicine Materia Medica, 3rd Edition, Seattle, Eastland Press, 1986, 1993, 2004, P 161
[1644] *Convenient Reader of Materia Medica*, Bensky, D, Clavey, S, Stöger, E & Gamble, A, Chinese Herbal Medicine Materia Medica, 3rd Edition, Seattle, Eastland Press, 1986, 1993, 2004, P 214
[1645] *Convenient Reader of Materia Medica*, Bensky, D, Clavey, S, Stöger, E & Gamble, A, Chinese Herbal Medicine Materia Medica, 3rd Edition, Seattle, Eastland Press, 1986, 1993, 2004, P 214
[1646] Zhang Bing Chen, *Convenient Reader of Materia Medica*, via Bensky, D, Clavey, S, Stöger, E & Gamble, A, Chinese Herbal Medicine Materia Medica, 3rd Edition, Seattle, Eastland Press, 1986, 1993, 2004, P 214
[1647] Bensky, D, Clavey, S, Stöger, E & Gamble, A, Chinese Herbal Medicine Materia Medica, 3rd Edition, Seattle, Eastland Press, 1986, 1993, 2004, P 166
[1648] Bensky, D, Clavey, S, Stöger, E & Gamble, A, Chinese Herbal Medicine Materia Medica, 3rd Edition, Seattle, Eastland Press, 1986, 1993, 2004, P 183
[1649] Brand, E & Wiseman, N, Concise Chinese Materia Medica, Taos, Paradigm Publications, 2008, P 114
[1650] Brand, E & Wiseman, N, Concise Chinese Materia Medica, Taos, Paradigm Publications, 2008, P 114, Bensky, D, Clavey, S, Stöger, E & Gamble, A, Chinese Herbal Medicine Materia Medica, 3rd Edition, Seattle, Eastland Press, 1986, 1993, 2004, P 147
[1651] Bensky, D, Clavey, S, Stöger, E & Gamble, A, Chinese Herbal Medicine Materia Medica, 3rd Edition, Seattle, Eastland Press, 1986, 1993, 2004, P 147

[1652] *Miscellaneous Records of Famous Physicians*, via Bensky, D, Clavey, S, Stöger, E & Gamble, A, Chinese Herbal Medicine Materia Medica, 3rd Edition, Seattle, Eastland Press, 1986, 1993, 2004, P 174
[1653] Tang Rong Chuan (Tang Zonghai), Ben Cao Wen Da, Personal Unpublished Translation, 2015, 2.3.5
[1654] Bensky, D, Clavey, S, Stöger, E & Gamble, A, Chinese Herbal Medicine Materia Medica, 3rd Edition, Seattle, Eastland Press, 1986, 1993, 2004, P 189
[1655] Brand, E & Wiseman, N, Concise Chinese Materia Medica, Taos, Paradigm Publications, 2008, P 116, Bensky, D, Clavey, S, Stöger, E & Gamble, A, Chinese Herbal Medicine Materia Medica, 3rd Edition, Seattle, Eastland Press, 1986, 1993, 2004, P 196
[1656] Bensky, D, Clavey, S, Stöger, E & Gamble, A, Chinese Herbal Medicine Materia Medica, 3rd Edition, Seattle, Eastland Press, 1986, 1993, 2004, P 215
[1657] Bensky, D, Clavey, S, Stöger, E & Gamble, A, Chinese Herbal Medicine Materia Medica, 3rd Edition, Seattle, Eastland Press, 1986, 1993, 2004, P 215
[1658] Bensky, D, Clavey, S, Stöger, E & Gamble, A, Chinese Herbal Medicine Materia Medica, 3rd Edition, Seattle, Eastland Press, 1986, 1993, 2004, P 215
[1659] Bensky, D, Clavey, S, Stöger, E & Gamble, A, Chinese Herbal Medicine Materia Medica, 3rd Edition, Seattle, Eastland Press, 1986, 1993, 2004, P 1010
[1660] Bensky, D, Clavey, S, Stöger, E & Gamble, A, Chinese Herbal Medicine Materia Medica, 3rd Edition, Seattle, Eastland Press, 1986, 1993, 2004, P 1010
[1661] Brand, E & Wiseman, N, Concise Chinese Materia Medica, Taos, Paradigm Publications, 2008, P 102
[1662] Zhang Bing Chen, *Convenient Reader of Materia Medica*, via Bensky, D, Clavey, S, Stöger, E & Gamble, A, Chinese Herbal Medicine Materia Medica, 3rd Edition, Seattle, Eastland Press, 1986, 1993, 2004, P 165
[1663] *Rectification of the Meaning of Materia Medica*, via Bensky, D, Clavey, S, Stöger, E & Gamble, A, Chinese Herbal Medicine Materia Medica, 3rd Edition, Seattle, Eastland Press, 1986, 1993, 2004, P 185
[1664] Bensky, D, Clavey, S, Stöger, E & Gamble, A, Chinese Herbal Medicine Materia Medica, 3rd Edition, Seattle, Eastland Press, 1986, 1993, 2004, P 193
[1665] Zhang Bing Chen, *Convenient Reader of Materia Medica*, via Bensky, D, Clavey, S, Stöger, E & Gamble, A, Chinese Herbal Medicine Materia Medica, 3rd Edition, Seattle, Eastland Press, 1986, 1993, 2004, P 193
[1666] Bensky, D, Clavey, S, Stöger, E & Gamble, A, Chinese Herbal Medicine Materia Medica, 3rd Edition, Seattle, Eastland Press, 1986, 1993, 2004, P 951
[1667] Miao Xi Yong, *Commentary on the Divine Husbandman's Classic of Materia Medica*, via Bensky, D, Clavey, S, Stöger, E & Gamble, A, Chinese Herbal Medicine Materia Medica, 3rd Edition, Seattle, Eastland Press, 1986, 1993, 2004, P 961
[1668] *Nanning City Medicines*, via Bensky, D, Clavey, S, Stöger, E & Gamble, A, Chinese Herbal Medicine Materia Medica, 3rd Edition, Seattle, Eastland Press, 1986, 1993, 2004, P 203
[1669] *Folk Medicines From Guizhou*, via Bensky, D, Clavey, S, Stöger, E & Gamble, A, Chinese Herbal Medicine Materia Medica, 3rd Edition, Seattle, Eastland Press, 1986, 1993, 2004, P 218
[1670] *Folk Medicines From Guizhou*, via Bensky, D, Clavey, S, Stöger, E & Gamble, A, Chinese Herbal Medicine Materia Medica, 3rd Edition, Seattle, Eastland Press, 1986, 1993, 2004, P 218

[1671] Brand, E & Wiseman, N, Concise Chinese Materia Medica, Taos, Paradigm Publications, 2008, P 120, Bensky, D, Clavey, S, Stöger, E & Gamble, A, Chinese Herbal Medicine Materia Medica, 3rd Edition, Seattle, Eastland Press, 1986, 1993, 2004, P 224
[1672] Bensky, D, Clavey, S, Stöger, E & Gamble, A, Chinese Herbal Medicine Materia Medica, 3rd Edition, Seattle, Eastland Press, 1986, 1993, 2004, P 224
[1673] Chen, JK & TT, Chinese Medical Herbology and Pharmacology, City of Industry, Art of Medicine Press, 2001/2004, P 247
[1674] Tang Rong Chuan (Tang Zonghai), Ben Cao Wen Da, Personal Unpublished Translation, 2015, 2.3.5
[1675] Brand, E & Wiseman, N, Concise Chinese Materia Medica, Taos, Paradigm Publications, 2008, P 121, Bensky, D, Clavey, S, Stöger, E & Gamble, A, Chinese Herbal Medicine Materia Medica, 3rd Edition, Seattle, Eastland Press, 1986, 1993, 2004, P 222
[1676] Chen, JK & TT, Chinese Medical Herbology and Pharmacology, City of Industry, Art of Medicine Press, 2001/2004, P 244
[1677] Brand, E & Wiseman, N, Concise Chinese Materia Medica, Taos, Paradigm Publications, 2008, P 119
[1678] Brand, E & Wiseman, N, Concise Chinese Materia Medica, Taos, Paradigm Publications, 2008, P 121
[1679] Brand, E & Wiseman, N, Concise Chinese Materia Medica, Taos, Paradigm Publications, 2008, P 132
[1680] Tang Rong Chuan (Tang Zonghai), Ben Cao Wen Da, Personal Unpublished Translation, 2015, 1.5.3
[1681] Bensky, D, Clavey, S, Stöger, E & Gamble, A, Chinese Herbal Medicine Materia Medica, 3rd Edition, Seattle, Eastland Press, 1986, 1993, 2004, P 239
[1682] Tang Rong Chuan (Tang Zonghai), Ben Cao Wen Da, Personal Unpublished Translation, 2015, 1.5.2
[1683] Maciocia, G, The Channels of Acupuncture, Philadelphia, 2006, P 446
[1684] Bensky, D, Clavey, S, Stöger, E & Gamble, A, Chinese Herbal Medicine Materia Medica, 3rd Edition, Seattle, Eastland Press, 1986, 1993, 2004, P 243
[1685] Chen, JK & TT, Chinese Medical Herbology and Pharmacology, City of Industry, Art of Medicine Press, 2001/2004, P 287
[1686] Brand, E & Wiseman, N, Concise Chinese Materia Medica, Taos, Paradigm Publications, 2008, P 139
[1687] *Seeking Accuracy in the Materia Medica*, via Bensky, D, Clavey, S, Stöger, E & Gamble, A, Chinese Herbal Medicine Materia Medica, 3rd Edition, Seattle, Eastland Press, 1986, 1993, 2004, P 254
[1688] *Seeking Accuracy in the Materia Medica*, via Bensky, D, Clavey, S, Stöger, E & Gamble, A, Chinese Herbal Medicine Materia Medica, 3rd Edition, Seattle, Eastland Press, 1986, 1993, 2004, P 254
[1689] Bensky, D, Clavey, S, Stöger, E & Gamble, A, Chinese Herbal Medicine Materia Medica, 3rd Edition, Seattle, Eastland Press, 1986, 1993, 2004, P 332
[1690] Bensky, D, Clavey, S, Stöger, E & Gamble, A, Chinese Herbal Medicine Materia Medica, 3rd Edition, Seattle, Eastland Press, 1986, 1993, 2004, P 332

[1691] Li Gao, via Bensky, D, Clavey, S, Stöger, E & Gamble, A, Chinese Herbal Medicine Materia Medica, 3rd Edition, Seattle, Eastland Press, 1986, 1993, 2004, P 332
[1692] Bensky, D, Clavey, S, Stöger, E & Gamble, A, Chinese Herbal Medicine Materia Medica, 3rd Edition, Seattle, Eastland Press, 1986, 1993, 2004, P 347
[1693] Bensky, D, Clavey, S, Stöger, E & Gamble, A, Chinese Herbal Medicine Materia Medica, 3rd Edition, Seattle, Eastland Press, 1986, 1993, 2004, P 347
[1694] Bensky, D, Clavey, S, Stöger, E & Gamble, A, Chinese Herbal Medicine Materia Medica, 3rd Edition, Seattle, Eastland Press, 1986, 1993, 2004, P 342
[1695] Bensky, D, Clavey, S, Stöger, E & Gamble, A, Chinese Herbal Medicine Materia Medica, 3rd Edition, Seattle, Eastland Press, 1986, 1993, 2004, P 342
[1696] Bensky, D, Clavey, S, Stöger, E & Gamble, A, Chinese Herbal Medicine Materia Medica, 3rd Edition, Seattle, Eastland Press, 1986, 1993, 2004, P 355
[1697] Bensky, D, Clavey, S, Stöger, E & Gamble, A, Chinese Herbal Medicine Materia Medica, 3rd Edition, Seattle, Eastland Press, 1986, 1993, 2004, P 354
[1698] Bensky, D, Clavey, S, Stöger, E & Gamble, A, Chinese Herbal Medicine Materia Medica, 3rd Edition, Seattle, Eastland Press, 1986, 1993, 2004, P 354
[1699] Brand, E & Wiseman, N, Concise Chinese Materia Medica, Taos, Paradigm Publications, 2008, P 154, Chen, JK & TT, Chinese Medical Herbology and Pharmacology, City of Industry, Art of Medicine Press, 2001/2004, P 312
[1700] Bensky, D, Clavey, S, Stöger, E & Gamble, A, Chinese Herbal Medicine Materia Medica, 3rd Edition, Seattle, Eastland Press, 1986, 1993, 2004, P 329
[1701] Bensky, D, Clavey, S, Stöger, E & Gamble, A, Chinese Herbal Medicine Materia Medica, 3rd Edition, Seattle, Eastland Press, 1986, 1993, 2004, P 329
[1702] Brand, E & Wiseman, N, Concise Chinese Materia Medica, Taos, Paradigm Publications, 2008, P 155
[1703] Brand, E & Wiseman, N, Concise Chinese Materia Medica, Taos, Paradigm Publications, 2008, P 155
[1704] Bensky, D, Clavey, S, Stöger, E & Gamble, A, Chinese Herbal Medicine Materia Medica, 3rd Edition, Seattle, Eastland Press, 1986, 1993, 2004, P 349
[1705] Chen, JK & TT, Chinese Medical Herbology and Pharmacology, City of Industry, Art of Medicine Press, 2001/2004, P 333
[1706] Ye Tian Shi, *Renewed Materia Medica*, via Bensky, D, Clavey, S, Stöger, E & Gamble, A, Chinese Herbal Medicine Materia Medica, 3rd Edition, Seattle, Eastland Press, 1986, 1993, 2004, P 351
[1707] Ye Tian Shi, *Renewed Materia Medica*, via Bensky, D, Clavey, S, Stöger, E & Gamble, A, Chinese Herbal Medicine Materia Medica, 3rd Edition, Seattle, Eastland Press, 1986, 1993, 2004, P 351
[1708] Bensky, D, Clavey, S, Stöger, E & Gamble, A, Chinese Herbal Medicine Materia Medica, 3rd Edition, Seattle, Eastland Press, 1986, 1993, 2004, P 360
[1709] Tang Rong Chuan (Tang Zonghai), Ben Cao Wen Da, Personal Unpublished Translation, 2015, 2.1.6
[1710] Chen, JK & TT, Chinese Medical Herbology and Pharmacology, City of Industry, Art of Medicine Press, 2001/2004, P 304, Bensky, D, Clavey, S, Stöger, E & Gamble, A, Chinese Herbal Medicine Materia Medica, 3rd Edition, Seattle, Eastland Press, 1986, 1993, 2004, P 323, Tang Rong Chuan (Tang Zonghai), Ben Cao Wen Da, Personal Unpublished Translation, 2015, 1.3.7
[1711] Maciocia, G, The Channels of Acupuncture, Philadelphia, 2006, P 446

[1712] Brand, E & Wiseman, N, Concise Chinese Materia Medica, Taos, Paradigm Publications, 2008, P 160

[1713] Li Zhong Zhi, *Penetrating the Mysteries of the Materia Medica*, via Bensky, D, Clavey, S, Stöger, E & Gamble, A, Chinese Herbal Medicine Materia Medica, 3rd Edition, Seattle, Eastland Press, 1986, 1993, 2004, P 358

[1714] Brand, E & Wiseman, N, Concise Chinese Materia Medica, Taos, Paradigm Publications, 2008, P 156

[1715] Brand, E & Wiseman, N, Concise Chinese Materia Medica, Taos, Paradigm Publications, 2008, P 156

[1716] Zhang, Jie Bin, *Rectification of the Meaning of Materia Medica*, via Bensky, D, Clavey, S, Stöger, E & Gamble, A, Chinese Herbal Medicine Materia Medica, 3rd Edition, Seattle, Eastland Press, 1986, 1993, 2004, P 352

[1717] Bensky, D, Clavey, S, Stöger, E & Gamble, A, Chinese Herbal Medicine Materia Medica, 3rd Edition, Seattle, Eastland Press, 1986, 1993, 2004, P 353

[1718] Bensky, D, Clavey, S, Stöger, E & Gamble, A, Chinese Herbal Medicine Materia Medica, 3rd Edition, Seattle, Eastland Press, 1986, 1993, 2004, P 356

[1719] Bensky, D, Clavey, S, Stöger, E & Gamble, A, Chinese Herbal Medicine Materia Medica, 3rd Edition, Seattle, Eastland Press, 1986, 1993, 2004, P 360

[1720] Brand, E & Wiseman, N, Concise Chinese Materia Medica, Taos, Paradigm Publications, 2008, P 163

[1721] Tang Rong Chuan (Tang Zonghai), Ben Cao Wen Da, Personal Unpublished Translation, 2015, 2.1.6

[1722] Bensky, D, Clavey, S, Stöger, E & Gamble, A, Chinese Herbal Medicine Materia Medica, 3rd Edition, Seattle, Eastland Press, 1986, 1993, 2004, P 337

[1723] Zhang, Jie Bin, *Rectification of the Meaning of Materia Medica*, via Bensky, D, Clavey, S, Stöger, E & Gamble, A, Chinese Herbal Medicine Materia Medica, 3rd Edition, Seattle, Eastland Press, 1986, 1993, 2004, P 352

[1724] Bensky, D, Clavey, S, Stöger, E & Gamble, A, Chinese Herbal Medicine Materia Medica, 3rd Edition, Seattle, Eastland Press, 1986, 1993, 2004, P 353

[1725] Bensky, D, Clavey, S, Stöger, E & Gamble, A, Chinese Herbal Medicine Materia Medica, 3rd Edition, Seattle, Eastland Press, 1986, 1993, 2004, P 278

[1726] Brand, E & Wiseman, N, Concise Chinese Materia Medica, Taos, Paradigm Publications, 2008, P 191

[1727] Brand, E & Wiseman, N, Concise Chinese Materia Medica, Taos, Paradigm Publications, 2008, P 200

[1728] Brand, E & Wiseman, N, Concise Chinese Materia Medica, Taos, Paradigm Publications, 2008, P 189

[1729] Bensky, D, Clavey, S, Stöger, E & Gamble, A, Chinese Herbal Medicine Materia Medica, 3rd Edition, Seattle, Eastland Press, 1986, 1993, 2004, P 304

[1730] Brand, E & Wiseman, N, Concise Chinese Materia Medica, Taos, Paradigm Publications, 2008, P 200

[1731] Brand, E & Wiseman, N, Concise Chinese Materia Medica, Taos, Paradigm Publications, 2008, P 212

[1732] Bensky, D, Clavey, S, Stöger, E & Gamble, A, Chinese Herbal Medicine Materia Medica, 3rd Edition, Seattle, Eastland Press, 1986, 1993, 2004, P 680

[1733] Tang Rong Chuan (Tang Zonghai), Ben Cao Wen Da, Personal Unpublished Translation, 2015, 1.2.4

[1734] Tang Rong Chuan (Tang Zonghai), Ben Cao Wen Da, Personal Unpublished Translation, 2015, 1.2.4

[1735] Maciocia, G, The Channels of Acupuncture, Philadelphia, 2006, P 446

[1736] Zhang Xi Chun, *Essays on Medicine Esteeming the Chinese and Respecting the Western*, via Bensky, D, Clavey, S, Stöger, E & Gamble, A, Chinese Herbal Medicine Materia Medica, 3rd Edition, Seattle, Eastland Press, 1986, 1993, 2004, P 545

[1737] Zhang, Jie Bin, *Rectification of the Meaning of Materia Medica*, via Bensky, D, Clavey, S, Stöger, E & Gamble, A, Chinese Herbal Medicine Materia Medica, 3rd Edition, Seattle, Eastland Press, 1986, 1993, 2004, P 515

[1738] Zhang, Jie Bin, *Rectification of the Meaning of Materia Medica*, via Bensky, D, Clavey, S, Stöger, E & Gamble, A, Chinese Herbal Medicine Materia Medica, 3rd Edition, Seattle, Eastland Press, 1986, 1993, 2004, P 515

[1739] Bensky, D, Clavey, S, Stöger, E & Gamble, A, Chinese Herbal Medicine Materia Medica, 3rd Edition, Seattle, Eastland Press, 1986, 1993, 2004, P 550

[1740] Bensky, D, Clavey, S, Stöger, E & Gamble, A, Chinese Herbal Medicine Materia Medica, 3rd Edition, Seattle, Eastland Press, 1986, 1993, 2004, P 550

[1741] Brand, E & Wiseman, N, Concise Chinese Materia Medica, Taos, Paradigm Publications, 2008, P 233

[1742] Brand, E & Wiseman, N, Concise Chinese Materia Medica, Taos, Paradigm Publications, 2008, P 233

[1743] Zhang, Shan Lei, *Rectification of the Meaning of Materia Medica,* via Bensky, D, Clavey, S, Stöger, E & Gamble, A, Chinese Herbal Medicine Materia Medica, 3rd Edition, Seattle, Eastland Press, 1986, 1993, 2004, P 528

[1744] Brand, E & Wiseman, N, Concise Chinese Materia Medica, Taos, Paradigm Publications, 2008, P 229

[1745] Bensky, D, Clavey, S, Stöger, E & Gamble, A, Chinese Herbal Medicine Materia Medica, 3rd Edition, Seattle, Eastland Press, 1986, 1993, 2004, P 527

[1746] Miao Xi Yong, *Commentary on the Divine Husbandman's Classic of Materia Medica*, via Bensky, D, Clavey, S, Stöger, E & Gamble, A, Chinese Herbal Medicine Materia Medica, 3rd Edition, Seattle, Eastland Press, 1986, 1993, 2004, P 512

[1747] Miao Xi Yong, *Commentary on the Divine Husbandman's Classic of Materia Medica*, via Bensky, D, Clavey, S, Stöger, E & Gamble, A, Chinese Herbal Medicine Materia Medica, 3rd Edition, Seattle, Eastland Press, 1986, 1993, 2004, P 512

[1748] Zhang Xi Chun, *Essays on Medicine Esteeming the Chinese and Respecting the Western*, via Bensky, D, Clavey, S, Stöger, E & Gamble, A, Chinese Herbal Medicine Materia Medica, 3rd Edition, Seattle, Eastland Press, 1986, 1993, 2004, P 494

[1749] Li Shi Zhen and Huang Gong Xiu, *Seeking Accuracy in the Materia Medica*, via Bensky, D, Clavey, S, Stöger, E & Gamble, A, Chinese Herbal Medicine Materia Medica, 3rd Edition, Seattle, Eastland Press, 1986, 1993, 2004, P 498

[1750] Bensky, D, Clavey, S, Stöger, E & Gamble, A, Chinese Herbal Medicine Materia Medica, 3rd Edition, Seattle, Eastland Press, 1986, 1993, 2004, P 1010
[1751] Bensky, D, Clavey, S, Stöger, E & Gamble, A, Chinese Herbal Medicine Materia Medica, 3rd Edition, Seattle, Eastland Press, 1986, 1993, 2004, P 1010
[1752] Zhang Lu, *Encountering the Sources of the Classic of Materia Medica*, via Bensky, D, Clavey, S, Stöger, E & Gamble, A, Chinese Herbal Medicine Materia Medica, 3rd Edition, Seattle, Eastland Press, 1986, 1993, 2004, P 1003
[1753] Bensky, D, Clavey, S, Stöger, E & Gamble, A, Chinese Herbal Medicine Materia Medica, 3rd Edition, Seattle, Eastland Press, 1986, 1993, 2004, P 590
[1754] Bensky, D, Clavey, S, Stöger, E & Gamble, A, Chinese Herbal Medicine Materia Medica, 3rd Edition, Seattle, Eastland Press, 1986, 1993, 2004, P 589
[1755] Chen, JK & TT, Chinese Medical Herbology and Pharmacology, City of Industry, Art of Medicine Press, 2001/2004, P 574
[1756] Brand, E & Wiseman, N, Concise Chinese Materia Medica, Taos, Paradigm Publications, 2008, P 267
[1757] Chen, JK & TT, Chinese Medical Herbology and Pharmacology, City of Industry, Art of Medicine Press, 2001/2004, P 587, Bensky, D, Clavey, S, Stöger, E & Gamble, A, Chinese Herbal Medicine Materia Medica, 3rd Edition, Seattle, Eastland Press, 1986, 1993, 2004, P 559
[1758] Brand, E & Wiseman, N, Concise Chinese Materia Medica, Taos, Paradigm Publications, 2008, P 264
[1759] Zhang Bing Chen, *Convenient Reader of Materia Medica*, via Bensky, D, Clavey, S, Stöger, E & Gamble, A, Chinese Herbal Medicine Materia Medica, 3rd Edition, Seattle, Eastland Press, 1986, 1993, 2004, P 560
[1760] Zhang Bing Chen, *Convenient Reader of Materia Medica*, via Bensky, D, Clavey, S, Stöger, E & Gamble, A, Chinese Herbal Medicine Materia Medica, 3rd Edition, Seattle, Eastland Press, 1986, 1993, 2004, P 560. In this section Bensky, D, Clavey, S, Stöger, E & Gamble, A, Chinese Herbal Medicine Materia Medica, 3rd Edition, Seattle, Eastland Press, 1986, 1993, 2004, P, et al. quote Zhang as saying that San Qi enters the Yang Ming and Jue Yin channels. For some reason they only include the large intestine in their assessment, but not the pericardium. I include it here as it is at least as reasonable a conclusion, and I have used clinically San Qi as a pericardium herb for many years with excellent effects.
[1761] Chen, JK & TT, Chinese Medical Herbology and Pharmacology, City of Industry, Art of Medicine Press, 2001/2004, P 568
[1762] Brand, E & Wiseman, N, Concise Chinese Materia Medica, Taos, Paradigm Publications, 2008, P 261
[1763] Huang Gong Xiu, *Seeking Accuracy in the Materia Medica*, via Bensky, D, Clavey, S, Stöger, E & Gamble, A, Chinese Herbal Medicine Materia Medica, 3rd Edition, Seattle, Eastland Press, 1986, 1993, 2004, P 576
[1764] Brand, E & Wiseman, N, Concise Chinese Materia Medica, Taos, Paradigm Publications, 2008, P 261
[1765] Brand, E & Wiseman, N, Concise Chinese Materia Medica, Taos, Paradigm Publications, 2008, P 269
[1766] Bensky, D, Clavey, S, Stöger, E & Gamble, A, Chinese Herbal Medicine Materia Medica, 3rd Edition, Seattle, Eastland Press, 1986, 1993, 2004, P 588

[1767] Bensky, D, Clavey, S, Stöger, E & Gamble, A, Chinese Herbal Medicine Materia Medica, 3rd Edition, Seattle, Eastland Press, 1986, 1993, 2004, P 588
[1768] Bensky, D, Clavey, S, Stöger, E & Gamble, A, Chinese Herbal Medicine Materia Medica, 3rd Edition, Seattle, Eastland Press, 1986, 1993, 2004, P 563
[1769] Bensky, D, Clavey, S, Stöger, E & Gamble, A, Chinese Herbal Medicine Materia Medica, 3rd Edition, Seattle, Eastland Press, 1986, 1993, 2004, P 562
[1770] Bensky, D, Clavey, S, Stöger, E & Gamble, A, Chinese Herbal Medicine Materia Medica, 3rd Edition, Seattle, Eastland Press, 1986, 1993, 2004, P 652
[1771] Chen, JK & TT, Chinese Medical Herbology and Pharmacology, City of Industry, Art of Medicine Press, 2001/2004, P 593
[1772] Brand, E & Wiseman, N, Concise Chinese Materia Medica, Taos, Paradigm Publications, 2008, P 266
[1773] Bensky, D, Clavey, S, Stöger, E & Gamble, A, Chinese Herbal Medicine Materia Medica, 3rd Edition, Seattle, Eastland Press, 1986, 1993, 2004, P 562
[1774] Zhang Bing Chen, *Convenient Reader of Materia Medica*, via Bensky, D, Clavey, S, Stöger, E & Gamble, A, Chinese Herbal Medicine Materia Medica, 3rd Edition, Seattle, Eastland Press, 1986, 1993, 2004, P 568
[1775] Bensky, D, Clavey, S, Stöger, E & Gamble, A, Chinese Herbal Medicine Materia Medica, 3rd Edition, Seattle, Eastland Press, 1986, 1993, 2004, P 567
[1776] Maciocia, G, The Channels of Acupuncture, Philadelphia, 2006, P 545
[1777] Brand, E & Wiseman, N, Concise Chinese Materia Medica, Taos, Paradigm Publications, 2008, P 260
[1778] Zhang Bing Chen, *Convenient Reader of Materia Medica*, via Bensky, D, Clavey, S, Stöger, E & Gamble, A, Chinese Herbal Medicine Materia Medica, 3rd Edition, Seattle, Eastland Press, 1986, 1993, 2004, P 569
[1779] Zhang Bing Chen, *Convenient Reader of Materia Medica*, via Bensky, D, Clavey, S, Stöger, E & Gamble, A, Chinese Herbal Medicine Materia Medica, 3rd Edition, Seattle, Eastland Press, 1986, 1993, 2004, P 569
[1780] Bensky, D, Clavey, S, Stöger, E & Gamble, A, Chinese Herbal Medicine Materia Medica, 3rd Edition, Seattle, Eastland Press, 1986, 1993, 2004, P 564
[1781] Brand, E & Wiseman, N, Concise Chinese Materia Medica, Taos, Paradigm Publications, 2008, P 288, Bensky, D, Clavey, S, Stöger, E & Gamble, A, Chinese Herbal Medicine Materia Medica, 3rd Edition, Seattle, Eastland Press, 1986, 1993, 2004, P 624
[1782] Bensky, D, Clavey, S, Stöger, E & Gamble, A, Chinese Herbal Medicine Materia Medica, 3rd Edition, Seattle, Eastland Press, 1986, 1993, 2004, P 655
[1783] Bensky, D, Clavey, S, Stöger, E & Gamble, A, Chinese Herbal Medicine Materia Medica, 3rd Edition, Seattle, Eastland Press, 1986, 1993, 2004, P 610
[1784] *Convenient Reader of Materia Medica*, Bensky, D, Clavey, S, Stöger, E & Gamble, A, Chinese Herbal Medicine Materia Medica, 3rd Edition, Seattle, Eastland Press, 1986, 1993, 2004, P 214
[1785] *Convenient Reader of Materia Medica*, Bensky, D, Clavey, S, Stöger, E & Gamble, A, Chinese Herbal Medicine Materia Medica, 3rd Edition, Seattle, Eastland Press, 1986, 1993, 2004, P 214
[1786] Zhang Bing Chen, *Convenient Reader of Materia Medica*, via Bensky, D, Clavey, S, Stöger, E & Gamble, A, Chinese Herbal Medicine Materia Medica, 3rd Edition, Seattle, Eastland Press, 1986, 1993, 2004, P 214

[1787] Zhang Bing Chen, *Convenient Reader of Materia Medica*, via Bensky, D, Clavey, S, Stöger, E & Gamble, A, Chinese Herbal Medicine Materia Medica, 3rd Edition, Seattle, Eastland Press, 1986, 1993, 2004, P 607
[1788] Bensky, D, Clavey, S, Stöger, E & Gamble, A, Chinese Herbal Medicine Materia Medica, 3rd Edition, Seattle, Eastland Press, 1986, 1993, 2004, P 653
[1789] Bensky, D, Clavey, S, Stöger, E & Gamble, A, Chinese Herbal Medicine Materia Medica, 3rd Edition, Seattle, Eastland Press, 1986, 1993, 2004, P 612
[1790] Brand, E & Wiseman, N, Concise Chinese Materia Medica, Taos, Paradigm Publications, 2008, P 293
[1791] Brand, E & Wiseman, N, Concise Chinese Materia Medica, Taos, Paradigm Publications, 2008, P 293
[1792] Brand, E & Wiseman, N, Concise Chinese Materia Medica, Taos, Paradigm Publications, 2008, P 300
[1793] Chen, JK & TT, Chinese Medical Herbology and Pharmacology, City of Industry, Art of Medicine Press, 2001/2004, P 655
[1794] Brand, E & Wiseman, N, Concise Chinese Materia Medica, Taos, Paradigm Publications, 2008, P 293
[1795] Bensky, D, Clavey, S, Stöger, E & Gamble, A, Chinese Herbal Medicine Materia Medica, 3rd Edition, Seattle, Eastland Press, 1986, 1993, 2004, P 605
[1796] Bensky, D, Clavey, S, Stöger, E & Gamble, A, Chinese Herbal Medicine Materia Medica, 3rd Edition, Seattle, Eastland Press, 1986, 1993, 2004, P 605
[1797] Brand, E & Wiseman, N, Concise Chinese Materia Medica, Taos, Paradigm Publications, 2008, P 284
[1798] Bensky, D, Clavey, S, Stöger, E & Gamble, A, Chinese Herbal Medicine Materia Medica, 3rd Edition, Seattle, Eastland Press, 1986, 1993, 2004, P 650
[1799] Bensky, D, Clavey, S, Stöger, E & Gamble, A, Chinese Herbal Medicine Materia Medica, 3rd Edition, Seattle, Eastland Press, 1986, 1993, 2004, P 650
[1800] Chen, JK & TT, Chinese Medical Herbology and Pharmacology, City of Industry, Art of Medicine Press, 2001/2004, P 659
[1801] Bensky, D, Clavey, S, Stöger, E & Gamble, A, Chinese Herbal Medicine Materia Medica, 3rd Edition, Seattle, Eastland Press, 1986, 1993, 2004, P 622
[1802] Bensky, D, Clavey, S, Stöger, E & Gamble, A, Chinese Herbal Medicine Materia Medica, 3rd Edition, Seattle, Eastland Press, 1986, 1993, 2004, P 622
[1803] Bensky, D, Clavey, S, Stöger, E & Gamble, A, Chinese Herbal Medicine Materia Medica, 3rd Edition, Seattle, Eastland Press, 1986, 1993, 2004, P 666
[1804] Brand, E & Wiseman, N, Concise Chinese Materia Medica, Taos, Paradigm Publications, 2008, P 298, Bensky, D, Clavey, S, Stöger, E & Gamble, A, Chinese Herbal Medicine Materia Medica, 3rd Edition, Seattle, Eastland Press, 1986, 1993, 2004, P 633
[1805] Tang Rong Chuan (Tang Zonghai), Ben Cao Wen Da, Personal Unpublished Translation, 2015, 1.5.18
[1806] Chen, JK & TT, Chinese Medical Herbology and Pharmacology, City of Industry, Art of Medicine Press, 2001/2004, P 646

[1807] Brand, E & Wiseman, N, Concise Chinese Materia Medica, Taos, Paradigm Publications, 2008, P 289, Bensky, D, Clavey, S, Stöger, E & Gamble, A, Chinese Herbal Medicine Materia Medica, 3rd Edition, Seattle, Eastland Press, 1986, 1993, 2004, P 614
[1808] *Grand Materia Medica*, via Bensky, D, Clavey, S, Stöger, E & Gamble, A, Chinese Herbal Medicine Materia Medica, 3rd Edition, Seattle, Eastland Press, 1986, 1993, 2004, P 127
[1809] Brand, E & Wiseman, N, Concise Chinese Materia Medica, Taos, Paradigm Publications, 2008, P 286
[1810] Wang, Hao Gu, *Harm and Benefit in the Materia Medica*, via Bensky, D, Clavey, S, Stöger, E & Gamble, A, Chinese Herbal Medicine Materia Medica, 3rd Edition, Seattle, Eastland Press, 1986, 1993, 2004, P 603
[1811] Chen, JK & TT, Chinese Medical Herbology and Pharmacology, City of Industry, Art of Medicine Press, 2001/2004, P 636 , Bensky, D, Clavey, S, Stöger, E & Gamble, A, Chinese Herbal Medicine Materia Medica, 3rd Edition, Seattle, Eastland Press, 1986, 1993, 2004, P 602
[1812] Tang Rong Chuan (Tang Zonghai), Ben Cao Wen Da, Personal Unpublished Translation, 2015, 1.2.3
[1813] Zhang, Shan Lei, *Rectification of the Meaning of Materia Medica,* via Bensky, D, Clavey, S, Stöger, E & Gamble, A, Chinese Herbal Medicine Materia Medica, 3rd Edition, Seattle, Eastland Press, 1986, 1993, 2004, P 628
[1814] Zhang, Shan Lei, *Rectification of the Meaning of Materia Medica,* via Bensky, D, Clavey, S, Stöger, E & Gamble, A, Chinese Herbal Medicine Materia Medica, 3rd Edition, Seattle, Eastland Press, 1986, 1993, 2004, P 628
[1815] Brand, E & Wiseman, N, Concise Chinese Materia Medica, Taos, Paradigm Publications, 2008, P 288
[1816] Chen, JK & TT, Chinese Medical Herbology and Pharmacology, City of Industry, Art of Medicine Press, 2001/2004, P 642
[1817] Brand, E & Wiseman, N, Concise Chinese Materia Medica, Taos, Paradigm Publications, 2008, P 296
[1818] Chen, JK & TT, Chinese Medical Herbology and Pharmacology, City of Industry, Art of Medicine Press, 2001/2004, P 1058
[1819] Bensky, D, Clavey, S, Stöger, E & Gamble, A, Chinese Herbal Medicine Materia Medica, 3rd Edition, Seattle, Eastland Press, 1986, 1993, 2004, P 656
[1820] Brand, E & Wiseman, N, Concise Chinese Materia Medica, Taos, Paradigm Publications, 2008, P 291
[1821] Zhang, Shan Lei, *Rectification of the Meaning of Materia Medica,* via Bensky, D, Clavey, S, Stöger, E & Gamble, A, Chinese Herbal Medicine Materia Medica, 3rd Edition, Seattle, Eastland Press, 1986, 1993, 2004, P 663
[1822] Tang Rong Chuan (Tang Zonghai), Ben Cao Wen Da, Personal Unpublished Translation, 2015, 1.2.3
[1823] Bensky, D, Clavey, S, Stöger, E & Gamble, A, Chinese Herbal Medicine Materia Medica, 3rd Edition, Seattle, Eastland Press, 1986, 1993, 2004, P 601
[1824] Chen, JK & TT, Chinese Medical Herbology and Pharmacology, City of Industry, Art of Medicine Press, 2001/2004, P 614
[1825] Brand, E & Wiseman, N, Concise Chinese Materia Medica, Taos, Paradigm Publications, 2008, P 285

[1826] Brand, E & Wiseman, N, Concise Chinese Materia Medica, Taos, Paradigm Publications, 2008, P 285

[1827] Huang Gong Xiu, *Seeking Accuracy in the Materia Medica*, via Bensky, D, Clavey, S, Stöger, E & Gamble, A, Chinese Herbal Medicine Materia Medica, 3rd Edition, Seattle, Eastland Press, 1986, 1993, 2004, P 652

[1828] Brand, E & Wiseman, N, Concise Chinese Materia Medica, Taos, Paradigm Publications, 2008, P 295

[1829] Miao Xi Yong, *Commentary on the Divine Husbandman's Classic of Materia Medica*, via Bensky, D, Clavey, S, Stöger, E & Gamble, A, Chinese Herbal Medicine Materia Medica, 3rd Edition, Seattle, Eastland Press, 1986, 1993, 2004, P 660

[1830] Bensky, D, Clavey, S, Stöger, E & Gamble, A, Chinese Herbal Medicine Materia Medica, 3rd Edition, Seattle, Eastland Press, 1986, 1993, 2004, P 660

[1831] Bensky, D, Clavey, S, Stöger, E & Gamble, A, Chinese Herbal Medicine Materia Medica, 3rd Edition, Seattle, Eastland Press, 1986, 1993, 2004, P 660

[1832] Bensky, D, Clavey, S, Stöger, E & Gamble, A, Chinese Herbal Medicine Materia Medica, 3rd Edition, Seattle, Eastland Press, 1986, 1993, 2004, P 432

[1833] Bensky, D, Clavey, S, Stöger, E & Gamble, A, Chinese Herbal Medicine Materia Medica, 3rd Edition, Seattle, Eastland Press, 1986, 1993, 2004, P 412

[1834] Brand, E & Wiseman, N, Concise Chinese Materia Medica, Taos, Paradigm Publications, 2008, P 312

[1835] Brand, E & Wiseman, N, Concise Chinese Materia Medica, Taos, Paradigm Publications, 2008, P 312, Bensky, D, Clavey, S, Stöger, E & Gamble, A, Chinese Herbal Medicine Materia Medica, 3rd Edition, Seattle, Eastland Press, 1986, 1993, 2004, P 421

[1836] Bensky, D, Clavey, S, Stöger, E & Gamble, A, Chinese Herbal Medicine Materia Medica, 3rd Edition, Seattle, Eastland Press, 1986, 1993, 2004, P 655

[1837] Brand, E & Wiseman, N, Concise Chinese Materia Medica, Taos, Paradigm Publications, 2008, P 322

[1838] Brand, E & Wiseman, N, Concise Chinese Materia Medica, Taos, Paradigm Publications, 2008, P 322

[1839] Chen, JK & TT, Chinese Medical Herbology and Pharmacology, City of Industry, Art of Medicine Press, 2001/2004, P 715

[1840] Chen, JK & TT, Chinese Medical Herbology and Pharmacology, City of Industry, Art of Medicine Press, 2001/2004, P 715

[1841] Bensky, D, Clavey, S, Stöger, E & Gamble, A, Chinese Herbal Medicine Materia Medica, 3rd Edition, Seattle, Eastland Press, 1986, 1993, 2004, P 404

[1842] Brand, E & Wiseman, N, Concise Chinese Materia Medica, Taos, Paradigm Publications, 2008, P 162

[1843] Bensky, D, Clavey, S, Stöger, E & Gamble, A, Chinese Herbal Medicine Materia Medica, 3rd Edition, Seattle, Eastland Press, 1986, 1993, 2004, P 428

[1844] Brand, E & Wiseman, N, Concise Chinese Materia Medica, Taos, Paradigm Publications, 2008, P 311

[1845] Chen, JK & TT, Chinese Medical Herbology and Pharmacology, City of Industry, Art of Medicine Press, 2001/2004, P 688

[1846] Chen, JK & TT, Chinese Medical Herbology and Pharmacology, City of Industry, Art of Medicine Press, 2001/2004, P 688
[1847] Brand, E & Wiseman, N, Concise Chinese Materia Medica, Taos, Paradigm Publications, 2008, P 311
[1848] Brand, E & Wiseman, N, Concise Chinese Materia Medica, Taos, Paradigm Publications, 2008, P 316
[1849] Bensky, D, Clavey, S, Stöger, E & Gamble, A, Chinese Herbal Medicine Materia Medica, 3rd Edition, Seattle, Eastland Press, 1986, 1993, 2004, P 377
[1850] Bensky, D, Clavey, S, Stöger, E & Gamble, A, Chinese Herbal Medicine Materia Medica, 3rd Edition, Seattle, Eastland Press, 1986, 1993, 2004, P 377
[1851] *Detailed Materia Medica*, via Bensky, D, Clavey, S, Stöger, E & Gamble, A, Chinese Herbal Medicine Materia Medica, 3rd Edition, Seattle, Eastland Press, 1986, 1993, 2004, P 409
[1852] *Detailed Materia Medica*, via Bensky, D, Clavey, S, Stöger, E & Gamble, A, Chinese Herbal Medicine Materia Medica, 3rd Edition, Seattle, Eastland Press, 1986, 1993, 2004, P 409
[1853] Brand, E & Wiseman, N, Concise Chinese Materia Medica, Taos, Paradigm Publications, 2008, P 321
[1854] Brand, E & Wiseman, N, Concise Chinese Materia Medica, Taos, Paradigm Publications, 2008, P 330
[1855] Chen Shi Duo, *New Edition of Materia Medica*, via Bensky, D, Clavey, S, Stöger, E & Gamble, A, Chinese Herbal Medicine Materia Medica, 3rd Edition, Seattle, Eastland Press, 1986, 1993, 2004, P 443
[1856] Chen, JK & TT, Chinese Medical Herbology and Pharmacology, City of Industry, Art of Medicine Press, 2001/2004, P 729
[1857] Chen Shi Duo, *New Edition of Materia Medica*, via Bensky, D, Clavey, S, Stöger, E & Gamble, A, Chinese Herbal Medicine Materia Medica, 3rd Edition, Seattle, Eastland Press, 1986, 1993, 2004, P 443
[1858] *Sichuan Chinese Materia Medica*, via Bensky, D, Clavey, S, Stöger, E & Gamble, A, Chinese Herbal Medicine Materia Medica, 3rd Edition, Seattle, Eastland Press, 1986, 1993, 2004, P 939
[1859] *Sichuan Chinese Materia Medica*, via Bensky, D, Clavey, S, Stöger, E & Gamble, A, Chinese Herbal Medicine Materia Medica, 3rd Edition, Seattle, Eastland Press, 1986, 1993, 2004, P 939
[1860] Bensky, D, Clavey, S, Stöger, E & Gamble, A, Chinese Herbal Medicine Materia Medica, 3rd Edition, Seattle, Eastland Press, 1986, 1993, 2004, P 543
[1861] Brand, E & Wiseman, N, Concise Chinese Materia Medica, Taos, Paradigm Publications, 2008, P 350, Bensky, D, Clavey, S, Stöger, E & Gamble, A, Chinese Herbal Medicine Materia Medica, 3rd Edition, Seattle, Eastland Press, 1986, 1993, 2004, P 928
[1862] Bensky, D, Clavey, S, Stöger, E & Gamble, A, Chinese Herbal Medicine Materia Medica, 3rd Edition, Seattle, Eastland Press, 1986, 1993, 2004, P 928
[1863] Bensky, D, Clavey, S, Stöger, E & Gamble, A, Chinese Herbal Medicine Materia Medica, 3rd Edition, Seattle, Eastland Press, 1986, 1993, 2004, P 928
[1864] Brand, E & Wiseman, N, Concise Chinese Materia Medica, Taos, Paradigm Publications, 2008, P 355
[1865] Brand, E & Wiseman, N, Concise Chinese Materia Medica, Taos, Paradigm Publications, 2008, P 355

[1866] Bensky, D, Clavey, S, Stöger, E & Gamble, A, Chinese Herbal Medicine Materia Medica, 3rd Edition, Seattle, Eastland Press, 1986, 1993, 2004, P 912
[1867] Wang, Hao Gu, *Harm and Benefit in the Materia Medica*, via Bensky, D, Clavey, S, Stöger, E & Gamble, A, Chinese Herbal Medicine Materia Medica, 3rd Edition, Seattle, Eastland Press, 1986, 1993, 2004, P 924
[1868] Chen, JK & TT, Chinese Medical Herbology and Pharmacology, City of Industry, Art of Medicine Press, 2001/2004, P 760, and Bensky, D, Clavey, S, Stöger, E & Gamble, A, Chinese Herbal Medicine Materia Medica, 3rd Edition, Seattle, Eastland Press, 1986, 1993, 2004, P 923
[1869] Chen, JK & TT, Chinese Medical Herbology and Pharmacology, City of Industry, Art of Medicine Press, 2001/2004, P 346, and *Thoroughly Revised Materia Medica*, via Bensky, D, Clavey, S, Stöger, E & Gamble, A, Chinese Herbal Medicine Materia Medica, 3rd Edition, Seattle, Eastland Press, 1986, 1993, 2004, P 916
[1870] Zhang Xi Chun, *Essays on Medicine Esteeming the Chinese and Respecting the Western*, via Bensky, D, Clavey, S, Stöger, E & Gamble, A, Chinese Herbal Medicine Materia Medica, 3rd Edition, Seattle, Eastland Press, 1986, 1993, 2004, P 911
[1871] Brand, E & Wiseman, N, Concise Chinese Materia Medica, Taos, Paradigm Publications, 2008, P 348
[1872] Bensky, D, Clavey, S, Stöger, E & Gamble, A, Chinese Herbal Medicine Materia Medica, 3rd Edition, Seattle, Eastland Press, 1986, 1993, 2004, P 910
[1873] Bensky, D, Clavey, S, Stöger, E & Gamble, A, Chinese Herbal Medicine Materia Medica, 3rd Edition, Seattle, Eastland Press, 1986, 1993, 2004, P 910
[1874] Brand, E & Wiseman, N, Concise Chinese Materia Medica, Taos, Paradigm Publications, 2008, P 347, Bensky, D, Clavey, S, Stöger, E & Gamble, A, Chinese Herbal Medicine Materia Medica, 3rd Edition, Seattle, Eastland Press, 1986, 1993, 2004, P 910
[1875] Maciocia, G, The Channels of Acupuncture, Philadelphia, 2006, P 545
[1876] Zhang Bing Chen, *Convenient Reader of Materia Medica*, via Bensky, D, Clavey, S, Stöger, E & Gamble, A, Chinese Herbal Medicine Materia Medica, 3rd Edition, Seattle, Eastland Press, 1986, 1993, 2004, P 919
[1877] Brand, E & Wiseman, N, Concise Chinese Materia Medica, Taos, Paradigm Publications, 2008, P 365
[1878] Bensky, D, Clavey, S, Stöger, E & Gamble, A, Chinese Herbal Medicine Materia Medica, 3rd Edition, Seattle, Eastland Press, 1986, 1993, 2004, P 920
[1879] Bensky, D, Clavey, S, Stöger, E & Gamble, A, Chinese Herbal Medicine Materia Medica, 3rd Edition, Seattle, Eastland Press, 1986, 1993, 2004, P 921
[1880] Yao Lan, *Materia Medica Arranged by Channel*, via Bensky, D, Clavey, S, Stöger, E & Gamble, A, Chinese Herbal Medicine Materia Medica, 3rd Edition, Seattle, Eastland Press, 1986, 1993, 2004, P 922
[1881] Brand, E & Wiseman, N, Concise Chinese Materia Medica, Taos, Paradigm Publications, 2008, P 365, and Wang, An, *Essentials of the Materia Medica*, via Bensky, D, Clavey, S, Stöger, E & Gamble, A, Chinese Herbal Medicine Materia Medica, 3rd Edition, Seattle, Eastland Press, 1986, 1993, 2004, P 914
[1882] Bensky, D, Clavey, S, Stöger, E & Gamble, A, Chinese Herbal Medicine Materia Medica, 3rd Edition, Seattle, Eastland Press, 1986, 1993, 2004, P 982

[1883] Chen, JK & TT, Chinese Medical Herbology and Pharmacology, City of Industry, Art of Medicine Press, 2001/2004, P 794, Bensky, D, Clavey, S, Stöger, E & Gamble, A, Chinese Herbal Medicine Materia Medica, 3rd Edition, Seattle, Eastland Press, 1986, 1993, 2004, P 982

[1884] Zhang Jie Gu via Li Shi Zhen, *Grand Materia Medica*, via Bensky, D, Clavey, S, Stöger, E & Gamble, A, Chinese Herbal Medicine Materia Medica, 3rd Edition, Seattle, Eastland Press, 1986, 1993, 2004, P 985

[1885] Brand, E & Wiseman, N, Concise Chinese Materia Medica, Taos, Paradigm Publications, 2008, P 84, and Huang Gong Xiu, *Seeking Accuracy in the Materia Medica*, via Bensky, D, Clavey, S, Stöger, E & Gamble, A, Chinese Herbal Medicine Materia Medica, 3rd Edition, Seattle, Eastland Press, 1986, 1993, 2004, P 112

[1886] Brand, E & Wiseman, N, Concise Chinese Materia Medica, Taos, Paradigm Publications, 2008, P 84

[1887] Bensky, D, Clavey, S, Stöger, E & Gamble, A, Chinese Herbal Medicine Materia Medica, 3rd Edition, Seattle, Eastland Press, 1986, 1993, 2004, P 991

[1888] Brand, E & Wiseman, N, Concise Chinese Materia Medica, Taos, Paradigm Publications, 2008, P 369, Bensky, D, Clavey, S, Stöger, E & Gamble, A, Chinese Herbal Medicine Materia Medica, 3rd Edition, Seattle, Eastland Press, 1986, 1993, 2004, P 970

[1889] Bensky, D, Clavey, S, Stöger, E & Gamble, A, Chinese Herbal Medicine Materia Medica, 3rd Edition, Seattle, Eastland Press, 1986, 1993, 2004, P 987

[1890] Zhang Bing Chen, *Convenient Reader of Materia Medica*, via Bensky, D, Clavey, S, Stöger, E & Gamble, A, Chinese Herbal Medicine Materia Medica, 3rd Edition, Seattle, Eastland Press, 1986, 1993, 2004, P 919

[1891] Brand, E & Wiseman, N, Concise Chinese Materia Medica, Taos, Paradigm Publications, 2008, P 365

[1892] Bensky, D, Clavey, S, Stöger, E & Gamble, A, Chinese Herbal Medicine Materia Medica, 3rd Edition, Seattle, Eastland Press, 1986, 1993, 2004, P 920

[1893] Bensky, D, Clavey, S, Stöger, E & Gamble, A, Chinese Herbal Medicine Materia Medica, 3rd Edition, Seattle, Eastland Press, 1986, 1993, 2004, P 921

[1894] Yao Lan, *Materia Medica Arranged by Channel*, via Bensky, D, Clavey, S, Stöger, E & Gamble, A, Chinese Herbal Medicine Materia Medica, 3rd Edition, Seattle, Eastland Press, 1986, 1993, 2004, P 922

[1895] Brand, E & Wiseman, N, Concise Chinese Materia Medica, Taos, Paradigm Publications, 2008, P 365, and Wang, An, *Essentials of the Materia Medica*, via Bensky, D, Clavey, S, Stöger, E & Gamble, A, Chinese Herbal Medicine Materia Medica, 3rd Edition, Seattle, Eastland Press, 1986, 1993, 2004, P 914

[1896] Bensky, D, Clavey, S, Stöger, E & Gamble, A, Chinese Herbal Medicine Materia Medica, 3rd Edition, Seattle, Eastland Press, 1986, 1993, 2004, P 980

[1897] Wang Zhen Qin, via Bensky, D, Clavey, S, Stöger, E & Gamble, A, Chinese Herbal Medicine Materia Medica, 3rd Edition, Seattle, Eastland Press, 1986, 1993, 2004, P 979

[1898] *Materia Medica of Toxic Herbs*, via Bensky, D, Clavey, S, Stöger, E & Gamble, A, Chinese Herbal Medicine Materia Medica, 3rd Edition, Seattle, Eastland Press, 1986, 1993, 2004, P 979

[1899] *Links to the Origins of the Records of Materia Medica*, via Bensky, D, Clavey, S, Stöger, E & Gamble, A, Chinese Herbal Medicine Materia Medica, 3rd Edition, Seattle, Eastland Press, 1986, 1993, 2004, P 805

[1900] Tang Rong Chuan (Tang Zonghai), Ben Cao Wen Da, Personal Unpublished Translation, 2015, 2.1.6
[1901] Tang Rong Chuan (Tang Zonghai), Ben Cao Wen Da, Personal Unpublished Translation, 2015, 2.1.6
[1902] Tang Rong Chuan (Tang Zonghai), Ben Cao Wen Da, Personal Unpublished Translation, 2015, 1.1.4
[1903] Bensky, D, Clavey, S, Stöger, E & Gamble, A, Chinese Herbal Medicine Materia Medica, 3rd Edition, Seattle, Eastland Press, 1986, 1993, 2004, P 986
[1904] Chen, JK & TT, Chinese Medical Herbology and Pharmacology, City of Industry, Art of Medicine Press, 2001/2004, P 825
[1905] Chen, JK & TT, Chinese Medical Herbology and Pharmacology, City of Industry, Art of Medicine Press, 2001/2004, P 825
[1906] Bensky, D, Clavey, S, Stöger, E & Gamble, A, Chinese Herbal Medicine Materia Medica, 3rd Edition, Seattle, Eastland Press, 1986, 1993, 2004, P 951
[1907] Miao Xi Yong, *Commentary on the Divine Husbandman's Classic of Materia Medica*, via Bensky, D, Clavey, S, Stöger, E & Gamble, A, Chinese Herbal Medicine Materia Medica, 3rd Edition, Seattle, Eastland Press, 1986, 1993, 2004, P 961
[1908] *High Plateau Handbook of Treatment with Chinese Materia Medica*, via Bensky, D, Clavey, S, Stöger, E & Gamble, A, Chinese Herbal Medicine Materia Medica, 3rd Edition, Seattle, Eastland Press, 1986, 1993, 2004, P 742
[1909] Li Shi Zhen, *Grand Materia Medica*, via Bensky, D, Clavey, S, Stöger, E & Gamble, A, Chinese Herbal Medicine Materia Medica, 3rd Edition, Seattle, Eastland Press, 1986, 1993, 2004, P 779
[1910] Li Shi Zhen says that Yin Yang Huo is an herb of the Arm and Leg Yang Ming, San Jiao and Ming Men, Li Shi Zhen, *Grand Materia Medica*, via Bensky, D, Clavey, S, Stöger, E & Gamble, A, Chinese Herbal Medicine Materia Medica, 3rd Edition, Seattle, Eastland Press, 1986, 1993, 2004, P 779
[1911] Brand, E & Wiseman, N, Concise Chinese Materia Medica, Taos, Paradigm Publications, 2008, P 418
[1912] Brand, E & Wiseman, N, Concise Chinese Materia Medica, Taos, Paradigm Publications, 2008, P 418
[1913] Brand, E & Wiseman, N, Concise Chinese Materia Medica, Taos, Paradigm Publications, 2008, P 418
[1914] Zhang Lu, *Encountering the Sources of the Classic of Materia Medica*, via Bensky, D, Clavey, S, Stöger, E & Gamble, A, Chinese Herbal Medicine Materia Medica, 3rd Edition, Seattle, Eastland Press, 1986, 1993, 2004, P 791
[1915] Bensky, D, Clavey, S, Stöger, E & Gamble, A, Chinese Herbal Medicine Materia Medica, 3rd Edition, Seattle, Eastland Press, 1986, 1993, 2004, P 762
[1916] Brand, E & Wiseman, N, Concise Chinese Materia Medica, Taos, Paradigm Publications, 2008, P 425
[1917] Brand, E & Wiseman, N, Concise Chinese Materia Medica, Taos, Paradigm Publications, 2008, P 425
[1918] Chen, JK & TT, Chinese Medical Herbology and Pharmacology, City of Industry, Art of Medicine Press, 2001/2004, P 883

[1919] Zhou Yan/Zhou Bo Du, *Records of Thoughtful Differentiation of Materia Medica*, via Bensky, D, Clavey, S, Stöger, E & Gamble, A, Chinese Herbal Medicine Materia Medica, 3rd Edition, Seattle, Eastland Press, 1986, 1993, 2004, P 809
[1920] Brand, E & Wiseman, N, Concise Chinese Materia Medica, Taos, Paradigm Publications, 2008, P 427
[1921] Zhang, Shan Lei, *Rectification of the Meaning of Materia Medica,* via Bensky, D, Clavey, S, Stöger, E & Gamble, A, Chinese Herbal Medicine Materia Medica, 3rd Edition, Seattle, Eastland Press, 1986, 1993, 2004, P 783
[1922] Chen, JK & TT, Chinese Medical Herbology and Pharmacology, City of Industry, Art of Medicine Press, 2001/2004, P 908
[1923] Chen, JK & TT, Chinese Medical Herbology and Pharmacology, City of Industry, Art of Medicine Press, 2001/2004, P 907, Brand, E & Wiseman, N, Concise Chinese Materia Medica, Taos, Paradigm Publications, 2008, P 423
[1924] *The Divine Husbandman's Classic of the Materia Medica*, via Bensky, D, Clavey, S, Stöger, E & Gamble, A, Chinese Herbal Medicine Materia Medica, 3rd Edition, Seattle, Eastland Press, 1986, 1993, 2004, P 796
[1925] Wang, An, *Essentials of the Materia Medica*, via Bensky, D, Clavey, S, Stöger, E & Gamble, A, Chinese Herbal Medicine Materia Medica, 3rd Edition, Seattle, Eastland Press, 1986, 1993, 2004, P 792, and Jeffrey Yuen San Francisco 6-26-2017
[1926] Brand, E & Wiseman, N, Concise Chinese Materia Medica, Taos, Paradigm Publications, 2008, P 427, Bensky, D, Clavey, S, Stöger, E & Gamble, A, Chinese Herbal Medicine Materia Medica, 3rd Edition, Seattle, Eastland Press, 1986, 1993, 2004, P 805
[1927] Tang Rong Chuan (Tang Zonghai), Ben Cao Wen Da, Personal Unpublished Translation, 2015, 1.3.6
[1928] Brand, E & Wiseman, N, Concise Chinese Materia Medica, Taos, Paradigm Publications, 2008, P 417
[1929] Zhang Lu, *Encountering the Sources of the Classic of Materia Medica*, via Bensky, D, Clavey, S, Stöger, E & Gamble, A, Chinese Herbal Medicine Materia Medica, 3rd Edition, Seattle, Eastland Press, 1986, 1993, 2004, P 781
[1930] Ye Tian Shi, *Case Records as a Guide to Clinical Practice*, via Bensky, D, Clavey, S, Stöger, E & Gamble, A, Chinese Herbal Medicine Materia Medica, 3rd Edition, Seattle, Eastland Press, 1986, 1993, 2004, P 767
[1931] Maciocia, G, The Channels of Acupuncture, Philadelphia, 2006, P 545
[1932] Brand, E & Wiseman, N, Concise Chinese Materia Medica, Taos, Paradigm Publications, 2008, P 432
[1933] Chen, JK & TT, Chinese Medical Herbology and Pharmacology, City of Industry, Art of Medicine Press, 2001/2004, P 928
[1934] Tang Rong Chuan (Tang Zonghai), Ben Cao Wen Da, Personal Unpublished Translation, 2015, 1.2.3
[1935] Maciocia, G, The Channels of Acupuncture, Philadelphia, 2006, P 545
[1936] Brand, E & Wiseman, N, Concise Chinese Materia Medica, Taos, Paradigm Publications, 2008, P 432

[1937] Brand, E & Wiseman, N, Concise Chinese Materia Medica, Taos, Paradigm Publications, 2008, P 432, Bensky, D, Clavey, S, Stöger, E & Gamble, A, Chinese Herbal Medicine Materia Medica, 3rd Edition, Seattle, Eastland Press, 1986, 1993, 2004, P 754 says, 'slightly Cold.'
[1938] Maciocia, G, The Channels of Acupuncture, Philadelphia, 2006, P 545
[1939] Chen, JK & TT, Chinese Medical Herbology and Pharmacology, City of Industry, Art of Medicine Press, 2001/2004, P 959, Bensky, D, Clavey, S, Stöger, E & Gamble, A, Chinese Herbal Medicine Materia Medica, 3rd Edition, Seattle, Eastland Press, 1986, 1993, 2004, P 763
[1940] Bensky, D, Clavey, S, Stöger, E & Gamble, A, Chinese Herbal Medicine Materia Medica, 3rd Edition, Seattle, Eastland Press, 1986, 1993, 2004, P 744
[1941] Brand, E & Wiseman, N, Concise Chinese Materia Medica, Taos, Paradigm Publications, 2008, P 447
[1942] Brand, E & Wiseman, N, Concise Chinese Materia Medica, Taos, Paradigm Publications, 2008, P 446, Bensky, D, Clavey, S, Stöger, E & Gamble, A, Chinese Herbal Medicine Materia Medica, 3rd Edition, Seattle, Eastland Press, 1986, 1993, 2004, P 841
[1943] Bensky, D, Clavey, S, Stöger, E & Gamble, A, Chinese Herbal Medicine Materia Medica, 3rd Edition, Seattle, Eastland Press, 1986, 1993, 2004, P 851
[1944] Bensky, D, Clavey, S, Stöger, E & Gamble, A, Chinese Herbal Medicine Materia Medica, 3rd Edition, Seattle, Eastland Press, 1986, 1993, 2004, P 846
[1945] Brand, E & Wiseman, N, Concise Chinese Materia Medica, Taos, Paradigm Publications, 2008, P 445
[1946] Bensky, D, Clavey, S, Stöger, E & Gamble, A, Chinese Herbal Medicine Materia Medica, 3rd Edition, Seattle, Eastland Press, 1986, 1993, 2004, P 846
[1947] *Materia Medica of Combinations*, via Bensky, D, Clavey, S, Stöger, E & Gamble, A, Chinese Herbal Medicine Materia Medica, 3rd Edition, Seattle, Eastland Press, 1986, 1993, 2004, P 844
[1948] Chen, JK & TT, Chinese Medical Herbology and Pharmacology, City of Industry, Art of Medicine Press, 2001/2004, P 959, Bensky, D, Clavey, S, Stöger, E & Gamble, A, Chinese Herbal Medicine Materia Medica, 3rd Edition, Seattle, Eastland Press, 1986, 1993, 2004, P 763
[1949] Ye Tian Shi, *Case Records as a Guide to Clinical Practice*, via Bensky, D, Clavey, S, Stöger, E & Gamble, A, Chinese Herbal Medicine Materia Medica, 3rd Edition, Seattle, Eastland Press, 1986, 1993, 2004, P 844
[1950] Bensky, D, Clavey, S, Stöger, E & Gamble, A, Chinese Herbal Medicine Materia Medica, 3rd Edition, Seattle, Eastland Press, 1986, 1993, 2004, P 839
[1951] Bensky, D, Clavey, S, Stöger, E & Gamble, A, Chinese Herbal Medicine Materia Medica, 3rd Edition, Seattle, Eastland Press, 1986, 1993, 2004, P 838
[1952] Chen, JK & TT, Chinese Medical Herbology and Pharmacology, City of Industry, Art of Medicine Press, 2001/2004, P 1003, Bensky, D, Clavey, S, Stöger, E & Gamble, A, Chinese Herbal Medicine Materia Medica, 3rd Edition, Seattle, Eastland Press, 1986, 1993, 2004, P 875
[1953] Bensky, D, Clavey, S, Stöger, E & Gamble, A, Chinese Herbal Medicine Materia Medica, 3rd Edition, Seattle, Eastland Press, 1986, 1993, 2004, P 875
[1954] Bensky, D, Clavey, S, Stöger, E & Gamble, A, Chinese Herbal Medicine Materia Medica, 3rd Edition, Seattle, Eastland Press, 1986, 1993, 2004, P 864
[1955] Ye Gui, *Renewed Materia Medica*, via Bensky, D, Clavey, S, Stöger, E & Gamble, A, Chinese Herbal Medicine Materia Medica, 3rd Edition, Seattle, Eastland Press, 1986, 1993, 2004, P 900

[1956] Ye Gui, *Renewed Materia Medica*, via Bensky, D, Clavey, S, Stöger, E & Gamble, A, Chinese Herbal Medicine Materia Medica, 3rd Edition, Seattle, Eastland Press, 1986, 1993, 2004, P 900
[1957] Bensky, D, Clavey, S, Stöger, E & Gamble, A, Chinese Herbal Medicine Materia Medica, 3rd Edition, Seattle, Eastland Press, 1986, 1993, 2004, P 904
[1958] Bensky, D, Clavey, S, Stöger, E & Gamble, A, Chinese Herbal Medicine Materia Medica, 3rd Edition, Seattle, Eastland Press, 1986, 1993, 2004, P 905
[1959] Bensky, D, Clavey, S, Stöger, E & Gamble, A, Chinese Herbal Medicine Materia Medica, 3rd Edition, Seattle, Eastland Press, 1986, 1993, 2004, P 900
[1960] Bensky, D, Clavey, S, Stöger, E & Gamble, A, Chinese Herbal Medicine Materia Medica, 3rd Edition, Seattle, Eastland Press, 1986, 1993, 2004, P 193
[1961] Bensky, D, Clavey, S, Stöger, E & Gamble, A, Chinese Herbal Medicine Materia Medica, 3rd Edition, Seattle, Eastland Press, 1986, 1993, 2004, P 883
[1962] Miao Xi Yong, *Commentary on the Divine Husbandman's Classic of Materia Medica*, via Bensky, D, Clavey, S, Stöger, E & Gamble, A, Chinese Herbal Medicine Materia Medica, 3rd Edition, Seattle, Eastland Press, 1986, 1993, 2004, P 859
[1963] Bensky, D, Clavey, S, Stöger, E & Gamble, A, Chinese Herbal Medicine Materia Medica, 3rd Edition, Seattle, Eastland Press, 1986, 1993, 2004, P 889
[1964] Maciocia, G, The Channels of Acupuncture, Philadelphia, 2006, P 545
[1965] Bensky, D, Clavey, S, Stöger, E & Gamble, A, Chinese Herbal Medicine Materia Medica, 3rd Edition, Seattle, Eastland Press, 1986, 1993, 2004, P 903
[1966] Maciocia, G, The Channels of Acupuncture, Philadelphia, 2006, P 545
[1967] Bensky, D, Clavey, S, Stöger, E & Gamble, A, Chinese Herbal Medicine Materia Medica, 3rd Edition, Seattle, Eastland Press, 1986, 1993, 2004, P 1017
[1968] Li Shi Zhen, *Grand Materia Medica*, via Bensky, D, Clavey, S, Stöger, E & Gamble, A, Chinese Herbal Medicine Materia Medica, 3rd Edition, Seattle, Eastland Press, 1986, 1993, 2004, P 1022
[1969] Chen, JK & TT, Chinese Medical Herbology and Pharmacology, City of Industry, Art of Medicine Press, 2001/2004, P 1045
[1970] Li Shi Zhen, *Grand Materia Medica*, via Bensky, D, Clavey, S, Stöger, E & Gamble, A, Chinese Herbal Medicine Materia Medica, 3rd Edition, Seattle, Eastland Press, 1986, 1993, 2004, P 1022
[1971] Chen, JK & TT, Chinese Medical Herbology and Pharmacology, City of Industry, Art of Medicine Press, 2001/2004, P 1039
[1972] Brand, E & Wiseman, N, Concise Chinese Materia Medica, Taos, Paradigm Publications, 2008, P 484
[1973] Brand, E & Wiseman, N, Concise Chinese Materia Medica, Taos, Paradigm Publications, 2008, P 484
[1974] Brand, E & Wiseman, N, Concise Chinese Materia Medica, Taos, Paradigm Publications, 2008, P 484
[1975] Bensky, D, Clavey, S, Stöger, E & Gamble, A, Chinese Herbal Medicine Materia Medica, 3rd Edition, Seattle, Eastland Press, 1986, 1993, 2004, P 655
[1976] Brand, E & Wiseman, N, Concise Chinese Materia Medica, Taos, Paradigm Publications, 2008, P 162
[1977] Chen, JK & TT, Chinese Medical Herbology and Pharmacology, City of Industry, Art of Medicine Press, 2001/2004, P 1056, Bensky, D, Clavey, S, Stöger, E & Gamble, A, Chinese Herbal Medicine Materia Medica, 3rd Edition, Seattle, Eastland Press, 1986, 1993, 2004, P 1040

[1978] Brand, E & Wiseman, N, Concise Chinese Materia Medica, Taos, Paradigm Publications, 2008, P 488
[1979] Brand, E & Wiseman, N, Concise Chinese Materia Medica, Taos, Paradigm Publications, 2008, P 492
[1980] Brand, E & Wiseman, N, Concise Chinese Materia Medica, Taos, Paradigm Publications, 2008, P 492
[1981] Brand, E & Wiseman, N, Concise Chinese Materia Medica, Taos, Paradigm Publications, 2008, P 492
[1982] Bensky, D, Clavey, S, Stöger, E & Gamble, A, Chinese Herbal Medicine Materia Medica, 3rd Edition, Seattle, Eastland Press, 1986, 1993, 2004, P 1023
[1983] Bensky, D, Clavey, S, Stöger, E & Gamble, A, Chinese Herbal Medicine Materia Medica, 3rd Edition, Seattle, Eastland Press, 1986, 1993, 2004, P 1026
[1984] Brand, E & Wiseman, N, Concise Chinese Materia Medica, Taos, Paradigm Publications, 2008, P 491
[1985] Bensky, D, Clavey, S, Stöger, E & Gamble, A, Chinese Herbal Medicine Materia Medica, 3rd Edition, Seattle, Eastland Press, 1986, 1993, 2004, P 1026
[1986] Miao Xi Yong, *Commentary on the Divine Husbandman's Classic of Materia Medica*, via Bensky, D, Clavey, S, Stöger, E & Gamble, A, Chinese Herbal Medicine Materia Medica, 3rd Edition, Seattle, Eastland Press, 1986, 1993, 2004, P 1032
[1987] Brand, E & Wiseman, N, Concise Chinese Materia Medica, Taos, Paradigm Publications, 2008, P 491
[1988] Brand, E & Wiseman, N, Concise Chinese Materia Medica, Taos, Paradigm Publications, 2008, P 296
[1989] Chen, JK & TT, Chinese Medical Herbology and Pharmacology, City of Industry, Art of Medicine Press, 2001/2004, P 1058
[1990] Brand, E & Wiseman, N, Concise Chinese Materia Medica, Taos, Paradigm Publications, 2008, P 120, Bensky, D, Clavey, S, Stöger, E & Gamble, A, Chinese Herbal Medicine Materia Medica, 3rd Edition, Seattle, Eastland Press, 1986, 1993, 2004, P 224
[1991] Bensky, D, Clavey, S, Stöger, E & Gamble, A, Chinese Herbal Medicine Materia Medica, 3rd Edition, Seattle, Eastland Press, 1986, 1993, 2004, P 224
[1992] Chen, JK & TT, Chinese Medical Herbology and Pharmacology, City of Industry, Art of Medicine Press, 2001/2004, P 247
[1993] Tang Rong Chuan (Tang Zonghai), Ben Cao Wen Da, Personal Unpublished Translation, 2015, 1.2.3
[1994] Bensky, D, Clavey, S, Stöger, E & Gamble, A, Chinese Herbal Medicine Materia Medica, 3rd Edition, Seattle, Eastland Press, 1986, 1993, 2004, P 601
[1995] Chen, JK & TT, Chinese Medical Herbology and Pharmacology, City of Industry, Art of Medicine Press, 2001/2004, P 614
[1996] Yao Lan, *Materia Medica Arranged by Channel*, via Bensky, D, Clavey, S, Stöger, E & Gamble, A, Chinese Herbal Medicine Materia Medica, 3rd Edition, Seattle, Eastland Press, 1986, 1993, 2004, P 922
[1997] Yao Lan, *Materia Medica Arranged by Channel*, via Bensky, D, Clavey, S, Stöger, E & Gamble, A, Chinese Herbal Medicine Materia Medica, 3rd Edition, Seattle, Eastland Press, 1986, 1993, 2004, P 922

[1998] Tang Rong Chuan (Tang Zonghai), Ben Cao Wen Da, Personal Unpublished Translation, 2015, 1.3.6
[1999] Brand, E & Wiseman, N, Concise Chinese Materia Medica, Taos, Paradigm Publications, 2008, P 417
[2000] Zhang Lu, *Encountering the Sources of the Classic of Materia Medica*, via Bensky, D, Clavey, S, Stöger, E & Gamble, A, Chinese Herbal Medicine Materia Medica, 3rd Edition, Seattle, Eastland Press, 1986, 1993, 2004, P 781
[2001] Bensky, D, Clavey, S, Stöger, E & Gamble, A, Chinese Herbal Medicine Materia Medica, 3rd Edition, Seattle, Eastland Press, 1986, 1993, 2004, P 846
[2002] Brand, E & Wiseman, N, Concise Chinese Materia Medica, Taos, Paradigm Publications, 2008, P 445
[2003] Bensky, D, Clavey, S, Stöger, E & Gamble, A, Chinese Herbal Medicine Materia Medica, 3rd Edition, Seattle, Eastland Press, 1986, 1993, 2004, P 846
[2004] *Materia Medica of Combinations*, via Bensky, D, Clavey, S, Stöger, E & Gamble, A, Chinese Herbal Medicine Materia Medica, 3rd Edition, Seattle, Eastland Press, 1986, 1993, 2004, P 844
[2005] Chen, JK & TT, Chinese Medical Herbology and Pharmacology, City of Industry, Art of Medicine Press, 2001/2004, P 455
[2006] Tang Rong Chuan (Tang Zonghai), Ben Cao Wen Da, Personal Unpublished Translation, 2015, 2.2.2
[2007] Bensky, D, Clavey, S, Stöger, E & Gamble, A, Chinese Herbal Medicine Materia Medica, 3rd Edition, Seattle, Eastland Press, 1986, 1993, 2004, P 83
[2008] Tang Rong Chuan (Tang Zonghai), Ben Cao Wen Da, Personal Unpublished Translation, 2015, 2.2.2
[2009] Tang Rong Chuan (Tang Zonghai), Ben Cao Wen Da, Personal Unpublished Translation, 2015, 2.2.2
[2010] Maciocia, G, The Channels of Acupuncture, Philadelphia, Elsevier, 2006, P 446
[2011] Bensky, D, Clavey, S, Stöger, E & Gamble, A, Chinese Herbal Medicine Materia Medica, 3rd Edition, Seattle, Eastland Press, 1986, 1993, 2004, P 39
[2012] Chen, JK & TT, Chinese Medical Herbology and Pharmacology, City of Industry, Art of Medicine Press, 2001/2004, P 62, Tang Rong Chuan (Tang Zonghai), Ben Cao Wen Da, Personal Unpublished Translation, 2015, 2.1.6
[2013] Maciocia, G, The Channels of Acupuncture, Philadelphia, Elsevier, 2006, P 446
[2014] Maciocia, G, The Channels of Acupuncture, Philadelphia, Elsevier, 2006, P 446
[2015] Maciocia, G, The Channels of Acupuncture, Philadelphia, Elsevier, 2006, P 585
[2016] Tang Rong Chuan (Tang Zonghai), Ben Cao Wen Da, Personal Unpublished Translation, 2015, 2.1.6
[2017] Tang Rong Chuan (Tang Zonghai), Ben Cao Wen Da, Personal Unpublished Translation, 2015, 2.1.3
[2018] Bensky, D, Clavey, S, Stöger, E & Gamble, A, Chinese Herbal Medicine Materia Medica, 3rd Edition, Seattle, Eastland Press, 1986, 1993, 2004, P 20/21
[2019] Maciocia, G, The Channels of Acupuncture, Philadelphia, Elsevier, 2006, P 446
[2020] Tang Rong Chuan (Tang Zonghai), Ben Cao Wen Da, Personal Unpublished Translation, 2015, 2.1.3

[2021] Chen, JK & TT, Chinese Medical Herbology and Pharmacology, City of Industry, Art of Medicine Press, 2001/2004, P 55, and Bensky, D, Clavey, S, Stöger, E & Gamble, A, Chinese Herbal Medicine Materia Medica, 3rd Edition, Seattle, Eastland Press, 1986, 1993, 2004, P 22

[2022] Tang Rong Chuan (Tang Zonghai), Ben Cao Wen Da, Personal Unpublished Translation, 2015, 1.5.3

[2023] Maciocia, G, The Channels of Acupuncture, Philadelphia, Elsevier, 2006, P 446

[2024] Brand, E & Wiseman, N, Concise Chinese Materia Medica, Taos, Paradigm Publications, 2008, P 132

[2025] Tang Rong Chuan (Tang Zonghai), Ben Cao Wen Da, Personal Unpublished Translation, 2015, 1.5.3

[2026] Bensky, D, Clavey, S, Stöger, E & Gamble, A, Chinese Herbal Medicine Materia Medica, 3rd Edition, Seattle, Eastland Press, 1986, 1993, 2004, P 239

[2027] Tang Rong Chuan (Tang Zonghai), Ben Cao Wen Da, Personal Unpublished Translation, 2015, 1.5.2

[2028] Maciocia, G, The Channels of Acupuncture, Philadelphia, Elsevier, 2006, P 446

[2029] Tang Rong Chuan (Tang Zonghai), Ben Cao Wen Da, Personal Unpublished Translation, 2015, 2.1.6

[2030] Chen, JK & TT, Chinese Medical Herbology and Pharmacology, City of Industry, Art of Medicine Press, 2001/2004, P 304, Bensky, D, Clavey, S, Stöger, E & Gamble, A, Chinese Herbal Medicine Materia Medica, 3rd Edition, Seattle, Eastland Press, 1986, 1993, 2004, P 323, Tang Rong Chuan (Tang Zonghai), Ben Cao Wen Da, Personal Unpublished Translation, 2015, 1.3.7

[2031] Maciocia, G, The Channels of Acupuncture, Philadelphia, Elsevier, 2006, P 446

[2032] Chen, JK & TT, Chinese Medical Herbology and Pharmacology, City of Industry, Art of Medicine Press, 2001/2004, P 455

[2033] Tang Rong Chuan (Tang Zonghai), Ben Cao Wen Da, Personal Unpublished Translation, 2015, 2.2.2

[2034] Bensky, D, Clavey, S, Stöger, E & Gamble, A, Chinese Herbal Medicine Materia Medica, 3rd Edition, Seattle, Eastland Press, 1986, 1993, 2004, P 83

[2035] Chen, JK & TT, Chinese Medical Herbology and Pharmacology, City of Industry, Art of Medicine Press, 2001/2004, P 441

[2036] Brand, E & Wiseman, N, Concise Chinese Materia Medica, Taos, Paradigm Publications, 2008, P 208

[2037] Zhang, Shan Lei, *Rectification of the Meaning of Materia Medica,* via Bensky, D, Clavey, S, Stöger, E & Gamble, A, Chinese Herbal Medicine Materia Medica, 3rd Edition, Seattle, Eastland Press, 1986, 1993, 2004, P 675

[2038] Tang Rong Chuan (Tang Zonghai), Ben Cao Wen Da, Personal Unpublished Translation, 2015, 2.2.2

[2039] Maciocia, G, The Channels of Acupuncture, Philadelphia, Elsevier, 2006, P 446

[2040] Ye Tian Shi, *Case Records as a Guide to Clinical Practice*, via Bensky, D, Clavey, S, Stöger, E & Gamble, A, Chinese Herbal Medicine Materia Medica, 3rd Edition, Seattle, Eastland Press, 1986, 1993, 2004, P 767

[2041] Brand, E & Wiseman, N, Concise Chinese Materia Medica, Taos, Paradigm Publications, 2008, P 120, Bensky, D, Clavey, S, Stöger, E & Gamble, A, Chinese Herbal Medicine Materia Medica, 3rd Edition, Seattle, Eastland Press, 1986, 1993, 2004, P 224

[2042] Bensky, D, Clavey, S, Stöger, E & Gamble, A, Chinese Herbal Medicine Materia Medica, 3rd Edition, Seattle, Eastland Press, 1986, 1993, 2004, P 224
[2043] Chen, JK & TT, Chinese Medical Herbology and Pharmacology, City of Industry, Art of Medicine Press, 2001/2004, P 247
[2044] Yao Lan, *Materia Medica Arranged by Channel*, via Bensky, D, Clavey, S, Stöger, E & Gamble, A, Chinese Herbal Medicine Materia Medica, 3rd Edition, Seattle, Eastland Press, 1986, 1993, 2004, P 922
[2045] Yao Lan, *Materia Medica Arranged by Channel*, via Bensky, D, Clavey, S, Stöger, E & Gamble, A, Chinese Herbal Medicine Materia Medica, 3rd Edition, Seattle, Eastland Press, 1986, 1993, 2004, P 922
[2046] Ye Tian Shi, *Case Records as a Guide to Clinical Practice*, via Bensky, D, Clavey, S, Stöger, E & Gamble, A, Chinese Herbal Medicine Materia Medica, 3rd Edition, Seattle, Eastland Press, 1986, 1993, 2004, P 844
[2047] Maciocia, G, The Channels of Acupuncture, Philadelphia, Elsevier, 2006, P 545
[2048] Zhang Xi Chun, *Essays on Medicine Esteeming the Chinese and Respecting the Western*, via Bensky, D, Clavey, S, Stöger, E & Gamble, A, Chinese Herbal Medicine Materia Medica, 3rd Edition, Seattle, Eastland Press, 1986, 1993, 2004, P 911
[2049] Brand, E & Wiseman, N, Concise Chinese Materia Medica, Taos, Paradigm Publications, 2008, P 348
[2050] Bensky, D, Clavey, S, Stöger, E & Gamble, A, Chinese Herbal Medicine Materia Medica, 3rd Edition, Seattle, Eastland Press, 1986, 1993, 2004, P 910
[2051] Bensky, D, Clavey, S, Stöger, E & Gamble, A, Chinese Herbal Medicine Materia Medica, 3rd Edition, Seattle, Eastland Press, 1986, 1993, 2004, P 910
[2052] Brand, E & Wiseman, N, Concise Chinese Materia Medica, Taos, Paradigm Publications, 2008, P 347, Bensky, D, Clavey, S, Stöger, E & Gamble, A, Chinese Herbal Medicine Materia Medica, 3rd Edition, Seattle, Eastland Press, 1986, 1993, 2004, P 910
[2053] Maciocia, G, The Channels of Acupuncture, Philadelphia, Elsevier, 2006, P 545
[2054] Maciocia, G, The Channels of Acupuncture, Philadelphia, Elsevier, 2006, P 545
[2055] Tang Rong Chuan (Tang Zonghai), Ben Cao Wen Da, Personal Unpublished Translation, 2015, 1.3.3
[2056] Maciocia, G, The Channels of Acupuncture, Philadelphia, Elsevier, 2006, P 545
[2057] Maciocia, G, The Channels of Acupuncture, Philadelphia, Elsevier, 2006, P 545
[2058] Tang Rong Chuan (Tang Zonghai), Ben Cao Wen Da, Personal Unpublished Translation, 2015, 1.2.3
[2059] Maciocia, G, The Channels of Acupuncture, Philadelphia, Elsevier, 2006, P 545
[2060] Brand, E & Wiseman, N, Concise Chinese Materia Medica, Taos, Paradigm Publications, 2008, P 432
[2061] Brand, E & Wiseman, N, Concise Chinese Materia Medica, Taos, Paradigm Publications, 2008, P 432, Bensky, D, Clavey, S, Stöger, E & Gamble, A, Chinese Herbal Medicine Materia Medica, 3rd Edition, Seattle, Eastland Press, 1986, 1993, 2004, P 754 says, 'slightly Cold.'
[2062] Maciocia, G, The Channels of Acupuncture, Philadelphia, Elsevier, 2006, P 545
[2063] Brand, E & Wiseman, N, Concise Chinese Materia Medica, Taos, Paradigm Publications, 2008, P 457, Bensky, D, Clavey, S, Stöger, E & Gamble, A, Chinese Herbal Medicine Materia Medica, 3rd Edition, Seattle, Eastland Press, 1986, 1993, 2004, P 860

[2064] Li Shi Zhen, *Grand Materia Medica*, via Bensky, D, Clavey, S, Stöger, E & Gamble, A, Chinese Herbal Medicine Materia Medica, 3rd Edition, Seattle, Eastland Press, 1986, 1993, 2004, P 861
[2065] Li Shi Zhen, *Grand Materia Medica*, via Bensky, D, Clavey, S, Stöger, E & Gamble, A, Chinese Herbal Medicine Materia Medica, 3rd Edition, Seattle, Eastland Press, 1986, 1993, 2004, P 861
[2066] Li Shi Zhen, *Grand Materia Medica*, via Bensky, D, Clavey, S, Stöger, E & Gamble, A, Chinese Herbal Medicine Materia Medica, 3rd Edition, Seattle, Eastland Press, 1986, 1993, 2004, P 861
[2067] Maciocia, G, The Channels of Acupuncture, Philadelphia, Elsevier, 2006, P 545
[2068] Maciocia, G, The Channels of Acupuncture, Philadelphia, Elsevier, 2006, P 545
[2069] Bensky, D, Clavey, S, Stöger, E & Gamble, A, Chinese Herbal Medicine Materia Medica, 3rd Edition, Seattle, Eastland Press, 1986, 1993, 2004, P 889
[2070] Maciocia, G, The Channels of Acupuncture, Philadelphia, Elsevier, 2006, P 545
[2071] Bensky, D, Clavey, S, Stöger, E & Gamble, A, Chinese Herbal Medicine Materia Medica, 3rd Edition, Seattle, Eastland Press, 1986, 1993, 2004, P 903
[2072] Maciocia, G, The Channels of Acupuncture, Philadelphia, Elsevier, 2006, P 545
[2073] Bensky, D, Clavey, S, Stöger, E & Gamble, A, Chinese Herbal Medicine Materia Medica, 3rd Edition, Seattle, Eastland Press, 1986, 1993, 2004, P 4
[2074] Tang Rong Chuan (Tang Zonghai), Ben Cao Wen Da, Personal Unpublished Translation, 2015, 1.4.6
[2075] Maciocia, G, The Channels of Acupuncture, Philadelphia, Elsevier, 2006, P 585
[2076] Tang Rong Chuan (Tang Zonghai), Ben Cao Wen Da, Personal Unpublished Translation, 2015, 2.2.2
[2077] Maciocia, G, The Channels of Acupuncture, Philadelphia, Elsevier, 2006, P 446
[2078] Maciocia, G, The Channels of Acupuncture, Philadelphia, Elsevier, 2006, P 585
[2079] Bensky, D, Clavey, S, Stöger, E & Gamble, A, Chinese Herbal Medicine Materia Medica, 3rd Edition, Seattle, Eastland Press, 1986, 1993, 2004, P 313
[2080] Bensky, D, Clavey, S, Stöger, E & Gamble, A, Chinese Herbal Medicine Materia Medica, 3rd Edition, Seattle, Eastland Press, 1986, 1993, 2004, P 313
[2081] Chen, JK & TT, Chinese Medical Herbology and Pharmacology, City of Industry, Art of Medicine Press, 2001/2004, P 308
[2082] Brand, E & Wiseman, N, Concise Chinese Materia Medica, Taos, Paradigm Publications, 2008, P 158
[2083] Maciocia, G, The Channels of Acupuncture, Philadelphia, Elsevier, 2006, P 585
[2084] '…circulates the Còu Lǐ-interstices and the Sān Jiāo.' Tang Rong Chuan (Tang Zonghai), Ben Cao Wen Da, Personal Unpublished Translation, 2015, 2.2.5
[2085] Maciocia, G, The Channels of Acupuncture, Philadelphia, Elsevier, 2006, P 585
[2086] Tang Rong Chuan (Tang Zonghai), Ben Cao Wen Da, Personal Unpublished Translation, 2015, 1.3.3
[2087] Maciocia, G, The Channels of Acupuncture, Philadelphia, Elsevier, 2006, P 585

Made in the USA
Monee, IL
13 November 2021